UPDATES IN THE UNDERSTANDING AND MANAGEMENT OF THYROID CANCER

Edited by **Thomas J. Fahey**

Updates in the Understanding and Management of Thyroid Cancer
Edited by Thomas J. Fahey

Published by InTech

Janeza Trdine 9, 51000 Rijeka, Croatia

Publishing Process Manager Masa Vidovic

Technical Editor Teodora Smiljanic

Cover Designer InTech Design Team

Additional hard copies can be obtained from orders@intechopen.com

Updates in the Understanding and Management of Thyroid Cancer,
Edited by Thomas J. Fahey
p. cm.
ISBN 978-953-51-0299-1

For EU product safety concerns:
IN TECH d.o.o., Prolaz Marije Krucifikse Kozulić 3, 51000 Rijeka, Croatia,
info@intechopen.com or visit our website at intechopen.com.

Contents

Chapter 1 **An Epidemiological Analysis of Thyroid Cancer in a Spanish Population: Presentation, Incidence and Survival 1**
A. Rego-Iraeta, L. Pérez-Mendez and R.V. García-Mayor

Chapter 2 **The Functionality of p53 in Thyroid Cancer 33**
Debolina Ray, Matthew T. Balmer and Susannah Gal

Chapter 3 **Glycosylation and Glycoproteins in Thyroid Cancer: A Potential Role for Diagnostics 53**
Anna Krześlak, Paweł Jóźwiak and Anna Lipińska

Chapter 4 **Insulin-Like Growth Factor Receptor Signaling in Thyroid Cancers: Clinical Implications and Therapeutic Potential 91**
Geetika Chakravarty and Debasis Mondal

Chapter 5 **Principles and Application of Microarray Technology in Thyroid Cancer Research 119**
Walter Pulverer, Christa Noehammer, Klemens Vierlinger and Andreas Weinhaeusel

Chapter 6 **Evaluation and Management of Pediatric Thyroid Nodules 147**
Melanie Goldfarb and John I. Lew

Chapter 7 **Papillary Thyroid Cancer in Childhood and Adolescence with Specific Consideration of Patients After Radiation Exposure 163**
Yuri Demidchik, Mikhail Fridman, Kurt Werner Schmid, Christoph Reiners, Johannes Biko and Svetlana Mankovskaya

Chapter 8 **Thyroid Cancer in the Pediatric Population 189**
Silva Frieda, Nieves-Rivera Francisco and Laguna Reinaldo

Chapter 9 **Current Innovations and Opinions in the Surgical Management of Differentiated Thyroid Carcinoma 199**
Brian Hung-Hin Lang

Chapter 10 **Sentinel Lymph Node Biopsy in Well Differentiated Thyroid Cancer 217**
Tamara Mijovic, Keith Richardson, Richard J. Payne and Jacques How

Chapter 11 **Preparing Patients for Radioiodine Treatment: Increasing Thyroid Cell Uptake and Accelerating the Excretion of Unbound Radioiodine 235**
Milovan Matović

Chapter 12 **Differentiation Therapy in Thyroid Carcinoma 251**
Eleonore Fröhlich and Richard Wahl

Chapter 13 **Using γ-Camera to Evaluate the *In Vivo* Biodistributions and Internal Medical Dosimetries of Iodine-131 in Thyroidectomy Patients 283**
Sheng-Pin Changlai, Tom Changlai and Chien-Yi Chen

Chapter 14 **Thyroid Cancer: The Evolution of Treatment Options 295**
Hitoshi Noguchi

1

An Epidemiological Analysis of Thyroid Cancer in a Spanish Population: Presentation, Incidence and Survival

A. Rego-Iraeta, L. Pérez-Mendez and R.V. García-Mayor
Department of Endocrinology, Diabetes, Nutrition and Metabolism,
University Hospital of Vigo
Spain

1. Introduction

Accurate statistics on cancer occurrence and outcome are essential both for the purposes of research and for planning and evaluation programmes for cancer control (Parkin, 2006). Although tumours of thyroid account for only 1% of the overall human cancer burden, they represent the most common malignancies of the endocrine system and pose a significant challenge to pathologists, surgeons and endocrinologists. Among epithelial tumors, carcinomas of follicular cell origin far outnumber those of C-cell origin. The vast majority of carcinomas of follicular cell origin are indolent malignancies with 10 year survivals in excess of 90 %.

1.1 Classification

Thyroid follicular epithelial-derived cancers are divided into three categories: papillary cancer, follicular cancer and anaplastic cancer. Papillary and follicular cancers are considered differentiated cancers, and patients with these tumours are often treated similarly despite numerous biologic differences. Most anaplastic (undifferentiated) cancers appear to arise from differentiated cancers. Other malignant diseases of the thyroid include medullary thyroid cancer (which can be familial, either as part of the multiple endocrine neoplasia type 2 syndrome or isolated familial medullary thyroid cancer), primary thyroid lymphoma, or metastases from breast, colon, or renal cancer or melanoma. In countries with adequate iodine intake, differentiated thyroid cancer accounts for more than 85% of all cases, being the most common type papillary (60-80%). Tumor histology is a critical determinant of patient outcomes; differentiated thyroid cancer is associated with the best survival rate and medullary and anaplastic have significantly poorer outcomes (Hundahl et al., 1998). Certain subtypes, such as the tall and columnar cell variants of papillary cancer and the insular variant of follicular cancer are more common in older patients with higher stage disease and have a worse prognosis than usual forms of thyroid cancer. The traditional separation of thyroid cancer into the major groups of papillary, follicular, medullary and undifferentiated (anaplastic) carcinoma, based on morphology and clinical features, is strongly supported by advances in molecular studies showing the involvement of distinct genes in these four groups, with little overlap (DeLellis & Williams, 2004).

1.2 Staging and prognostic factors

Numerous staging systems have been created in an attempt to accurately prognosticate outcomes for individual patients; two careful studies have compared the efficacy of the various staging systems and found that none is superior (Brierley et al., 1997; Sherman et al., 1998). Consequently, the European Thyroid Association (ETA) (Pacini et al., 2006) and the American Thyroid Association (ATA) (Cooper et al., 2009) have recommended the use of the Tumour, Node, Metastasis (TNM) classification of the American Joint Commission on Cancer (AJCC) and the International Union Against Cancer because it is universally available and widely accepted for other disease sites. An interesting feature of the TNM staging system compared to other classifications is the age factor. While the staging of head and neck cancers relies exclusively in the anatomical extent of disease, it is not possible to follow this pattern for the particular group of malignant tumors that arise in the thyroid gland. The effect of age is such significance in behavior and prognosis, that both the histologic diagnosis and the age of the patient are included in the staging system for these tumors. The AJCC classification is based on the TNM system, which relies on assessing three components: (1) extent of the primary tumour (T), (2) absence or presence of regional lymph node metastases (N), and (3) absence or presence of distant metastases (M). The fifth edition (Fleming et al., 1997), (Table 1) was revised as the sixth edition (Greene et al., 2002), (Table 2). A major alteration was the reclassification of tumour staging (T). For differentiated (papillary and follicular) and medullary tumours confined to the parenchyma of the thyroid gland without extrathyroidal extension, there is no evidence to suggest that using a size cut-off of 1 cm provides better prognostic stratification compared with the 2-cm cut-off used for

	Papillary or Follicular		Medullary	Anaplastic
Stage	Age < 45 years	Age > 45 years	Any age	
I	Any T Any N M0	T1 N0 M0	T1 N0 M0	
II	Any T Any N M1	T2 N0 M0 T3 N0 M0	T2 N0 M0 T3 N0 M0 T4 N0 M0	
III		T4 N0 M0 Any T N1 M0	Any T N1 M0	
IV		Any T Any N M1	Any T Any N M0	Any T Any N Any M

Table 1. AJCC TNM classification for thyroid cancer (fifth edition). **T1** - Tumor 1 cm or less in greatest dimension limited to the thyroid. **T2** - Tumour more than 1 cm, but not more than 4 cm, in greatest dimension limited to the thyroid. **T3** - Tumour more than 4 cm in greatest dimension limited to the thyroid. **T4** - Tumour of any size extending beyond the thyroid capsule. **T4a** - Excluded. **T4b** - Excluded. Regional lymph nodes are the cervical and upper mediastinal lymph nodes. **N1a** - Metastasis in ipsilateral cervical lymph node(s). **N1b** - Metastasis in bilateral, midline, or contralateral cervical or mediastinal lymph node (s). **M0-** no distance metastases; **M1-** distance metastases.

other head and neck sites. Therefore, fifth edition T1 (≤1 cm) and T2 (between 1 and 4 cm) were redefined as sixth edition T1 (≤2 cm) and T2 (between 2 and 4 cm). In the sixth edition, T3 includes not only large tumours (4 cm or more) but also tumours with minimal extension, and T4 consists of T4a and T4b. The fact that diverse outcomes may be expected in these two groups of patients is now recognized in the sixth edition: tumors that involve the sternothyroid muscle are classified as T3, while extension to larynx, trachea, oesophagus, recurrent laryngeal nerve, or subcutaneous soft tissue, all of which are surgically resectable, is classified as T4a. Tumours that invade the prevertebral fascia or encase the carotid artery or mediastinal great vessels are not resectable for cure, and these patients are staged T4b. Thus, the sixth edition divides fifth edition T4 tumors into T3 (minimal invasion), T4a (extended invasion), and T4b (more extensive unresectable invasion) tumours according to the degree of extrathyroid extension. The degree of extension has been closely related to adverse prognoses. Therefore, the sixth edition is expected to predict more accurately different outcomes in patients with extrathyroid extension compared with the fifth edition.

	Papillary or Follicular		**Medullary**	**Anaplastic**
Stage	**Age < 45 years**	**Age > 45 years**	**Any age**	
I	Any T, Any N, M0	T1 N0 M0	T1 N0 M0	
II	Any T Any N M1	T2 N0 M0	T2 N0 M0	
III		T3 N0 M0 T1 N1a M0 T2 N1a M0 T3 N1a M0	T3 N0 M0 T1 N1a M0 T2 N1a M0 T3 N1a M0	
IVA		T4a N0 M0 T4a N1a M0 T1 N1b M0 T2 N1b M0 T3 N1b M0 T4a N1b M0	T4a N0 M0 T4a N1a M0 T1 N1b M0 T2 N1b M0 T3 N1b M0 T4a N1b M0	T4a Any N M0
IVB		T4b Any N M0	T4b Any N M0	T4b Any N M0
IVC		Any T Any N M1	Any T Any N M1	Any T Any N M1

Table 2. AJCC TNM classification for thyroid cancer (sixth edition). **T1** - Tumor 2 cm or less in greatest dimension limited to the thyroid. **T2** - Tumour more than 2 cm, but not more than 4 cm, in greatest dimension limited to the thyroid. **T3** - Tumour more than 4 cm in greatest dimension limited to the thyroid or any tumour with minimal extrathyroid extension (extension to sternothyroid muscle or perithyroid soft tissues). **T4** - Excluded. **T4a** - Tumour of any size extending beyond the thyroid capsule to invade subcutaneous soft tissues, larynx, trachea, oesophagus, or recurrent laryngeal nerve. **T4b** - Tumour invades prevertebral fascia or encases carotid artery or mediastinal vessels. **T4a** - Intrathyroidal anaplastic carcinoma—surgically resectable. **T4b** - Extrathyroidal anaplastic carcinoma—surgically unresectable. Regional lymph nodes are the central compartment, lateral cervical, and upper mediastinal lymph nodes. **N1a** - Metastasis to Level IV (pretracheal, paratracheal, and prelaryngeal/Delphian lymph nodes). **N1b** - Metastasis to unilateral, bilateral, or contralateral cervical or superior mediastinal lymph nodes. **M0-** no distance metastases; **M1-** distance metastases.

TNM classification is also used for hospital cancer registries and epidemiologic studies. One of the greatest inadequacies of TNM system is that it is a static representation of the patient's disease at the time of presentation; it does not allow for modification of risk during lifelong follow-up. Most patients with papillary cancer in the TNM system are classified as stage I disease (Hundahl et al., 1998), with an associated mortality rate of 1.7% (Loh et al., 1997). It is important to note, however, that there is a 15% recurrence rate 10 years after initial treatment (Loh et al., 1997). Recurrent or persistent disease, therefore, may necessitate additional therapy and can certainly affect the patient's quality of life. Further limitations of tumour staging include the lack of consideration of tumour histology, extracapsular extension of the tumour or molecular characteristics of the primary tumour. As is well known, these factors can predict poorer outcomes for individual patients. As TNM staging was developed to predict risk of death and not recurrence, the ATA (Cooper et al., 2009) has created a more functional definition of risk stratification for individual patients that is similar to one outlined by the ETA (Pacini et al., 2006). Patients are classified as low-risk if they have the following characteristics: no local or distant metastases, resection of all macroscopic tumour, no tumour invasion into locoregional tissues, tumour that is not an aggressive histological variant, no vascular invasion, and no uptake outside the thyroid bed on the post-treatment whole body scan (if ^{131}I is given). Intermediate-risk patients are those with any of the following criteria: microscopic tumour invasion into the perithyroidal tissues at initial surgery, cervical lymph node metastases or ^{131}I uptake outside the thyroid bed on the initial post-treatment scan, or tumour with aggressive histology or vascular invasion. Finally, high-risk patients have macroscopic tumour invasion, incomplete tumour resection, distant metastases or elevated thyroglobulin out of proportion to what is seen on the post-treatment scan (Cooper et al., 2009). This stratification was designed to help identify patients who are at higher risk for recurrent disease and may benefit from more aggressive postoperative management (Cooper et al., 2009). Such a definition of risk is more intuitive for the management of patients with thyroid cancer and is more in accordance with the clinical behaviour of these tumours.

1.3 Epidemiology

Epidemiology has shown the influence of factors such as age and sex on thyroid cancer incidence. Thyroid cancer is rare in children below 16 years, with an annual incidence between 0.02 and 0.3 cases per 100,000 children and occurs exceptionally before age 10. In adults, the mean age of diagnosis is the mid 40´s to early 50´s for the papillary type, 50´s for the follicular and medullary types and 60´s for the less common undifferentiated types. It is well established that thyroid cancer is 2 to 4 times more common in women than in men, although this will differ among countries. Nevertheless, this sex difference is far less pronounced before puberty and after menopause. Several epidemiological studies have examined several reproductive traits, but the cause of this increased prevalence of thyroid cancer in women is unclear. The annual incidence of thyroid cancer varies considerably in different registries, with the highest incidence rates in the world reported in Hawaii and Iceland (Ferlay et al., 2007; Kolonel et al., 1990). In Europe, the highest incidence occurs in Iceland, followed by Finland, while relatively low incidence characterizes the United Kingdom and Denmark (Ferlay et al., 2007,). These differences have been attributed to ethnic or environmental factors, but different standards of health care may also play a role in the efficiency of cancer detection. Although thyroid cancer incidence is low in general when compared with other diseases and tumours, over the last few decades, increasing rates have been reported in several countries, including Europe (Akslen et al., 1993; Colonna et al., 2002 ; dos Santos Silva et al., 1993; Gomez-Segovia et al., 2004; Petterson et al., 1991; Reynolds et al., 2005; Szybinski et al., 2003), the United States (Davies & Welch, 2006; Merhy et al., 2001; Zheng et al., 1996), Canada (Liu et al., 2001), and Australia (Burgess, 2002). Curiously, this increase has occurred almost exclusively in papillary thyroid cancer, with an epidemic of micropapillary thyroid carcinoma (MPTC) representing up to 43% of operated cancers in the present series (Leenhart et al., 2004a). The reasons for the rise in thyroid cancer incidence are not completely understood and considerable controversy exists now about whether this increase is real or only apparent due to an increase in diagnostic activity (Leenhart et al., 2004a; Leenhart et al., 2004b; Colonna et al., 2007). Recently, some researchers (Colonna et al., 2007; Davies & Welch, 2006; Kent et al., 2007) have suggested that this increase is predominantly due to the increased detection of small, subclinical tumours through the use of medical imaging. Moreover, thyroid surgery is constantly increasing, with more systematic use of total thyroidectomies even for benign pathologies, which makes it easier to detect MPTC. According to the World Health Organization (WHO), the term MPTC is used for a papillary carcinoma of the thyroid no larger than 1 cm in diameter (Hedinger et al., 1988). With the new classification published in 2004, the previous definition of MPTC now includes the additional criteria of being found incidentally (LiVolsi, 2004). MPTC seems to be present in a significant proportion of the general population with large variations in the prevalence rate between different geographic areas (6–35%) (Sampson et al., 1974), which may also be due to differences in the depth of the pathological examination (Martinez-Tello et al., 1993). Although the mortality risk for an individual patient with thyroid cancer is the greatest concern for patients and clinicians alike, most patients have excellent 10-20-year disease specific survival (Hundahl et al., 1998). EUROCARE (European Cancer Registry-based Study on Survival and Care of Cancer Patients) is a collaborative project between European cancer registries (Capocaccia et al., 2003). A major aim of EUROCARE is to estimate and compare cancer survival in European populations. EUROCARE-2 (Teppo & Hakulinen, 1998) was the first publication on thyroid cancer survival in Europe. This study included all malignant thyroid tumors (excluding lymphomas) in patients 15 or older. Relative survival was analyzed using population-based EUROCARE -2 data from 1985-1989. The overall 5-year relative survival rate, standardized by age (Table 3), was 67% for men and 78% for women across Europe. Substantial variation in this 5-year rate was observed between countries ranging from 56% in Slovenia to 100% in Austria (men), (Teppo & Hakulinen, 1998). Higher than average survival rates were observed in Finland, Iceland, The Netherlands and Sweden. Relative survival was higher in the younger population group. In the age group 15 - 44 years, for men the rate was at least 86% and for women at least 94 %. In contrast, much lower rates were seen in the the group of older population (75 + years). EUROCARE-3 study (Sant et al., 2003) analyzed the survival of adult cancer diagnosed from 1990 to 1994 in 22 European countries and followed them until the end of 1998. Neoplasms in situ were collected but not included in the analysis of survival. The overall relative survival of patients diagnosed with thyroid cancer in this period was 83% at 5 years. Austria, Finland, France, Iceland, Italy, Norway, Malta, Spain, Switzerland and Sweden had rates above the European average. Most of these countries also had high survival for this cancer in EUROCARE-2. Denmark, Germany, The Netherlands,

England, Scotland, Wales and the countries of Eastern Europe had survival below the European average (Table 3). Again, the most favorable outcomes were observed in patients aged 15-44 years; for the oldest patient's survival was five times lower. Part of variation in thyroid cancer survival was attributed to variations in the distribution of histological types. Other likely factors contributing to this are differences in the stage distribution and varying efficacy of treatment (Sant et al., 2003; Teppo & Hakulinen, 1998).

	EUROCARE-2		EUROCARE-3	
	female	**male**	**female**	**male**
Iceland	90	88	85	87,4
Austria	87	100	88	81
Sweden	84	74	85	80
The Netherlands	84	77	79	68,6
Finland	82	77	86	79
France	81	61	85	74
Switzerland	78	-	90	-
Spain	**78**	**70,6**	**85,7**	**82**
Italy	77	66	85	72,6
Germany	77	62	77	69,4
Estonia	76	57	77	58
England	74	64	79	71
Scotland	73	67	76	73
Denmark	72	63	80	76,6
Slovakia	71	63	76	-
Eslovenia	70	56	77	83
Poland	66	64	66	57
EUROPE	**78**	**67**	**81,4**	**71,8**

Table 3. Thyroid cancer 5-year Relative Survival (%) from 1985 to 1989 (EUROCARE-2) and from 1990 to 1994 (EUROCARE-3) in European countries.

In the U.S., the National Cancer Data Base (NCDB) represents a national electronic registry system of incident cancers. Between 1985 and 1995, NCDB captured demographic, patterns-of-care, stage, treatment, and outcome information for a sample of 53,856 thyroid carcinoma cases. The 10-year overall relative survival rates for U. S. patients with papillary, follicular, Hürthle cell, medullary, and undifferentiated/anaplastic carcinoma was 93%, 85%, 76%, 75%, and 14%, respectively (Hundahl et al., 1998). Relative survival, the survival analogue of excess mortality, is commonly used in population-based studies of cancer survival although its utility is not restricted to this area. Relative survival is the ratio of the observed survival in a group of patients to the survival probability estimated over the same period in a group of people in the general population of similar age and sex. It is usual to estimate the expected survival proportion from nationwide population life tables stratified by age, sex, calendar time, and, where applicable, race (Berkson & Gage, 1950). In order to be comparable between different populations, relative survival figures must be either age-specific or age-adjusted. A major advantage of relative survival is that information on cause of death is not required, thereby circumventing problems with the inaccuracy or no availability of death certificates (Percy et al., 1981). However, our interest is typically in net survival rather than all-cause survival, that is, we are interested in mortality due to cancer. Cause-specific survival is commonly estimated in cancer clinical trials and only those deaths which can be attributed to the cancer in question are considered to be events, while all other deaths are considered censorings. Using cause-specific survival to estimate net survival requires that reliably coded information on cause of death is available. The distinguishing feature of survival analysis is that at the end of the follow-up period the event (such as death due to cancer) will probably not have occurred for all patients. For these patients the survival time is said to be censored, indicating that the observation period was cut off before the event occurred. For example, a person who had the cancer and died 10 years later of car accident would be censored at death, having contributed 10 person-year of survival to the analysis. A person who had the cancer and died 10 years later of the cancer would contribute an event, a death due to the cancer, having also contributed 10 person-years of survival time. A 90 % cancer specific survival at 10 years would mean that 90 % of patients had not died from their cancer, while 10 % had died from their cancer (Kaplan, 1958). Calculation of cause-specific survival is especially important when studying diseases with a favorable prognosis, as is the case at hand, where the patients live long enough to be exposed to other causes of death. The indolent course of thyroid cancer requires very large cohorts of patients followed over several decades to confirm significant differences in prognostic factors and treatment efficacy. Neither randomized clinical trials nor meta-analysis are available and evidence is based on a number of retrospective studies with multivariate for mortality risk factors or data from national cancer registries (Gilliland et al., 1997; Hundahl et al., 1998). Unfortunately, very remarkable differences in patient's selection, staging systems, and clinical management affect the available studies. In particular, radioiodine treatment is not routinely carried out in a standard manner and outcome results of different studies are thus not comparable (Sciuto et al., 2009). Since scarce data exist on the epidemiology of thyroid cancer in Spain, the main aim of this study was to analyze changes in thyroid cancer presentation, incidence, prevalence and survival in South Galicia (north-western Spain) over a 24-year period (1978–2001) and compare these results with those described in the leading international series. The people of this region are homogeneous in terms of ethnicity. This period spans the population's transition from mild iodine deficiency to iodine sufficiency after beginning iodine prophylaxis in 1985 (Garcia-Mayor et al., 1999; Rego-Iraeta et al., 2007). As a high incidence of thyroid cancer owing to improved screening procedures is generally associated with an elevated proportion of small carcinomas, we have specifically considered the impact of MPTC on thyroid cancer incidence and trends in tumour size over time as an indicator of enhanced medical procedures for thyroid cancer. We have also studied the proportion of our population undergoing thyroid surgery over the study period and the percentage of thyroid cancers found per thyroidectomy performed.

2. Materials and methods

2.1 Identification of thyroid cancer cases

Data on thyroid cancer incidence in the period from 1978 to 2001 (inclusive) were obtained from the Pathology Registry of the University Hospital of Vigo which belongs to the Spanish public health system and collects data on about 97% of the cancerous lesions verified by microscopic examination. This ensures virtually complete ascertainment for all the new cases of thyroid cancer diagnosed in our population during the study period. Over the observation period, a total of 329 cases of thyroid cancer were registered. Seven cases (six lymphomas and one Angiosarcoma) were excluded from the study based on rarity. The remaining 322 cases of primary thyroid cancer were assigned to one of the four major diagnostic categories: papillary thyroid carcinoma; follicular thyroid carcinoma, including Hürthle carcinomas; medullary thyroid carcinoma; and anaplastic thyroid carcinoma, diagnosed according to the WHO classification (Hedinger et al., 1988). Original histology slides for all cases of follicular carcinomas (53 cases) were reviewed by two hystopathologists blinded to the original diagnosis. Nine of them were reclassified as papillary carcinomas and 44 cases were classified as true follicular carcinomas. All tumour stages were classified according to fifth edition of AJCC (Fleming et al., 1997) since most studies reported having used this classification. In the present study all papillary carcinomas of the thyroid <1 cm in diameter were classified as MPTC (Hedinger et al., 1988). All thyroid cancer cases were also characterized by sex, date of birth, and date of diagnosis. We also recorded data on number of thyroidectomies recorded in the registry which were almost exclusively performed by two senior surgeons during the study period. Near-total thyroidectomy has been used as standard treatment protocol for thyroid cancer and comprises neck dissection if confirmed lymph node involvement; one course of ablative radioiodine treatment with 100 mC, further radioiodine therapies with 100 mC if needed, with an interval of 6 months-1 year and thyrotropin-suppressive thyroid hormone therapy with levothyroxine lifetime.

2.2 Follow up the vital status of patients

Active follow-up of patients was carried-out through searches in medical records and phone contacts. A detailed review of the medical record to ascertain the cause of death was made. Mortality data were taken into account only when primary cause of death was directly related to thyroid cancer and all other deaths were considered censorings. Cause-specific 1-, 5-, 10-, 20- and 25 year survival rates were used as measures of survival.

2.3 Study population

The studied population had an average of 500,000 inhabitants. Corresponding population data by size, age, sex, and year were available from official statistics. Data during the period 1978–2001 show that Vigo's population increased by 6.3%. The male to female ratio remained stable at about 0.92. The people of the region are homogeneous in terms of ethnicity. For studies of genetic characteristics, the Spanish Galician region is considered a relatively isolated European population at the westernmost continental edge (Salas et al., 1998).

2.4 Statistical analysis

Trends in age, sex, histological type, and tumour size (differentiated thyroid carcinoma) at diagnosis were analyzed. Data on number of thyroidectomies performed were also recorded. The general descriptive analyses were performed using Microsoft Excel and SPSS

12.0 software (SPSS, Inc., Chicago, IL). Data were analyzed using the chi-square test for nonparametric data. A p value below 0.05 was considered to be statistically significant. Results were expressed as mean± standard deviation of the mean (mean±SD) for quantitative variables. Data were analyzed using the Student t test for normally distributed variables and the chi-square test for nonparametric data. Crude incidence rates, expressed per 100,000 inhabitants each year were calculated. In order to compare incidence rates between populations that differ with respect to age (since age has such a powerful influence on the risk of cancer), age standardized incidence rates were also calculated; standardization was performed using the World Standard Population (direct method) (Bray, 2002). For the whole group of thyroid cancer, the overall incidence by sex for each year from 1978 to 2001 was calculated. Due to the small sample size, which produces unstable rates for individual years, rates were calculated for several years combined (1978 to 1985, 1986 to 1993, and 1994 to 2001). Incidence trends for each of the distinct histological categories, including MPTC incidence, were also examined. The prevalence of thyroid cancer was defined as the number of persons in our defined population whom have been diagnosed of thyroid cancer, and who were still alive in three cross-sectional surveys performed in December 1985, December 1993, and December 2001. The prevalence rates have been reported per 100,000 inhabitants. A 95% confidence interval (CI) for the rates was determined to compare incidence and prevalence rates. Survival from the data of initial surgery to each endpoint, i.e. cancer specific survival, was estimated by the Kaplan–Meier product-limit method at 1, 5, 10, and 20 and, in some cases, at 25 years of diagnosis. The log-rank test was used to assess difference between subgroups. Age at diagnosis was grouped into the same five categories used by previous EUROCARE studies: 15-44, 45-54, 55-64, 65-74 and 75-99 years. We used multivariate Cox analysis to calculate those independent variables related to the survival of differentiated thyroid cancer.

3. Results

A total of 322 cases of primary differentiated thyroid cancer were diagnosed in our area between 1978 and 2001. The mean age at diagnosis was 46.6 years (range, 8–91 years). Eight patients were younger than 18 years at diagnosis. The female to male ratio was 3.6/1.

3.1 General characteristics on thyroid cancer

3.1.1 Histological distribution

Out of 322 cases of primary thyroid cancer, papillary was the predominant tumour type with 245 cases (76%), followed by follicular with 44 cases (13.7%), medullary with 23 cases (7.1%), and anaplastic with 10 cases (3.1%), (Table 1). The papillary to follicular ratio in the entire period was as high as 5.8; when MPTC cases were excluded, this ratio was 2.

3.1.2 Age and sex distribution

The youngest age at presentation corresponded to medullary and papillary cancers of the thyroid. Anaplastic cancer and Hürthle cells occurred at older ages. Of the total of thyroid cancers, 78.3% of the cases were females and 21.7% outstanding men. This female predominance is maintained in all histologic types (Table 4).

3.1.3 Pathologic Tumor-Node-Metastases (pTNM) distribution

Altogether, 73% of the primary tumours presented with T1 to T3 tumor size; 15 % were locally invasive to extrathyroidal soft tissues (T4), 22% had metastatic involvement of cervical lymph nodes and 4.7% had distant metastases. Of 11.8% of cases the tumor size was unknown. Among all tumors, medullary and papillary carcinomas were the most commonly presented with cervical lymphadenopathy while follicular carcinoma the most often presented distant metastasis (Table 4). In our series, we identified 95 MPTC out of a total of 245 papillary thyroid cancers (38.7%). Of these, 87 cases (91%) were incidentally diagnosed in thyroidectomies performed for thyroid pathologies other than thyroid cancer.

	Papillary	Follicular	Hürthle	Medullary	Anaplastic	Total
N° cases (%)	245 (76%)	32 (10%)	12 (3.7%)	23 (7.1%)	10 (3.1 %)	322
Mean age (range)	44 (8-91)	50 (23-78)	61 (33-91)	43.8 (19-78)	71 (52-89)	46.6 (8-91)
Female/Male	4	3.5	5	2.28	1.5	3.6
T_1-T_3	80 %	56 %	78 %	52 %	0 %	73 %
T_4	10.6 %	22 %	8 %	17.4 %	100 %	15 %
N_1	23 %	12.5 %	8 %	39 %	20 %	22 %
M_1	2.4 %	19 %	0 %	13 %	0 %	4.7 %

Table 4. Thyroid cancer characteristics at diagnosis (1978-2001).

3.1.4 Distribution of pTNM stages of thyroid cancer at diagnosis (1978-2001)

Most of thyroid cancer patients (75 %) presented low pathological tumor-node,-metastases (stages I and II). Most papillary cancers presented with either stage I (63 %) or stage II (18 %). Stage III accounted for fewer than 12 % of cases. Few (1.2 %) patients presented with distant metastases and had stage IV disease. For follicular and Hürthle cancers these figures were 37, 28, 15, 6% and 25, 58, 8 and 0 % respectively. Most patients with medullary thyroid cancer (43.5 %) had stage II; patients with stage I accounted for only 4 %; and stages III and IV, 26 % and 13 % respectively. Figure 1, illustrates the distribution of pTNM stage and histologic subgroup of thyroid cancer patients.

3.1.5 Trends in thyroid cancer presentation: Tumour size

Table 1 shows no significant change over time for sex distribution and age between the three time periods (1978–1985, 1986–1993, and 1994–2001). The proportion of MPTC among total papillary thyroid cancers cases increased significantly over time: 16.7% (1978 to 1985), 23% (1986 to 1993), and 43% (1994 to 2001). The papillary to follicular ratio significantly increased over time from 2.3 to 3.6 and 11.5. When MPTC was excluded, the papillary to follicular ratios were 1.9, 2.7, and 6.6, respectively. Besides MPTC cases, no significant variations were observed with respect to tumour size (pT) at presentation, in papillary and follicular over time. For some patients there was no precise pathological description about tumour size (pTx), (Table 5).

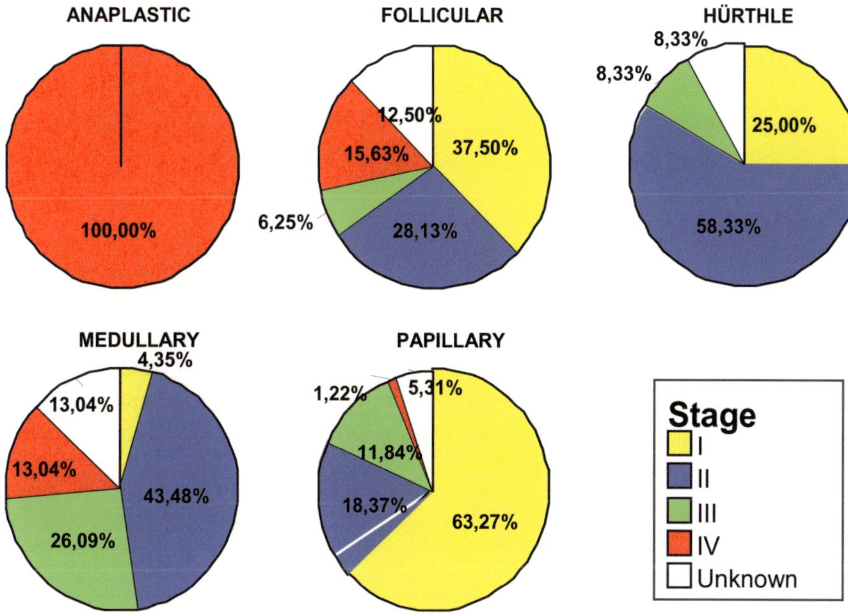

Fig. 1. Thyroid cancer pTNM stages and histologic distribution at diagnosis (1978-2001).

		1° Period 1978-1985	2°Period 1986-1993	3°Period 1994-2001	p
Female/Male		4.3	3.6	3.4	0.854
Mean age ± DT (years)		42.2±16.5	46.8±17.2	47.6±16.7	0.601(1° vs 3°)
Papillary/Follicular		2.3	3.6	11.5	0.000*
Papillary (no-MPTC)/Follicular		1.9	2.7	6.6	0.013*
(%) MPTC/ Total Papillary		16.7 %	23 %	43 %	0.010*
Papillary (no- MPTC)	$T_{2\ (n=81)}$	47.8 %	45.8 %	60 %	0.360
	$T_{3(n=20)}$	8.7 %	20.8 %	10 %	
	$T_{4(n=27)}$	17.4 %	18.8 %	17.5 %	
	$T_{x\ (n=22)}$	26.1 %	14.6 %	12.5 %	
Follicular	$T_{1\ (n=4)}$	7.7 %	16.7 %	0 %	0.213
	$T_{2\ (n=20)}$	38.5%	38.9%	61.5 %	
	$T_{3\ (n=4)}$	0 %	11.1 %	15.4 %	
	$T_{4\ (n=8)}$	15.4 %	16.7 %	23.1 %	
	$T_{x\ (n=8)}$	38.5 %	16.7 %	0 %	

Table 5. Time trend of thyroid cancer presentation (1978-2001).

3.2 Trends in thyroid surgery

A total of 2345 thyroidectomies were performed during the studied period. During this period the percentage of the population undergoing a thyroid surgery significantly increased from 13.76 per 100,000 each year (95% CI 12.35-14.56) to 23.83 (95% CI 22.17-

24.73) and 45.01 (95% CI 42.45–46.39) in 1978–1985, 1986–1993, and 1994–2001, respectively. The proportion of thyroid carcinomas among operated patients rose from 9.92% in 1978–1985 to 12.31% in 1986–1993 and to 15.35% in 1994–2001, respectively ($p < 0.015$). Total thyroidectomy accounted for 48% of initial surgical procedures (1978–1985) and 74% during 1994–2001.

3.3 Trends in thyroid cancer incidence

As shown in Fig. 2 and Table 6, incidence rates were considerably lower for males than for females. Overall crude incidence of thyroid cancer in women increased significantly from 1.61 per 100,000 each year (1978 to 1985) to 4.43 (1986 to 1993) and 10.29 (1994 to 2001). These figures in men were 0.35, 1.31, and 3.24, respectively. Age-standardized incidence rates (ASR) over this period show the same tendency, with a significant increase in females: 1.56 per 100,000 each year (1978 to 1985) to 3.83 (1986 to 1993) and 8.23 (1994 to 2001); and males: 0.33, 1.19, and 2.65, respectively (Table 6).

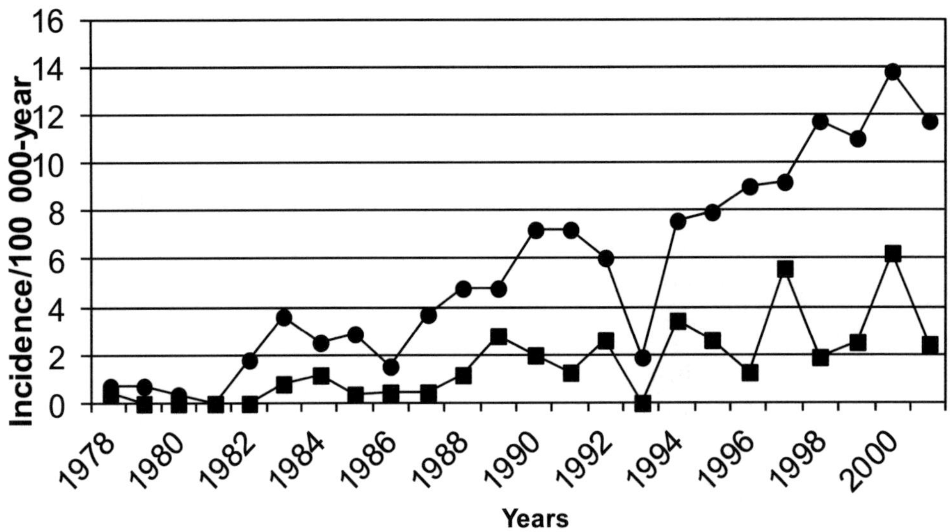

Fig. 2. Annual crude incidence of thyroid cancer, by sex (1978-2001); females (circles) and males (squares).

	Females			Males		
Period (years)	Crude Incidence	ASR *	IC (95 %)	Crude Incidence	ASR *	IC (95 %)
1978-1985	1.61	1.56	1.03-2.08	0.35	0.33	0.08-0.58
1986-1993	4.43	3.83	2.93-4.71	1.31	1.19	0.67-1.70
1994-2001	10.29	8.23	6.82-9.63	3.24	.65	1.82-3.46

Table 6. Time trend of crude and age-standardized incidence rates of thyroid cancer, by sex. (*) Age-standardized incidence rate (ASR).

3.3.1 Trends in thyroid cancer incidence by histopathology: Incidence of MPTC

Figure 3 displays the overall (males and females) crude incidence rates of thyroid cancer in relation to the histological types; the increase in the incidence of thyroid cancer over the three periods of time was primarily due to an increase in papillary cancer incidence. After the second period, the incidence of follicular cancer decreased and there was no significant change in the incidence of MTC and anaplastic cancer. Table 7 shows that the increase in the incidence of PTC was the result of an increased incidence of both MPTC and papillary measuring more than 1 cm (Papillary non-MPTC). This occurred both in males and females.

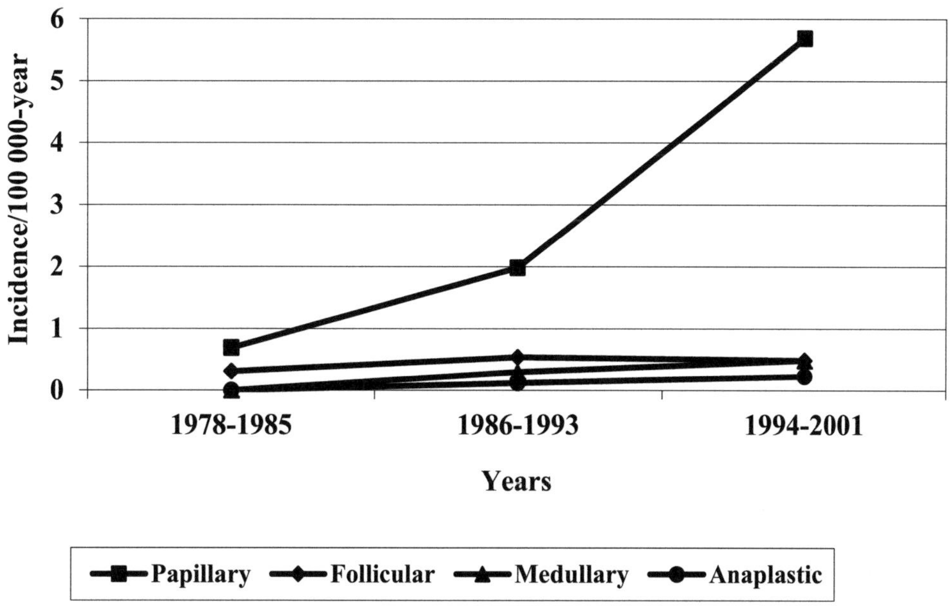

Fig. 3. Time trend of crude incidence rates of thyroid cancer, by histology.

	Females				Males			
Period	Papillary No-MPTC Incidence	CI (95%)	MPTC Incidence	CI (95%)	Papillary No-MPTC Incidence	CI (95%)	MPTC Incidence	CI (95%)
1978-1985	0.97	0.55-1.38	0.14	-0.02-0.29	0.15	-0.02-0.32	0.10	-0.04-0.24
1986-1993	2.19	1.49-2.88	0.81	0.38-1.23	0.75	0.32-1.17	0.12	-0.05-0.30
1994-2001	4.82	3.65-5.98	3.94	2.89-4.99	1.58	0.89-2.27	0.79	0.30-1.28

Table 7. Time trend of papillary thyroid cancer crude incidence rates, by sex
(CI: Confidence Interval)

3.4 Trends in thyroid cancer prevalence

Table 8 shows that prevalence of thyroid cancer increased substantially between 1985 and 2001 in both sexes. Thyroid cancer was significantly more prevalent in female than in male subjects.

Year	Sex	Prevalence	CI (95%)
1985	Female	**12.53**	8.38-16.68
1993	Female	**65.89**	53.23-78.56
2001	Female	**128.34**	111.75-144.92
1985	Male	**2.72**	0.70-4.73
1993	Male	**17.85**	10.99-24.71
2001	Male	**35.66**	26.56-44.77

Table 8. Time trend of thyroid cancer prevalence, by sex.

3.5 Thyroid cancer survival

We followed a total of 321 cases of thyroid cancer. The median follow-up was 7.7 years, ranging between 4 and 27.8 years. We recorded a total of 43 deaths, of which 30 (70%) were directly related to thyroid cancer, yielding a cancer- specific mortality rate of 9. 3 % for the whole cohort. Over 4 %(4.3) of cancer -specific deaths was represented by patients with differentiated thyroid carcinomas. Among the remaining 13 deaths not attributable to thyroid cancer, 9 (69%) were due to second malignancies (three breast cancer case, 1 prostate cancer case, 1 case of sigmoid colon cancer, 1 case of liver cancer, 1 case of glioblastoma multiform, 1 case of pancreatic cancer , 1 case of multiple myeloma) and 4 (31%) were attributed to other causes. Overall survival of patients diagnosed with thyroid cancer in the period 1978-2001 was 88 % at 25 years, being 90 % for women and 80% for men; although survival was higher in women, there were no significant differences between both genders (p = 0, 097), (Table 9). When excluding MPTC, we observed a decrease in thyroid cancer survival. Thus, the overall survival of thyroid cancer was 84% at 25 years, being 87% in women and 76% in men, again without significant differences between genders (p = 0.15), (Table 10).

Gender	**Patients**			**Survival**		
		1 year	**5 years**	**10 years**	**20 years**	**25 years**
Female	251	97%	93%	91%	90%	90%
Male	75	95%	91%	84%	80%	80%
Total	321	96%	93%	89%	88%	88%

Table 9. Overall cause-specific survival of thyroid cancer (1978-2001).

Gender	**Patients**			**Survival**		
		1 year	**5 years**	**10 years**	**20 years**	**25 years**
Female	180	96%	91%	89%	87%	87%
Male	56	94%	89%	81%	76%	76%
Total	236	95%	90%	86%	84%	84%

Table 10. Overall cause-specific survival of thyroid cancer (1978-2001), excluding MPTC.

3.5.1 Cause –specific survival according to age

Table 11 and Figure 4, reflect the cause-specific survival by age group (excluding MPTC) and emphasizes the influence of age on the prognosis of patients with thyroid carcinoma. As can be seen there is one more striking decline in survival after 55 years of age.

Age	Patients	Survival				
		1 year	5 years	10 years	20 years	25 years
ago-44	117	100%	98%	96%	94%	94%
45-54	45	97%	95%	95%	95%	95%
55-64	34	90%	84%	74%	63%	-
65-74	22	86%	77%	69%	57%,18 years	-
75-91	18	83%	59%	47%	47%,18 years	-

Table 11. Cause-specific survival of thyroid cancer by age group, excluding MPTC (1978-2001).

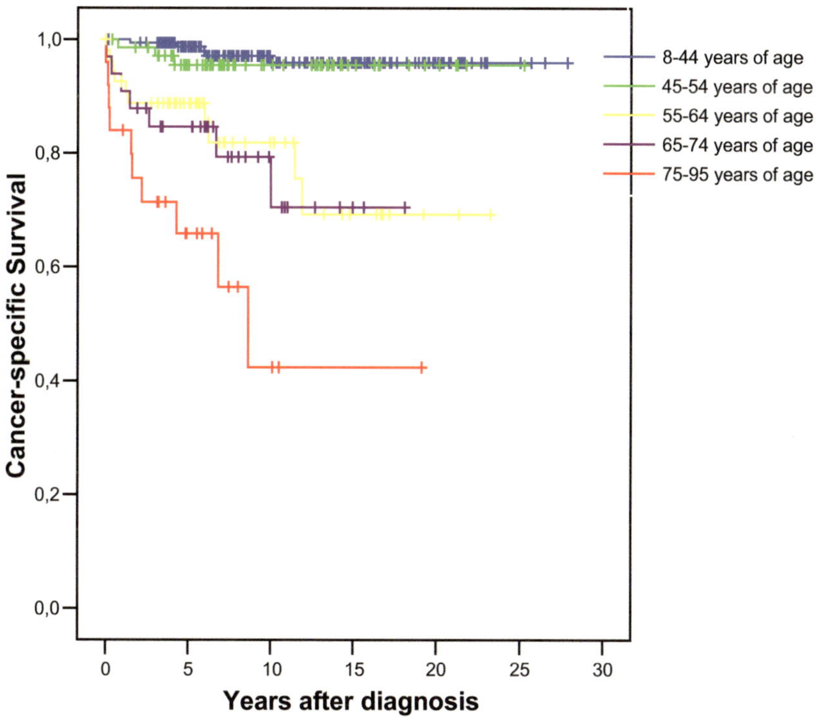

Fig. 4. Cause-specific survival of thyroid cancer by age group, excluding MPTC (1978-2001).

3.5.2 Cause -specific survival according to histological type

As known, histologic type is a strong determinant of thyroid cancer survival. In our series, papillary thyroid cancer patients had 25-year specific-survival greater than 93 %, even when excluding MPTC. The survival of MPTC was 100% at 25 years in the present study. Follicular and medullary carcinoma patients had lower survivals (83% at 25 years and %at 20 years, respectively). However, the prognosis was is ominous for anaplastic thyroid carcinoma (Table 12 and Figure 5).

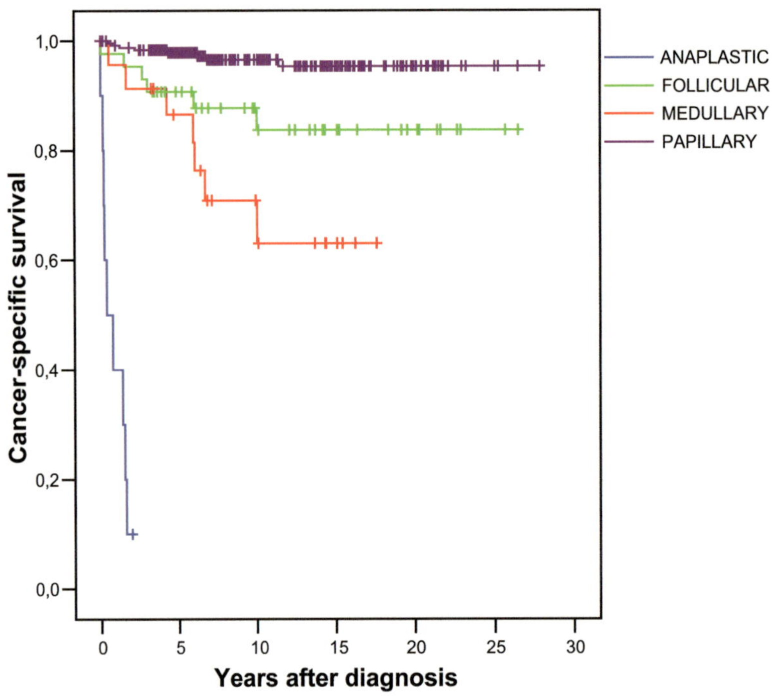

Fig. 5. Cause-specific survival of thyroid cancer according to histological type (1978-2001).

Histologic type	Patients	Survival				
		1 year	5 years	10 years	20 years	25 years
Papillary (total)	245	99%	97%	96%	95%	95%
Papilar (no MPTC)	160	98%	96%	95%	93%	93%
Follicular (including Hürthle)	43	97%	90%	87%	83%	83%
Medullary	23	95%	86%	70%	63%	-
Anaplastic	10	40%	10%	-	-	-

Table 12. Cause-specific survival of thyroid cancer according to histological type (1978-2001).

3.5.3 Cause –specific survival according to p TNM stage distribution

Stage at diagnosis is a strong prognostic factor for thyroid cancer survival. Thus, cause specific-survival vas 100% at 25 years of follow- up in stage I. At more advanced stages survival decreases progressively (Table 13).

Stage	Patients	Survival				
		1 year	5 years	10 years	20 years	25 years
I	171	100%	100%	100%	100%	100%
II	71	100%	100%	97%	94%	-
III	38	97%	88%	69%	69%	69%
IV	21	37%	15%	15%	0%	-
Unknown	20	100%	100%	94%	94%	94%

Table 13. Cause-specific survival of thyroid cancer by pTNM stage (1978-2001).

3.5.4 Prognostic analysis in differentiated thyroid carcinoma

Risk factors associated with differentiated thyroid cancer mortality were identified by Cox regression analysis. Univariate and multivariate analysis results for thyroid cancer mortality are illustrated in Table 14. In the univariate analysis, the following factors were significantly associated with mortality for differentiated thyroid cancer: age, follicular histology, local tumor extension and distant metastases at presentation. Neither sex nor the presence of lymph node metastases contributed to mortality risk. Multivariate analysis confirmed as independent predictor variables of increased risk of cancer mortality-only age and presence of distant metastases.

Variables	Variables	Univariate Analysis RR (CI 95 %)	Multivariate Analysis. RR (CI 95 %)
Sex	Female	1	
	Male	1,5 (0,48-4,95)	
	8 - 44	1	
	45 - 54	2,3 (0,14-36,7)	3,17 (0,2-51,6)
Age (years)	55 - 64	20,7 (2,42-178)	17,8 (2,12-150)
	65 - 74	30,5 (3,4-274)	15,6 (1,6-147)
	> 75	38,5 (3,90-377)	38,5 (3,30-338)
Histology	Papillary	1	
	Follicular	4,07 (1,41-11,76)	
	T1	1	
Tumoral size	T2	2,75 (0,26-24,5)	
	T3	3,33 (0,20-53,5)	
	T4	24,80 (3,1-198)	
Regional extension	N0	1	
	N1	2,5 (0,78-8,40)	
Distance extension.	M0	1	
	M1	29,9 (10,4-85)	17,68 (6,11-51,1)

Table 14. Univariate and Multivariate survival analysis of prognostic factors of differentiated thyroid cancer (1978-2001).

4. Discussion

The main objective of epidemiological studies is to measure the frequency of disease. Prevalence measures are particularly useful in the healthcare planning. Furthermore, incidence reflects the "flow" from health to illness in populations and therefore constitutes the basis of causative research. On the other hand, survival measures are an indicator of the global efficiency of healthcare services. These questions are also fundamentally important in thyroid cancer, since an understanding of the basic causes and related risk factors may lead to novel interventions and preventive measures. The reason why we carried out this work was the paucity of data on the major epidemiological features of thyroid cancer in our country (Spain) and particularly in our region (Galicia). In this study we conducted an epidemiologic survey in our community, to evaluate time trends in presentation, incidence, prevalence and survival of thyroid cancer between January 1978 and December 2001; a period that spans our community transition from mild iodine deficiency to iodine sufficiency after beginning iodine prophylaxis (iodized salt) in 1985. Several factors could have an impact on the epidemiology of thyroid cancer in our area. On the one hand, the eradication of iodine deficiency in our population in the last decades (Garcia-Mayor et al., 1999; Rego-Iraeta et al., 2007; Rodriguez I et al., 2002), on the other hand, the progressive increase in the use of diagnostic techniques and the preference for carrying out near-total thyroidectomy since the nineties, (compared to the "lumpectomy" or hemithyroidectomy) which is known to increase the likelihood of detecting microscopic carcinomas incidentally, mainly papillary lineage. In Galicia, like in the rest of Spain, 97% of the population receives health care through the public health system, with other kinds of medical care being negligible (Etxabe & Vazquez, 1994). This ensures virtually complete case ascertainment for diagnosed thyroid cancer in the population. Given that practically the whole population of Galicia is registered with the social security system, our study is representative of the Galician population (North-western Spain).

The general characteristics of our patients with thyroid cancer such as the mean age at diagnosis (46.6 years old) and the predominance of females to males (3.6/1) were similar to those reported in other studies around the world (Blanco Carrera et al., 2005; Gilliland et al., 1997; Sant et al. 2003; Scheiden et al., 2006; Sciuto et al., 2009). Agree with this, the youngest age at presentation corresponded to medullary and papillary thyroid carcinomas, followed by follicular carcinoma, Hürthle cell cancer and finally by the anaplastic carcinoma. The histological distribution of thyroid cancer in the present series was similar to that reported in iodine-sufficient areas, with a higher proportion of papillary thyroid cancer (76% over overall thyroid carcinomas). It represents the same pattern that was reported in the USA (Hundahl et al., 1998; Scheiden et al., 2006; Schlumberger et al., 2008) and some European countries (Blanco Carrera et al., 2005; Farahati et al., 2004; Sant et al. 2003; Scheiden et al., 2006). Likewise, in our series the ratio papillary/follicular was high, which is the predominant pattern reported in the Western world (Sant et al., 2003; Teppo & Hakulinen, 1998). This happened even in the first period of our study when there was a mild iodine deficiency in our population (median iodine of 60μg/l) (Garcia-Mayor et al., 1999). This ratio increased over time, even when MPTC were excluded from the calculation. We speculate that the amelioration of iodine nutrition, which happened in our population over the last decades (Garcia-Mayor et al., 1999; Rego-Iraeta et al., 2007), may explain this finding to some degree. However, an increase in the incidence of papillary thyroid cancer has also been reported in Luxemburg, considered an iodine deficient area (Sant et al., 2003), and in Tasmania (Australia), in spite of the recurrence of mild iodine deficiency (Burgess et al., 2000). This phenomenon may be related with a dose-threshold effect for iodine nutrition and modulation of tumour genesis (Burgess et al., 2000), or alternatively, environmental factors other than iodine nutrition may be contributing.

In our study, most of patients (75 %) had low pathological p-TNM stages (stages I and II) at presentation. These results are similar to those described in a cohort of more than 2700 patients with thyroid cancer at the Mayo Clinic of Rochester who underwent thyroidectomy from 1940 to 1997 (Schlumberger et al., 2008). Among papillary carcinoma cases, this series reported extrathyroidal invasion in 15 % (range 5 to 34%), and clinically evident lymphadenopathy at presentation in about one third of cases. Only 1 to 7% of papillary carcinomas had metastases at diagnosis. However, it is noteworthy that about 35 to 50 % of removed neck nodes have histologic evidence of involvement (Schlumberger et al., 2008), so that our low rate of lymph node involvement may reflect the fact that node dissection is not performed routinely in our environment. Regional lymph node metastases from follicular carcinomas are uncommon (4 to 6% of patients). Indeed, wherever they are observed, other alternative diagnoses, should be considered. Around 5 to 20% of these tumors have distant metastases at presentation (Schlumberger et al., 2008). In our series, 12.5% of follicular carcinomas and 8% of Hürthle cell carcinomas had lymph nodes at diagnosis. In accordance with previous observations, we found distant metastases in 19% of follicular carcinomas, although we found no distant metastases in the group of the Hürthle cell carcinomas. In relation to staging at presentation, we compared our results with the case material of the Mayo Clinic, between 1940 and 1997.

The distribution of pathological stages I, II, III and IV for papillary carcinoma at the Mayo Clinic was respectively 60, 22, 17 and 1%, very similar to the corresponding in our study, which was 63, 18, 12 and 1.2% for the same stages. With regard to follicular carcinomas, the Mayo Clinic study found that the distribution of stages I, II, III and IV was 22, 53, 4 and 17% for follicular carcinoma and 17, 69, 9 and 5% for the Hürthle cell carcinoma. Curiously, stage I was more frequent among our follicular carcinomas (the distribution of stages I, II, III and IV for follicular carcinoma was 37, 28, 6.2 and 15.6% and for Hürthle carcinoma 25, 58, 8 and 0%; respectively). With reference to medullary carcinoma, the Mayo Clinic cohort data revealed a predominance of stage I (stage I, II, III and IV; 57, 19, 22 and 2% respectively), while in our study only 4.3 % of patients presented with stage I. This is probably due to earlier introduction of RET proto-oncogene testing at the Mayo Clinic.

Thyroid cancer has increased dramatically in most countries in the last 30 years (Kilfoy et al., 2009), excluding countries such as Iceland, Sweden and Norway (Engholm et al., 2009). In the present study, the incidence of thyroid cancer is increasing over time. When comparing incidence rates among different populations there are two points to bear in mind; first, since a rapid increase in thyroid cancer incidence is seen, it is important to consider the period of time the rate refers to, and secondly due to the differences in the age distribution among different populations, it is necessary to display an age-standardized rate of incidence (ASR). Most of the series, report ASR referred to world population. In the present investigation, both crude incidences and ASR show an increasing trend over time. In comparison with other European countries, our ASR in the final period of time, 1994-2001, (8.2 per 100,000-year in women and 2.65 in men) is similar to the reports from our neighbouring countries such as Portugal, France and Italy and is higher than that reported by the IARC for Spain (period 1997- 1999) (Ferlay et al., 2004). A previous study in our community (Garcia-Mayor et al., 1997), reported a decrease in the number of patients requiring surgical treatment with an increase in the frequency of malignancy in the surgical specimens after the introduction of FNAB in the management of nodular thyroid disease in 1991. However, when we studied the total number of thyroid surgeries performed in our population, we found that the rate of population undergoing thyroid surgery significatively increased over time with an increase in the ratio of total thyroidectomy for other kind of thyroidectomy. Undeniable, this trend makes it easier to detect MPTC. In fact, 43 % of our operated cancers were MPTCs in the latter period studied versus a 16.7 % in the first period. A similar trend has been reported in France where there was an increase in thyroid cancer incidence, mainly due to the papillary type, with an epidemic of microcarcinomas (43% of operated cancers, for the period 1998–2001) (Leenhardt et al., 2004a). This trend has been reported in many other studies (Chow et al., 2003; Colonna et al., 2007; Scheiden et al., 2006; Verkooijen et al., 2003). The improvement in diagnostic tools (image procedures and fine-needle aspiration biopsy) (Colonna et al., 2007; Scheiden et al., 2006) and greater extensiveness and number of thyroidectomies performed, which makes it easier to detect MPTCs (Leenhardt et al., 2004a), has been suspected to be of etiological importance in the observed increase of papillary thyroid cancer. One study (Kovacs et al., 2005) estimated the prevalence of thyroid microcarcinomas found at autopsies is 100–1000 times higher than in clinical cancer; they were not related to iodine intake and were exclusively of the papillary type (MPTC). It suggests that a large proportion of the population probably lives with undetected thyroid cancer and fits with the hypothesis of an apparent increase in thyroid cancer incidence. Any interpretation of reports of the incidence of papillary thyroid carcinoma must take into account the remarkably high prevalence of MPTC in thyroids removed for reasons other than thyroid cancer and in autopsy series (Hedinger & Sobin 1988). In this sense, it is noteworthy, that many cancer registries do not specify the contribution of MPTC to the incidence of thyroid cancer, so differences in the inclusion criteria can cause mistakes in the comparison of the incidences (Teppo & Hakulinen 1998). For these reasons we have separately analyzed the incidence of MPTC and the incidence of papillary cancer not including MPTC (Papillary non MPTC). In the present investigation, we found 245 cases of papillary cancer, of which 95 cases (38.7 %) were MPTC carcinomas (pT1). Remarkably, most of these tumours (91%) were detected incidentally after thyroid surgery performed for reasons other than thyroid cancer. Although the incidence of MPTC is increasing in our population, also an increase in the incidence of tumours greater than 1 cm (Papillary non MPTC) was evident in both sexes. Similar findings have been reported in studies performed by Burgess in Australia (Burgess, 2002; Burgess & Tucker 2006). We also observed an increase in the ratio of total thyroidectomy for other kind of thyroidectomy over time. A recent study performed by Mitchell et al. in USA (Mitchell et al., 2007), examined trends in surgical therapy for thyroid cancer. They hypothesized that if a true increase occurs in the incidence of thyroid cancer, then thyroidectomy, as the primary treatment for thyroid cancer, should also increase during the same period. This study reported a regional difference in the incidence of thyroid cancer with an increase in North-eastern and Southern and an actual decrease in the Midwest United States. Newly papillary thyroid cancer accounted for most of this increase. Furthermore, thyroidectomy, in these areas seemed to mirror their respective regional changes in incidence. Supporting the hypotheses of recent changes in medical practice as the cause of the increase in thyroid cancer incidence, some authors (Davies & Welch, 2006; Kent et al., 2007) found a shift in the tumour size distribution of thyroid cancer toward smaller papillary cancers in recent years, suggesting an apparent (not real) increase in thyroid cancer incidence due to increased detection of subclinical tumours. However, besides MPTC, we did not observe a significant change in tumour size over time in differentiated thyroid carcinomas at presentation with a percentage of pT_2, pT_3 and pT_4 lesions which remain stable over time. Moreover, there are three questions to be in mind; firstly, the increase in thyroid cancer incidence in our area has happened equally in the incidence of MPTC and in the incidence of PTC greater than 1 cm.; secondly, there has not been a shift over time in thyroid cancer tumour size, besides MPTC, and thirdly, there is no similar increase in the incidence of other histological types of thyroid cancer (Rego-Iraeta et al., 2009). Interestingly, Kent and colleagues (Kent et al., 2007) found that the incidence of medium-sized tumours (2-4 cm) remained stable over time, but were surprised to discover a slight increase in large tumours (larger than 4 cm). Several others papers from U.S. support the notion that the increase in incidence is not entirely due to increased screening and detection. Thus, Enewold and colleagues found, among white women, the rate of increase for cancers larger than 5 cm. almost equaled that for the smallest papillary cancers. Chen et al. similarly reported an increase in differentiated thyroid cancer of all sizes with the most rapid increase occurring in females. Cramer et al. showed an increase in the incidence of papillary thyroid cancers with a significant increase in all size categories. A report by Morris & Myssiorek drew similar conclusions based on data demonstrating significant rises in the incidence of large (>4 cm), and well-differentiated cancers with clinically significant pathological adverse features (Chen et al., 2009; Cramer et al., 2010; Enewold et al., 2009; Hodgson et al., 2004; Morris & Myssiorek, 2004). Improved detection has undoubtedly occurred and may explain much of the increase in small well-differentiated cancers. However, the most important evidence that increased diagnostic activity is not the sole cause for this increase is that large and more advanced cancers are increasing as well as small tumours. This trend suggest than some environmental factor, besides increased diagnostic activity, may be contributing to the increase in thyroid cancer incidence. Thyroid cancer can be induced in experimental animals directly by mutagenic carcinogens and indirectly through hormone imbalance.

The only well established risk factor for thyroid cancer in humans is ionizing radiation. Sex hormones, iodine deficiency and other factors (nutritional, volcanoes) have been proposed as risk factors for thyroid cancer, but the findings are inconsistent (Nagataki & Nystrom, 2002). The increase in thyroid cancer risk could be attributed to ionizing radiation exposure. Studies of individuals living in the Chernobyl areas have shown an increased risk among those exposed as children (Cardis et al., 2006). In our study, only 8 cases of thyroid cancer in people of 18 years of age or less could be identified, so ionizing radiation exposure cannot explain the recent increase in incidence of thyroid cancer in our community. However, a longer latency period for low doses of radiation could not be ruled out (Yamashita, 2006). Some authors have suggested that iatrogenic exposure to radiation during imaging by computed tomography, especially in children when radiation sensitivity of the thyroid gland is greater, could contribute to the increase in thyroid cancer (Baker & Bhatti, 2006); however this link remains unproven at the moment. Nutritional factors such as a low fruit and vegetable and selenium consumption have been linked to thyroid cancer and cancer in general (Clark et al., 1996; Franceschi et al, 1990; Rayman, 2000). The role of Brassica vegetable in cancer protection (Keck & Finley, 2004; Verhoeven et al., 1996) has also been reported. Remarkably, our soils are acidic with low selenium content and the consumption of these Brassica vegetables (cabbage), traditional in our community of the North-West of Spain, has decreased over the last decades due to the globalization of our diet and loss of the popularity of these foods because of their goitrogenous potential.

Contrary to what happened with reports on the incidence of thyroid cancer, reports on prevalence are scarce. In the USA, the prevalence estimate for thyroid cancer was 310,000 in 2001 (Sherman & Fagin 2005), averaging about 105 cases per 100,000 population. In our study, we observed an increase in the prevalence of thyroid cancer from 8 cases per 100,000 population in 1985 to 83 cases in 2001. The prevalence varied for both sexes, with the figure being greater in women (128 cases per 100,000 in 2001). The increase in thyroid cancer incidence seen in our area together with the good prognosis of this neoplasia can explain the increase in the prevalence of thyroid cancer. These data should be taken into account when planning health resources for the management of these patients.

In the present study, we also performed an analysis of cause–specific survival in our patients diagnosed of thyroid cancer between 1978-2001. In the case of deceased patients, we investigated the exact cause of death by reviewing the medical records to carry out the calculation of cause-specific survival. Throughout the follow-up period, we recorded in our series a total of 43 deaths, of which 70% were directly related to thyroid cancer. Among the remaining deaths not attributable to thyroid cancer, 69% were due to second malignancies. A high percentage of secondary neoplasms as the cause of death in thyroid cancer patients is also reflected in other series, for example, a Norwegian and a Dutch study found a 38% and 58% of deaths, respectively, attributable to other malignancies (Akslen et al., 1991; Eustatia-Rutten et al., 2006). In Europe we have data on thyroid cancer survival from the EUROCARE database. As the first publication on cancer survival in Europe, EUROCARE-1 (1978-1985) (Berrino et al., 1995) did not involved thyroid cancer, EUROCARE-2 (1985-1989) (Teppo et al., 1998) was the first publication on thyroid cancer survival. We also have more recent data from the EUROCARE-3 (1990-1994) (Sant et al., 2003). Both studies were population-based and used relative survival, i.e. an estimate of excess mortality. Five-year relative survival collected for Spain in the EUROCARE-3 (85.7% women and 82% in men) places it slightly above the European average (81.4% females and 71.8% in men). In our study, we observed an overall thyroid cancer cause-specific survival after excluding MPTC (91% in women, 89% in men) that is better than those previously reported over European countries as was reflected in the EUROCARE 2 and 3. As expected, we observed that survival decreases gradually with age in our study. We found a 5-year survival of 65% in the group older than 75 years (59% when excluding the MPTC). With regard to the histologic distribution, cause-specific survival at 25 years in our series is 95% for papillary thyroid carcinoma (93% if we exclude MPTC) and 83% for follicular carcinoma (including Hürthle cell). In the case of medullary carcinoma, the 20-year survival rate was 63%. As expected, anaplastic carcinoma was an ominous prognosis with a 5-year survival rate of 10%. We can compare these results with those of the cohort of patients with thyroid cancer at the Mayo Clinic (Schlumberger et al., 2008), where the cause-specific survival at 25 years for papillary thyroid carcinoma was 95%, wich was significantly higher than the rates found for medullary, Hürthle and follicular thyroid carcinoma, wich were 79, 71 and 66%, respectively. Curiously, patients with medullary thyroid carcinoma at the Mayo Clinic have similar or better outcomes than those patients with non papillary follicular thyroid carcinoma; as more patients have been diagnosed by genetic testing, most of them have curable disease and better survival. With regard to survival by histologic type, we found very similar results to those published in the U.S. series (Hundahl et al., 1998) where 10-year overall relative survival rates for patients with papillary, follicular, Hürthle cell, medullary, and undifferentiated/anaplastic carcinoma were 93, 85, 76, 75 and 14%, respectively (Hundahl et al., 1998). In our series, 10-year cause-specific survival for papillary thyroid carcinoma was 96% (95% if we exclude the MPTC, 87% for follicular carcinoma (including Hürthle cell), 70 % for medullary carcinoma and 0% for anaplastic carcinoma. A similar distribution of histologic types and pTNM stages may be one explanation for these similar results. With regard to staging, as expected, we found a survival of 100% at 25 years for tumors which were presented in stage I. Accordingly; we did not record any deaths due to thyroid cancer in our 95 cases of MPTC. Survival gradually worsened with more advanced staging at presentation, being only 15% at 10 years for stage IV tumors. In our study, the stage of tumors at presentation was generally favorable, which may have contributed positively to overall survival. Despite being a relatively benign disease, a continual decline in cancer-specific survival is noted in all tumor stages at successive follow-up intervals. This underscores the need of life-long surveillance for thyroid cancer patients.

Another objective of this study was to describe the prognostic factors associated with thyroid cancer survival. Because these variables are often strongly interrelated, we have identified risk factors associated with mortality from differentiated thyroid cancer using the Cox regression analysis. This was determined only in the group of differentiated thyroid carcinomas, as the rest of the tumors represent a little large in total thyroid cancers and they have a different clinical behavior. Age, follicular histotype, local tumor extension as well as distant metastases were found to have a significant negative influence on survival in the univariate analysis. However, in the multivariate analysis, only age and distant metastases were found to retain their independent prognostic values. Multiple studies have identified several prognostic factors, but overall the findings have been inconsistent, possibly due to bias introduced by the use of different institutional series with different distributions of histologic types and differences in follow-up and histologic classification of disease. Therefore, we do not know the relative importance of each of these features as prognostic factors and whether the findings in one population can be generalized to other populations (Gilliland et al., 1997). Although the majority of studies reported the effect of age on the prognosis of patients with differentiated thyroid carcinoma, data from some studies (Elisei et al. 2010; Gilliland et al., 1997; Hundahl et al., 1998; Sciuto et al. 2009) also suggest an effect on other thyroid histologies as well. The association between age and survival is not explained by differences in stage at diagnosis, differentiation, socio-demographic variables, or treatment. It has been speculated that other age-dependent factors such as nutritional or immune status, or differences in the spectrum of genetic alterations in tumors in the elderly, may play a role in survival (Gilliland et al., 1997). In this sense, several studies have found that survival does not differ for patients of similar ages and stages diagnosed with papillary or follicular carcinoma (Thoresen et al. 1989; Torres et al., 1985). Children and people younger than 20 years tend to present with higher stage disease and greater likelihood of locoregional and distant metastases, despite it, children generally have excellent survival rates, the exception to this rule is the disease in children aged < 10 years (Sipos & Mazzaferri, 2010). In the same line as most of the studies (Beenken et al., 2000; Eichhorn et al., 2003; Gilliland et al., 1997; Lerch et al., 1997; Mazzaferri, 1999; Shah et al., 1992), we found that the presence of distant metastases at presentation is an independent risk factor in the prognosis of differentiated thyroid carcinoma. The main cause of death from differentiated thyroid cancer is distant metastases (Mazzaferri, 1993). Mortality is high with distant disease, with 50 % survival at 3.5 years according to one recent study (Sampson et al., 2007). However, survival is improved in younger patients (Sampson et al., 2007), patients with microscopic rather than macroscopic disease (Durante et al. 2006), and patients with iodine-avid tumours (Durante et al. 2006; Sampson et al., 2007). Furthermore, the ability to achieve a negative post-treatment scan after multiple doses of radioiodine was associated with 92% overall 10-year survival, compared with 19% survival for patients who did not achieve a negative post-treatment scan (Durante et al. 2006). Numerous factors affect outcome of patients with thyroid cancer; in spite of these various factors, only a few are considered in the currently recommended TNM staging system. The clinician must therefore have a complete understanding of the various prognostic factors and how they contribute to the outcome, so that the patient can be counselled accordingly about treatment and long-term surveillance decisions (Sipos & Mazzaferri, 2010).

5. Conclusions

In conclusion, we have analyzed for the first time, the descriptive epidemiology of thyroid cancer in Vigo, Galicia (Spain), between 1985 and 2001. Long term follow-up ascertainment was practically complete, providing valid information on thyroid cancer prognosis. The results of this study can be summarized as follows: the first point to note is the histologic distribution of thyroid cancer in our population; wich is similar to that found in areas with high iodine intake, with a clear predominance of differentiated thyroid carcinoma and a high ratio of papillary to follicular carcinomas. As in many other regions and countries, the incidence of thyroid cancer is increasing and this trend is primarily caused by an increase in the incidence of papillary type. Our data showing an increase in papillary cancers larger than 1 cm suggest that some environmental factor may be contributing to this trend. There is a significant increase in the prevalence of thyroid cancer over time, especially among women. These data should be taken into account when planning health resources for management of this disease. Cause-specific survival of thyroid cancer in our study is higher than the European average, similar to that found in the U.S. series of thyroid cancer. Possible explanations for these results are: a high proportion of differentiated carcinoma, particularly papillary thyroid carcinoma, and a favorable stage (I and II) of the tumors at presentation. This study has some limitations: the relatively limited number of cases, particularly for selected histologic type; the study is merely descriptive, so it is not possible to give a definitive explanation for the observed increase in the incidence of thyroid cancer. His strength is also limited because we could not continue the study beyond 2001 in order to see if this trend continues or instead, the incidence of thyroid cancer reaches a plateau. Furthermore, information on a number of variables, such as vascular invasion, tumour recurrence and treatment (dose and frequency of I-131) were not controlled and may have influenced on survival. Further studies in these areas seem prudent.

6. References

Akslen, L., Haldorsen, T., Thoresen, SO., Glattre, E. (1993). Incidence pattern of thyroid cancer in Norway: influence of birth cohort and time period. *International Journal of Cancer,* Vol.53, pp. 183-187, ISNN 0020-7136

Baker, S. & Bhatti, WA. (2006). The thyroid cancer epidemic: is it the dark side of the CT revolution? *European Journal of Radiology,* Vol.60, No.1, pp. 67-69, ISNN 0720-048X

Beenken, S., Roye, D., Weiss, H., Sellers, M., Urist, M., Diethelm, A., Goepfert, H. (2000). Extent of surgery for intermediate-risk well-differentiated thyroid cancer. *American Journal of Surgery,* Vol.179, pp. 51- 56, ISNN 0002-9610.

Berkson, J. & Gage, RP. (1950). Calculation of survival rates for cancer. *Proceedings of the Staff Meeting.* Vol.25 No.11, pp. 270-286, ISNN 0092-699X

Berrino, F., Sant, M., Capocaccia, R., Hakulinen, T., Esteve, J. (Eds). (1995). *Survival of cancer patients in Europe: the EUROCARE study,* International Agency for Research on Cancer, ISBN 92 832 2132 X, Lyon.

Blanco Carrera, C., Pelaez Torres, N., Garcia-Diaz, JD., Maqueda Villaizan, E., Sanz JM., Alvarez Hernandez, J. (2005). Epidemiological and clinicopathological study of thyroid cancer in east Madrid. *Revista Clínica Española,* Vol.205, pp. 307-310, ISNN 0014-2565

Bray F. (2002). Age-standardization, In: *Cancer Incidence in Five Continents,* Parkin DM, Whelan SL, Ferlay J, Teppo L, Thomas DB (Eds), pp. 87-91, International Agency for Research on Cancer (IARC) Scientific Publications, ISBN 92 832 2155 9, Lyon.

Brierley, J., Panzarella, T., Tsang, RW., Gopodarowicz, MK., O'Sullivan, B. (1997). A comparison of different staging systems predictability of patient outcome. Thyroid carcinoma as an example. *Cancer,* Vol.79, pp. 2414-2423, ISNN 0008-543X

Burgess, J., Dwyer, T., McArdle, K., Tucker, P., Shugg, D. (2000). The changing incidence and spectrum of thyroid carcinoma in Tasmania (1978-1998) during a transition from iodine sufficiency to iodine deficiency. *The Journal of Clinical Endocrinology and Metabolism,* Vol.85, pp. 1513-1517, ISNN 0021-972X

Burgess, J. (2002). Temporal trends for thyroid carcinoma in Australia: an increasing incidence of papillary thyroid carcinoma (1982-1997). *Thyroid,* Vol.12, pp. 141-149, ISNN 1050-7256

Burgess, J. & Tucker, P. (2006). Incidence trends for papillary thyroid carcinoma and their correlation with thyroid surgery and thyroid fine-needle aspirate cytology. *Thyroid,* Vol.16, pp. 47-53, ISNN 1050-7256

Capocaccia, R., Gatta, G., Roáis, P., Carrani, E., Santaquilani, M., De Angelis, R., Tavilla, A. and the Eurocare Working Group. (2003). The EUROCARE-3 methodology of data collection, standardisation, quality control and statistical analysis. *Annals of Oncology,* Vol.14, pp. 14-27, ISNN 0923-7534

Cardis, E., Howe, G., Ron, E., Bebeshko, V., Bogdanova, T., Bouville., A, Carr, Z., Chumak, V., Davis, S., Demidchik, Y., Drozdovitch, V., Gentner, N., Gudzenko, N., Hatch, M., Ivanov, V., Jacob, P., Kapitonova, E., Kenigsberg, Y., Kesminiene, A., Kopecky, KJ., Kryuchkov, V., Loos, A., Pinchera, A., Reiners, C., Repacholi, M., Shibata, Y., Shore, RE., Thomas, G., Tirmarche, M., Yamashita, S., Zvonova, I. (2006). Cancer consequences of the Chernobyl accident: 20 years on. *Journal of Radiological Protection,* Vol.26, pp. 127-140, ISNN 0952-4746

Chen, A., Jemal, A., Ward, EM. (2009). Increasing incidence of differentiated thyroid cancer in the United States, 1988-2005. *Cancer,* Vol.115, No.16, pp. 3801-3807, ISNN 0008-543X

Chow, S., Law, SC., Au, SK., Mang, O., Yau, S., Yuen, KT., Lau, WH. (2003). Changes in clinical presentation, management and outcome in 1348 patients with differentiated thyroid carcinoma: experience in a single institute in Hong Kong, 1960-2000. *Clinical Oncology (Royal College of Radiologists (Great Britain)),* Vol.15, pp. 329-336, ISNN 0936-6555

Clark, L., Combs, GF Jr., Turnbull, BW., Slate, EH., Chalker, DK., Chow, J., Davis, LS., Glover, RA., Graham, GF., Gross, EG., Krongrad, A., Lesher, JL Jr., Park, HK., Sanders, BB Jr., Smith, CL., Taylor, JR . (1996). Effects of selenium supplementation for cancer prevention in patients with carcinoma of the skin. A randomized controlled trial. Nutritional Prevention of Cancer Study Group. *Journal of the American Medical Association,* Vol.276, pp. 1957-1963, ISNN 0098-7484

Colonna, M., Grosclaude, P., Remontet, L., Schvartz, C., Mace-Lesech, J., Velten, M., Guizard, A., Tretarre, B., Buemi, AV., Arveux, P., Esteve, J. (2002). Incidence of thyroid cancer in adults recorded by French cancer registries (1978-1997). *European Journal of Cancer,* Vol.38, pp. 1762-1768, ISNN 0959-8049

Colonna, M., Guizard, AV., Schvartz, C., Velten, M., Raverdy, N., Molinie, F., Delafosse, P., Franc, B., Grosclaude, P. (2007). A time trend analysis of papillary and follicular cancers as a function of tumour size: a study of data from six cancer registries in France (1983-2000). *European Journal of Cancer* Vol.43, pp. 891-900, ISNN 0959-8049

Cooper, D., Doherty, GM., Haugen, BR., Kloos, RT., Lee, SL., Mandel, SJ., Mazzaferri, EL., McIver, B., Sherman, SI., Tuttle, RM. (2006). American Thyroid Association Guidelines Taskforce. Management guidelines for patients with thyroid nodules and differentiated thyroid cancer. *Thyroid,* Vol.16, No.2, pp. 109-142, ISNN 1050-7256

Cramer, J., Fu, P., Harth, KC., Margevicius, S., Wilhelm, SM. (2010). Analysis of the rising incidence of thyroid cancer using the Surveillance, Epidemiology and End Results national cancer data registry. *Surgery,* Vol.148, No.6, pp. 1147-1152, discussion: pp. 1152-1143, ISNN 0263-9319

Davies, L. & Welch, HG. (2006). Increasing incidence of thyroid cancer in the United States, 1973-2002. *Journal of the American Medical Association,* Vol. 295, pp. 2164-2167, ISNN 0098-7484

DeLellis RA. & Willliams ED. (2004). Thyroid and parathyroid tumours, In *World Health Organization Classification of Tumours. Pathology and Genetics of Tumours of Endocrine Organs.* DeLillis RA, Lloyd RV, Heitz PU, Eng C. (Eds), pp. 49-133, IARC Press, ISBN 92 832 2416 7, Lyon

dos Santos Silva, I., Swerdlow, AJ. (1993). Thyroid cancer epidemiology in England and Wales: time trends and geographical distribution. *British Journal of Cancer,* Vol. 67, pp. 330-340, ISNN 0007-0920

Durante, C., Haddy, N., Baudin, E. et al. (2006). Long-term outcome of 444 patients with distant metastases from papillary and follicular thyroid carcinoma: benefits and limits of radioiodine therapy. *The Journal of Clinical Endocrinology and Metabolism,* Vol.91, pp. 2892-2899, ISNN 0021-972X

Eichhorn, W., Tabler, H., Lippold, R., Lochmann, M., Schreckenberger, M., Bartenstein, P. (2003). Prognostic factors determining long-term survival in well-differentiated thyroid cancer: an analysis of four hundred eighty-four patients undergoing therapy and aftercare at the same institution. *Thyroid,* Vol.13, No.10, pp. 949-958, ISNN 1050-7256

Elisei, R., Molinaro, E., Agate, L., Bottici, V., Masserini, L., Ceccarell,i C., Lippi, F., Grasso, L., Basolo, F., Bevilacqua, G., Miccoli, P, Di Coscio, G., Vitti P, Pacini, F., Pinchera, A. (2010). Are the clinical and pathological features of differentiated thyroid carcinoma really changed over the last 35 years? Study on 4187 patients from a single Italian institution to answer this question. *The Journal of Clinical Endocrinology and Metabolism,* Vol.95, No.4, pp. 1516-1527, ISNN 0021-972X

Enewold, L., Zhu, K., Ron, E., Marrogi, AJ., Stojadinovic, A., Peoples, GE., Devesa, SS. (2009). Rising thyroid cancer incidence in the United States by demographic and tumor characteristics, 1980-2005. *Cancer Epidemiology and Biomarkers Prevention,* Vol.18, No.3, pp. 784-791, ISNN 055-9965

Engholm, G., Ferlay, J., Christensen, N., Bray, F., Gjerstorff, M., Klint, A., Køtlum, J., Ólafsdóttir, E., Pukkala, E.,Storm, H. (2009). NORDCAN: Cancer Incidence, Mortality, Prevalence and Prediction in the Nordic Countries, Version 3.5. Association of the Nordic Cancer Registries. Danish Cancer Society. Available from: http://www.ancr.nu.

Etxabe, J., Vazquez, JA. (1994). Morbidity and mortality in Cushing's disease: an epidemiological approach. *Clinical Endocrinology (Oxford),* Vol.40, pp. 479-484, ISNN 0300-0664

Eustatia-Rutten, C., Corssmit, EPM, Biermasz, NR., Pereira, AM-, Romjin, JA., Smit, JW. (2006). Survival and death causes in differentiated thyroid carcinoma. *The Journal of Clinical Endocrinology and Metabolism,* Vol. 91, pp. 313-319, ISNN 0021-972X

Farahati, J., Geling, M., Mader, U., Mortl, M., Luster, M., Muller, JG., Flentje, M., Reiners, C. (2004). Changing trends of incidence and prognosis of thyroid carcinoma in lower Franconia, Germany, from 1981-1995. *Thyroid,* Vol.14, pp. 141-147, ISNN 1050-7256

Ferlay, J., Bray, F., Pisani, P., Parkin, DM. (2004). GLOBOCAN 2002: Cancer Incidence, Mortality and Prevalence Worldwide. IARC CancerBase N°5, version 2.0 Lyon: IARC Press. Available from: http://www-dep.iarc.fr/

Ferlay, J., Autier, P., Boniol, M., Heanue, M., Colombet, M., Boyle, P. (2007). Estimates of the cancer incidence and mortality in Europe in 2006. *Annals of Oncology,* Vol.18, pp. 581-592, ISNN 0923-7534

Fleming, ID., Cooper, JS., Henson, DE., Hutter, RVP., Kennedy, BJ., Murphy, GP., O´Sullivan, B., Sobin, LH., Yarbro, JW. (Eds). (1997). *AJCC Cancer Staging Manual,* Lippincott-Raven Publishers, ISBN 0-397-584114-8. Philadelphia.

Franceschi, S., Talamini, R., Fassina, A., Bidoli, E. (1990). Diet and epithelial cancer of the thyroid gland. *Tumori,* Vol. 76, pp. 331-338, ISNN 0300-8916

Garcia-Mayor, R., Perez Mendez, LF., Paramo, C., Luna Cano, R., Rego-Iraeta, A., Regal, M., Sierra, JM., Fluiters, E. (1997). Fine needle aspiration biopsy of thyroid nodules: impact on clinical practice. *Journal of Endocrinological Investigation,* Vol.20, pp. 482-487, ISNN 0391-4097

Garcia-Mayor, R., Rios, M., Fluiters, E., Perez Mendez, LF., Garcia- Mayor, EG., Andrade, A. (1999). Effect of iodine supplementation on a pediatric population with mild iodine deficiency. *Thyroid,* Vol.9, pp. 1089-1093, ISNN 1050-7256

Gilliland, F., Hunt, WC., Morris, DM, Key CR (1997). Prognostic factors for thyroid carcinoma. A population-based study of 15,698 cases from the Surveillance, Epidemiology and End Results (SEER) program 1973-1991. *Cancer,* Vol.79, pp. 564-573, ISNN 0008-543X

Gomez Segovia I., GH, Kresnik E, Kumnig G, Igerc I, Matschnig S, Stronegger WJ, Lind P. (2004). Descriptive epidemiology of thyroid carcinoma in Carinthia, Austria: 1984-2001. Histopathologic features and tumor classification of 734 cases under elevated general iodination of table salt since 1990: population-based age-stratified analysis on thyroid carcinoma incidence. *Thyroid,* Vol.14, 277-286, ISNN 1050-7256

Greene, FL., Page, DL., Fleming, ID., Fritz, A., Balch, CM., Haller, DG., Morrow, M. (Eds). (2002). *American Joint Committte on Cancer: AJCC Staging Manual*. Springer-Verlag, ISBN 978-0387952710, New York.

Hedinger, CE., Williams, ED., Sobin, LH. (1988). Histological typing of thyroid tumours, In: *International Histological Classification of Tumours,* World Health Organization (Ed), pp. 1-20 Springer-Verlag, ISBN 0387192441, New York.

Hodgson, N., Button J., Solorzano CC. (2004). Thyroid cancer: is the incidence still increasing?. *Annals of Surgical Oncology* Vol.11, No.12, pp. 1093-1097, ISNN 1068-9265

Hundahl, S., Fleming, ID., Fremgen, AM., Menck, HR. (1998). A National Cancer Data Base report on 53,856 cases of thyroid carcinoma treated in the U.S.1985-1995. *Cancer,* Vol.83, pp. 2638-2648, ISNN 0008-543X

Kaplan, E. (1958). Nonparametric estimation from incomplete observations. *Journal of the American Statistical Association,* Vol.53, pp. 457-481, ISNN 0162-1459

Keck, A. & Finley, JW. (2004). Cruciferous vegetables: cancer protective mechanisms of glucosinolate hydrolysis products and selenium. *Integrative Cancer Therapies,* Vol.3, pp. 5-12, ISNN 1534-7354

Kent, W., Hall, S., Isotalo, PA., Houlden, RL., George, RL., Groome, PA. (2007). Increased incidence of differentiated thyroid carcinoma and detection of subclinical disease. *Canadian Medical Association Journal,* Vol.177, No.11, pp. 1357-1361, ISNN 0820-3946

Kilfoy, B., Zheng, T., Holford, TR. et al. (2009). International patterns and trends in thyroid cancer incidence, 1973-2002. *Cancer Causes Control* Vol.20, No.5, pp. 525-531, ISNN 0957-5243

Kolonel, L., Hankin, JH., Wilkens, LR., Fukunaga, FH., Hinds, MW. (1990). An epidemiologic study of thyroid cancer in Hawaii. *Cancer Causes Control,* Vol.1, No.3, pp. 223-234, ISNN 0957-5243

Kovacs, G., Gonda, G., Vadasz, G., Ludmany, E., Uhrin, K., Gorombey, Z., Kovacs, L., Hubina, E., Bodo, M., Goth, MI., Szabolcs, I. (2005). Epidemiology of thyroid microcarcinoma found in autopsy series conducted in areas of different iodine intake. *Thyroid,* Vol.15, pp. 152-157, ISNN 1050-7256

Leenhardt, L., Grosclaude, P., Cherie-Challine, L. (2004). Increased incidence of thyroid carcinoma in France: a true epidemic or thyroid nodule management effects? Report from the French Thyroid Cancer Committee. *Thyroid,* Vol.14, pp. 1056-1060 (a), ISNN 1050-7256

Leenhardt, L., Bernier, MO., Boin-Pineau, MH., Conte Devolx, B., Marechaud, R., Niccoli-Sire, P., Nocaudie, M., Orgiazzi, J., Schlumberger, M., Wemeau, JL., Cherie-Challine, L., De Vathaire, F. (2004). Advances in diagnostic practices affect thyroid cancer incidence in France. *European Journal of Endocrinology,* Vol.150, pp. 133-139. (b), ISNN 0804-4643

Lerch, H., Schober, O., Kuwert, T., Saur, HB. (1997). Survival of differentiated thyroid carcinoma studied in 500 patients. *Journal of Clinical Oncology,* Vol.15, pp. 2067-2075, ISNN 0732-183X

Liu, S., Semenciw, R., Ugnat, AM., Mao, Y. (2001). Increasing thyroid cancer incidence in Canada, 1970-1996: time trends and age-period-cohort effects. *British Journal of Cancer,* Vol. 85, pp. 1335-1339, ISNN 0007-0920

LiVolsi, VA. (2004). Papillary carcinoma, In *World Health Organization Classification of Tumours. Pathology and Genetics of Tumours of Endocrine Organs.* DeLillis RA, Lloyd RV, Heitz PU, Eng C. (Eds), pp. 57-66, IARC Press, ISBN 92 832 2416 7, Lyon.

Loh, K., Greenspan, FS., Gee, L., Miller, TR., Yeo, PP. (1997). Pathological tumor-node-metastasis (pTNM) staging for papillary and follicular thyroid carcinomas: a retrospective analysis of 700 patients. *The Journal of Clinical Endocrinology and Metabolism,* Vol.82, pp. 3553-3562, ISNN 0021-972X

Martinez-Tello, F., Martinez-Cabruja, R., Fernandez-Martin, J., Lasso-Oria, C., Ballestin-Carcavilla, C. (1993). Occult carcinoma of the thyroid. A systematic autopsy study from Spain of two series performed with two different methods. *Cancer,* Vol.71, pp. 4022-4029, ISNN 0008-543X

Mazzaferri, EL. (1993). Thyroid carcinoma: papillary and follicular, In: *Endocrine tumors.* Mazzaferri EL, Samaan N. (Eds), pp. 278-333, Blackwell Scientific Publications, ISBN 0865422672, Cambridge, MA.

Mazzaferri, EL. (1999). An overview of the management of papillary and follicular thyroid carcinoma. *Thyroid* Vol. 9, pp. 421-427, ISNN 1050-7256

Merhy, J., Driscoll, HK., Leidy, JW., Chertow, BS. (2001). Increasing incidence and characteristics of differentiated thyroid cancer in Huntington, West Virginia. *Thyroid,* Vol.11, pp. 1063-1069, ISNN 1050-7256

Mitchell, I., Livingston, EH., Chang, AY., Holt, S., Snyder, WH. 3rd., Lingvay, I., Nwariaku, FE. (2007). Trends in thyroid cancer demographics and surgical therapy in the United States. *Surgery,* Vol.142, pp. 823-828; discussion 828-821, ISNN 0263-9319

Morris, L. & Myssiorek, D. (2010). Improved detection does not fully explain the rising incidence of well-differentiated thyroid cancer: a population-based analysis. *American Journal of Surgery,* Vol.200, No.4, pp. 454-461, ISNN 0002-9610

Nagataki, S. & Nystrom. E. (2002). Epidemiology and primary prevention of thyroid cancer. *Thyroid,* Vol.12, pp. 889-896, ISNN 1050-7256

Pacini, F., Schlumberger, M., Dralle, H., Elisei, R., Smit, JW., Wiersinga, W. (2006). European Thyroid Cancer Taskforce. European consensus for the management of patients with differentiated thyroid carcinoma of the follicular epithelium. *European Journal of Endocrinology,* Vol.154, No.6, pp. 787-803. Erratum in: Eur J Endocrinol. 2006 Aug; 2155 (2002):2385, ISNN 0804-4643

Parkin, DM. (2006). The evolution of the population-based cancer registry. *Nature Reviews. Cancer,* Vol.6, pp. 603-612, ISNN 1474-175X

Percy, C., Stanek, E 3rd., Gloeckler L. (1981). Accuracy of cancer death certificates and its effect on cancer mortality statistics. *American Journal of Public Health,* Vol.71, No.3, *pp.* 242-250, ISNN 0090-0036

Pettersson, B., Adami, HO., Wilander, E., Coleman, MP. (1991). Trends in thyroid cancer incidence in Sweden, 1958-1981, by histopathologic type. *International Journal of Oncology,* Vol.48, pp. 28-33, ISNN 1019-6439

Rayman, M. (2000). The importance of selenium to human health. *The Lancet,* Vol. 356, pp. 233-241, ISNN 0099-5355

Rego-Iraeta, A., Perez-Fdez, R., Cadarso-Suarez, C., Tome, M., Fdez-Marino, A., Mato, JA., Botana, M., Solache, I. (2007). Iodine nutrition in the adult population of Galicia (Spain). *Thyroid,* Vol.17, pp. 161-167, ISNN 1050-7256

Rego-Iraeta, A., Perez-Mendez, LF., Mantinan, B., Garcia-Mayor, RV. (2009). Time trends for thyroid cancer in northwestern Spain: true rise in the incidence of micro and larger forms of papillary thyroid carcinoma. *Thyroid,* Vol.19, pp. 333-340, ISNN 1050-7256

Reynolds, R., Weir, J., Stockton D., Brewster, DH., Sandeep, TC., Strachan, MW. (2005). Changing trends in incidence and mortality of thyroid cancer in Scotland. *Clinical Endocrinology (Oxford),* Vol. 62, pp. 156-162, ISNN 0300-0664

Rodríguez, I., Luna, R., Ríos, M., Fluiters, E., Páramo, C., García-Mayor, RV. (2002). Iodine deficiency in pregnant and fertile women in an area of normal iodine intake. *Medicina Clínica,* Vol.18, pp. 217-218, ISNN 0025-7753

Salas, A., Comas, D., Lareu, MV., Bertranpetit, J., Carracedo, A. (1998). mtDNA analysis of the Galician population: a genetic edge of European variation. *European Journal of Human Genetics,* Vol. 6, pp. 365-375, ISNN 1018-4813

Sampson, E., Brierley, JD., Le, LW., Rotstein, L., Tsang, RW. (2007). Clinical management and outcome of papillary and follicular (differentiated) thyroid cancer presenting with distant metastasis at diagnosis. *Cancer,* Vol.110, pp. 1451-1456, ISNN 0008-543X

Sampson, R., Woolner, LB., Bahn, RC., Kurland, LT. (1974). Occult thyroid carcinoma in Olmsted County, Minnesota: prevalence at autopsy compared with that in Hiroshima and Nagasaki, Japan. *Cancer,* Vol.34, pp. 2072-2076, ISNN 0008-543X

Sant, M., Aareleid, T., Berrino, F., Bielska Lasota, M., Carli, PM., Faivre, J., Grosclaude, P., Hedelin, G., Matsuda, T., Moller, H., Moller, T., Verdecchia, A., Capocaccia, R., Gatta, G., Micheli, A., Santaquilani, M., Roazzi, P., Lisi, D. (2003). EUROCARE-3: survival of cancer patients diagnosed 1990-94-results and commentary. *Annals of Oncology,* Vol.14, No.Suppl 5, pp.61-118, ISNN 0923-7534

Scheiden, R., Keipes, M., Bock, C., Dippel, W., Kieffer, N., Capesius, C. (2006). Thyroid cancer in Luxembourg: a national population-based data report (1983-1999). *British Medical Cancer,* Vol.6, pp.102, ISNN 1471-2407

Schlumberger, M., Filetti, S., Hay, ID. (2008). Nontoxic diffuse and nodular goiter and thyroid neoplasia, In: *Williams Textbook of Endocrinology.* Kronenberg HM, Melmed S, L Polonsky KS, Larsen PR (Eds), pp. 411–442, Saunders, ISBN 978-1-4160-2911-3, Philadelphia.

Sciuto, R., Romano, L., Rea, S., Marandino, F., Sperduti, I., Maini, CL. (2009). Natural history and clinical outcome of differentiated thyroid carcinoma: a retrospective analysis of 1503 patients treated at a single institution. *Annals of Oncology,* No.10, pp. 1728-1735, ISNN 0923-7534

Shah, J., Loree, TR., Dharker, D., Strong, EW., Begg, C., Vlamis, V. (1992). Prognostic factors in differentiated carcinoma of the thyroid gland. *American Journal of Surgery,* Vol.164, pp. 658- 661, ISNN 0002-9610

Sherman, S., Brierley, JD., Sperling, M., et al. (1998). Prospective multicenter study of thyroid carcinoma treatment: initial analysis of staging and outcome. National Thyroid Cancer Treatment Cooperative Study Registry Group. *Cancer,* Vol.83, pp. 1012-1021, ISNN 0008-543X

Sherman, S. & Fagin, J. (2005). Why thyroid cancer? *Thyroid,* Vol.15, pp. 303-304, ISNN 1050-7256

Sipos, J., Mazzaferri, EL. (2010). Thyroid cancer epidemiology and prognostic variable. *Clinical Oncology (Royal College of Radiologists (Great Britain)),* Vol.22, No.6, pp. 395-404, ISNN 0936-6555

Szybinski, Z., Huszno, B., Zemla, B., Bandurska-Stankiewicz, E., Przybylik-Mazurek, E., Nowak, W., Cichon, S., Buziak-Bereza, M., Trofimiuk, M., Szybinski, P. (2003). Incidence of thyroid cancer in the selected areas of iodine deficiency in Poland. *Journal of Endocrinological Investigation,* Vol.26, pp. 63-70, ISNN 0391-4097

Teppo, L. & Hakulinen, T. (1998). Variation in survival of adult patients with thyroid cancer in Europe. *European Journal of Cancer,* Vol. 34, pp. 2248-2252, ISNN 0959-8049

Thoresen, S., Akslen, LA., Glattre, E., Haldorsen, T., Lund, EV., Schoultz, M. (1989). Survival and prognostic factors in differentiated thyroid cancer-a multivariate analysis of 1,055 cases. *British Journal of Cancer,* Vol.59, No.2, pp. 231-235, ISNN 0007-0920

Torres, J., Volpato, RD., Power, EG., Lopez, EC., Dominguez, ME., Maira, JL., Ugarte, JA., Martinez, VC. (1985). Thyroid cancer. Survival in 148 cases followed for 10 years or more. *Cancer,* Vol.56, No.9, pp. 2298-2304, ISNN 0008-543X

Verhoeven, D., Goldbohm, RA., van Poppel, G., Verhagen, H., van den Brandt, PA. (1996). Epidemiological studies on brassica vegetables and cancer risk. Cancer Epidemiology, Biomarkers & Prevention, Vol.5, pp. 733-748, ISNN 1055-9965

Verkooijen, H., Fioretta, G., Pache, JC., Franceschi, S., Raymond, L., Schubert, H., Bouchardy, C. (2003). Diagnostic changes as a reason for the increase in papillary thyroid cancer incidence in Geneva, Switzerland. *Cancer Causes Control,* Vol.14, pp. 13-17, ISNN 0957-5243

Yamashita, S. (2006). Radiation-induced thyroid cancer. *Nippon Rinsho,* Vol.Suppl 1, pp. 493-496, ISNN 0047-1852

Zheng, T., Holford, TR., Chen, Y., Ma, JZ., Flannery, J., Liu, W., Russi, M., Boyle, P. (1996). Time trend and age-period-cohort effect on incidence of thyroid cancer in Connecticut, 1935-1992. *International Journal of Oncology,* Vol. 67, pp. 504-509, ISNN 1019-6439

2

The Functionality of p53 in Thyroid Cancer

Debolina Ray, Matthew T. Balmer and Susannah Gal
Department of Biological Sciences, Binghamton University
Binghamton, NY
USA

1. Introduction

Abnormalities in several important cellular pathways and processes are often a major contributing factor to the progression of cancer. The cell cycle is regulated by checkpoint proteins, including the cyclins and cyclin dependent protein kinases (cdk), which play an important role in the prevention of aberrant cell division. Normal cells have the ability to stop cell division and initiate DNA repair or apoptosis (programmed cell death) when genomic abnormalities cannot be repaired. Apoptotic signaling is necessary for the elimination of unwanted cells arising from exposure to stress or toxins or as a function of normal tissue development and senescence. Proteins regulating these pathways are critical to maintain genomic integrity by controlling normal cell division and cell death; one of the most important of these is the tumor suppressor p53. The p53 protein plays a critical role in maintaining genomic integrity through control of cell division, apoptosis, DNA repair and angiogenesis, and thus is known as the "guardian of the genome" (Lane, 1992). Cancer cells have evolved the ability to bypass the cell cycle checkpoints, to favor anti-apoptotic pathways and thus, proliferate uncontrollably. Many anti-tumor drugs and treatments such as radiation are designed to target the induction of pro-apoptotic pathways in cancer cells in an effort to stop cell division and ultimately kill these aberrant cells. In many cases, these drugs and treatments activate p53 which can then regulate the expression of genes controlling the cell cycle and apoptotic pathways. Understanding the role of the tumor suppressor p53 in the regulation of these processes is the focus of many laboratories around the world.

Many cancer cells have incorporated genetic alterations that allow the cells to evade the normal control of cell cycle and apoptotic processes and gain survival advantage. Oncogenic activation of the RAS/RAF/MEK/ERK pathway is considered the most common molecular alteration in thyroid cancer. Loss of function of tumor suppressors, such as PAX-8/PPARγ, PTEN, β-catenin and p53 has been observed in thyroid cancers, so these changes are likely involved in the progression of the disease (Hunt, 2005; Kroll, 2004). p53 is found to be mutated in 50% of human cancers, yet mutations in this gene are found in only 10% of thyroid cancers, primarily in poorly differentiated and aggressive types (Olivier et al., 2002). Based on these data, it is probable that the majority of thyroid cancers activate an alternative pathway that compromises the function of wild-type p53. Well-differentiated thyroid cancers generally do not express a mutation in p53 (Fagin et al., 1993). This suggests that mutation in the *p53* gene is a late stage event in the progression of thyroid cancer. The function of mutant p53 in thyroid cancer is not well understood.

1.1 p53 structure and regulation

p53 is a tumor suppressor protein transcribed by the *TP53* gene. The p53 protein is composed of 393 amino acids which span 5 conserved regions, including (1) an acidic N-terminus transcription-activation domain (residues 1-75); (2) a proline-rich domain (residues 64-92); (3) a DNA-binding domain (DBD) (residues 100-292); (4) an oligomerization domain (residues 324-355); and (5) a basic C-terminal regulatory domain (residues 360-393). Also of importance are the nuclear localization signal, NLS (residues 316-325) and the nuclear export signal, NES (residues 356-362), in the oligomerization domain and the C-terminal regulatory domain, respectively. Oligomerization of each p53 monomer and subsequent dimerization is a prerequisite to the formation of functionally active tetrameric p53 protein (Jeffrey et al., 1999); therefore, the tumor suppressor activity of p53 is dependent on tetramerization of each dimeric p53 molecule. Although p53 proteins that harbor a missense mutation in the oligomerization domain are known, these mutant monomers are generally functionally inactive and therefore these are not likely to play a role in altered DNA binding specificity. The full crystal structure of the wild-type p53 protein bound to DNA has been elucidated and well analyzed, and a list of "hot spot" mutations within the DBD associated with cancer are at sites that make contact with DNA. The structural complexity of these mutations and their altered activity in DNA binding are not well understood, although studies show that mutations are frequent at certain residues (i.e. R175, R273) in the DBD and may affect thermodynamic stability of the protein, or lead to steric interference and conformational changes at the DNA binding surface (Joerger et al., 2006).

The amount of p53 in normal cells is maintained at a very low level (Collavin et al., 2010). p53 activation in response to environmental challenges results in an overall increase in the accumulation and stabilization of p53, as well as qualitative changes in the protein, culminating in regulation of p53 target genes in the cell. p53 is activated under conditions of cellular stress and binds DNA within the promoters of target genes. p53 is capable of arresting the cell cycle at G1, G2 or in S phase, largely by induction of the *p21* gene whose protein product subsequently blocks the cdk's responsible for checkpoint regulation and progression of the cell cycle (Bai & Zhu, 2006). This allows the cell adequate time to repair damage to replicating DNA, or if this damage cannot be repaired, higher levels of p53 may signal a different set of genes that induce cell death through up or down-regulation of p53 targets that control apoptosis. Through these and other mechanisms, p53 works to maintain genomic stability. Transcriptional activity of the p53 protein is highly regulated by post-translational modification (PTM), particularly phosphorylation of serine (S) residues in both the N-terminal transactivation domain and the C-terminal regulatory domain, as well as acetylation of multiple lysine (K) residues in the C-terminal regulatory domain (Xu, 2003). Acetylation at residues K372, K373, K381 and K382 has been implicated in blocking the ubiquitin ligase activity of Mdm2, while other research suggests that phosphorylation at S15 and S392 results in accumulation of p53 in cancer cells by inhibiting interaction with Mdm2 (S15) and by blocking the Mdm2-ubiquitin degradation pathway (S392) (Kubbutat et al., 1998). As p53 is an activator of the *mdm2* gene, there is a negative auto-regulatory feedback loop between p53 and Mdm2, which works to maintain low levels of p53 in normal cells.

Once activated, p53 upregulates the gene which encodes the ubiquitin ligase that induces its degradation. This feedback pathway restricts the growth inhibitory actions of p53 in unstressed cells (Kubbutat et al., 1997). When p53 loses its ability to induce the *mdm2* gene and propagate the aforementioned negative feedback loop, the p53 protein accumulates in cells. This has been associated with poor clinical outcome (Vogelstein et al., 2000). Jung and colleagues (2011) recently reported that they observed a time and dose-dependent effect when treating adenocarcinoma cells (Ishikawa cells) with hydrogen peroxide, resulting in an increase in the amount of p53 protein and an increase in Bax, a pro-apoptotic member of the *bcl2* gene family. High levels of p53 staining observed in previous immunohistochemistry (IHC) studies of biopsy samples indicate that mutant p53 accumulates in tumors (Alsner et al., 2008). Interestingly, we and others have observed an accumulation of wild-type as well as mutant p53 in the nucleus of various cancer cell lines (Chandrachud & Gal, 2009; Olivier et al., 2005; Ray & Gal, unpublished). Hence, it becomes important to understand the functional significance of the p53 found in tumor samples, irrespective of the type of cancer.

1.2 The role of p53 in thyroid carcinoma

The role of *TP53* mutation in anaplastic thyroid cancer has been documented through research over the years. Mutation of *TP53* has been implicated as a late event in thyroid carcinomas (Pollina et al., 1996; Blagosklonny et al., 1998). In various experiments performed thus far, only about 14% of the thyroid tumors studied harbor p53 mutations (Shehdain, 2001). Mutations in p53 are found in poorly differentiated thyroid tumors (Shehdain, 2001) as well as in thyroid tumors displaying distant metastasis (Pavelic et al., 2006). Among the benign thyroid lesions, 100% of the cases of adenomatous goiter, thyroiditis and Grave's disease in this study showed the presence of wild-type *TP53* gene, 5% of follicular adenoma tumors display p53 mutation and 5% of the Hurtle adenomas show loss of heterozygosity (LOH) of the *TP53* gene. Among the malignant thyroid tumors analyzed in one study, advanced cases show LOH and mutation at the *TP53* locus, whereas the initial stages harbor the wild-type *TP53* gene (Pavelic et al., 2006). Immunohistochemical investigations of thyroid tumor samples have indicated the accumulation of both wild-type and mutant p53. p53 accumulation is observed not only in anaplastic and poorly differentiated forms where p53 mutation has been widely noticed, but also in well differentiated tumors in the absence of any p53 mutation (Soares et al., 1994). In both instances, the function of the accumulated protein is compromised. One of the accepted mechanisms of p53 inactivation is the altered interaction with Mdm2 used in the degradation of the p53 (see section 1.1 above). In the presence of the wild-type p53 protein, other mechanisms for inactivating p53 in thyroid cancers include cytoplasmic retention of the protein and over expression of *mdm2*. The enhanced expression of the *mdm2* gene is correlated with poor clinical outcome (Horie et al., 2001). Mutations in different locations of p53 appear to have different biological consequences that may lead to the development and progression of tumors through a range of mechanisms. In other cancers, the vast majority of the mutants create a p53 protein with an altered amino acid in the DNA binding domain (Soussi et al., 2005). Mutation at codons 213 and 238 are common in malignant thyroid cancers, while anaplastic carcinomas show most of the *TP53* gene mutations occurring at codons 238, 248 and 273 (Fagin et al., 1993). The patients carrying those mutations show lower survival rates, as well as lower rates of apoptosis in isolated tumor cells (Pavelic et al., 2006). Any of these changes in the *TP53* gene could affect the function of the p53 protein in thyroid cancer cells.

1.3 p53 functions as a transcription factor

Sequence specific transactivation of genes is an essential function of p53 as a tumor suppressor. The genes for several members of the cell cycle and cell death regulatory pathways are under the control of p53 in cells causing either their activation or repression of expression. The regulation of these genes is highly variable among different cancer cell lines (Yu et al., 1999). Literature suggests that aberrant regulation of target genes by p53 may lead to oncogenic activation or suppression of the expression of important genes leading to an imbalance in cell division or cell death and ultimately cancer (Vogelstein et al., 2000; Vousden & Lu, 2002). The p53 protein is known to regulate more than 50 different genes. A small subset of those genes in pathways regulating the cell cycle and apoptosis were studied here and are listed in Table 1.

Gene containing p53 regulatory sequence	Pathway involved	Gene up-regulated or down regulated by wild-type p53	Sequence of top strand used for DNA binding analysis (5'→3')
p21-5' site	Cell cycle	Up	CGAGGAACATGTCCCAACATGTTGCTCGAG
bax	Apoptosis	Up	GGGCTCACAAGTTAGAGACAAGCCTGGGCG
noxa	Apoptosis	Up	ATCTGAGGCTTGCCCCGGCAAGTTGCGCTC
survivin	Apoptosis	Down	AAGAGGGCGTGCGCTCCCGACATGCCCCGCG
cdc25c	Cell cycle	Down	GGGCAAGTCTTACCATTTCCAGAGCAAGCAC

Table 1. The p53 genes and their regulatory sequences used for this study. Information presented here is from the IARC web site: http://www-p53.iarc.fr/index.html and Lacroix et al., 2006. One strand of the biotinylated double-stranded DNA sequences used for the binding studies is given.

For this study, we focused on the regulatory regions of 5 genes; 3 regulating apoptosis and 2 regulating the cell cycle (Table 1). **p21** is an important cell cycle regulatory protein which inhibits a wide variety of cyclin/cdk complexes essential for the transition between the phases of the cell cycle (Xiong et al., 1993). Expression of the *p21* gene is induced in a p53- dependent manner in response to cell stress, such as radiation (Dulic et al., 1994) or drug treatment (i.e. 5-fluorouracil) (Hernandez-Vargas et al., 2006). It has also been found that *p21* is activated in a p53-independent manner (Parker et al., 1995). **Bax** is one of the major members of the apoptotic pathway of cells whose gene is upregulated by wild-type p53 (Milhara et al., 2003). Bax is a pro-apoptotic member of the Bcl2 family, which functions on the mitochondrial membrane to promote cytochrome c release into the cell cytoplasm and subsequent events of apoptosis (Lindsten et al., 2000). Wild–type p53 has been shown to down-regulate ***survivin*** in cancer cells in response to chemotherapeutic agents (Hoffman et al., 2002; Mirza et al., 2002). In turn, this results in depletion of cells in the G2/M phase and induction of apoptosis (Zhou et al., 2002). Similarly ***cdc25C*** is an important gene associated with cell cycle regulation and its gene product belongs to the family of protein phosphatases that activates the cdk's by dephosphorylating a specific serine that promotes the entry of cells into the mitotic phase. In a normal cell, Cdc25C suppresses the inhibitory effect exerted by p53 on mitotic entry of cells. It has been shown that the tumor suppressor p53 down-regulates the expression of the *cdc25A* gene, preventing abnormal cell proliferation (Nilson & Hoffman, 2000). The **Noxa** protein is an important mediator of apoptotic response induced by p53. This candidate encodes for BH3-only protein and is a pro-apoptotic member of the Bcl2 family, needed to initiate apoptosis in response to DNA damage (Huntington et al., 2009). As DNA binding is an essential component of transcriptional activation of a gene and the contribution of altered DNA binding by mutant p53 to its target gene sequences has not been fully elucidated, our present analysis of this function of p53 should provide insight into the expected regulation of gene expression.

1.4 Methods of studying protein-DNA binding

DNA binding by the p53 protein is known to regulate the expression of genes. We and others hypothesize that altered protein structure of mutant p53 might result in differential p53-DNA binding which could translate into abnormal target gene expression. The study of the DNA–protein interaction is done using a number of methods and each has its own advantages and disadvantages. The most common among them is the **Electrophoretic Mobility Shift Assay** (EMSA). In this assay, there is a shift in the migration of a DNA band on a gel in the presence of a DNA binding protein. Park and his colleagues (1994) demonstrated that the p53 mutant with changes at codon 273 (like the anaplastic thyroid cancer cell line ARO) has the ability to bind to the p53 consensus DNA sequence and activate transcription, whereas all the other mutants (at positions 156, 175, 223, 248 and 280) bound to the DNA, but did not transactivate the reporter gene. Their research also found that the p53 from the follicular thyroid cancer cell line WRO with mutation at codon 223 was able to bind to DNA, but was unable to activate transcription. It was concluded that cancer cells with mutation at codon 273 of p53 are very different from cells with mutations at other sites in the protein. One of the challenges faced with EMSA is that it does not easily provide quantitative values for the binding of protein to the DNA sequence. A study by Namba and colleagues (1995) utilized EMSA to show that wild-type p53 in nuclear extracts from cells exposed to radiation bound to *p21* and *gadd45* regulatory sequences and induced G_1 arrest through the accumulation of the p21 protein. **Scintillation Proximity Assay** (SPA) uses a radioactively labeled DNA sequence of interest that binds to p53 immobilized on scintillant containing beads and generates light which can be quantified. The intensity of binding is reflected as a higher number of counts (Gal et al., 2006; Chandrachud & Gal, 2009). The authors here have developed the SPA method to quantitate p53 DNA binding from baculovirus-expressed p53, as well as in extracts from human cancer cell lines. It has been shown that wild-type p53 from MCF-7 breast cancer cells treated with hydrogen peroxide and WRO (a thyroid cancer cell line with mutant p53) show greater affinity for the *cyclin G* gene regulatory sequence when compared to extracts from other cancer cell lines. **Fluorescence anisotropy** has also been utilized to study sequence specific DNA binding to several of the p53 target gene sequences by p53 protein obtained from bacterial expression (Weinberg et al., 2004, 2005). Fluorescence anisotropy measures the presence of the DNA binding protein as it alters the mobility of the fluorescently labeled DNA and as such, affects the polarity of the emitted light by the fluorophor. Heterologously expressed p53 protein forms (wild-type and truncated) have been shown to bind to gene regulatory sequences with differential affinities, particularly the genes within the apoptosis pathway. The **Streptavidin Magnetic Bead Assay** (SA) utilizes biotinylated DNA sequences and protein extracts containing wild-type or mutant p53. This assay requires the use of streptavidin magnetic beads to separate the p53 DNA complex with the help of a magnet. DNA binding with p53 protein from tissue lysates of frozen breast cancer specimens has been carried out using streptavidin and biotinylated DNA. The results showed that some of the extracts demonstrated binding to the consensus sequence, whereas others failed to show such binding (Liu et al., 2001). Studies by Chandrachud and Gal (2009) demonstrated variable binding of wild-type and mutant p53 from MCF-7 and thyroid cancer cells, respectively, to different gene regulatory sequence by SA.

In order to better understand the role of p53 in thyroid cancer, we have analyzed the sub-cellular localization, post-translational modifications and the DNA binding specificity of the p53 from 3 cell lines; 2 thyroid cancer cell lines, ARO and WRO, both with mutant p53 and a breast cancer cell line, MCF-7, carrying wild-type p53 protein. We also studied the effects of oxidative stress (in the form of H_2O_2 treatment) on p53 level, localization and DNA binding activity in all 3 cell lines.

2. Materials and methods

2.1 Cell culture and hydrogen peroxide treatment

Thyroid cancer cell lines ARO and WRO (originally provided by Frances Carr Professor of Pharmacology, University of Vermont) were grown in RPMI-1640 (ATCC, Manassas, VA) supplemented with 10% fetal bovine serum (Thermofisher Scientific, Rockford, IL), 100U/ml penicillin and 100µg/ml streptomycin (Lonza, Walkersville,MD) at 37° C and 5% CO_2. MCF-7 cells (American Type Culture Collection (ATCC), Manassas, VA) were cultured following the same conditions as mentioned above except that they were grown in Minimum Essential Medium (ATCC). At about 80-85% confluence, the cells were treated with 0.2mM freshly prepared hydrogen peroxide (H_2O_2) (J. T Baker Inc., Phillipsburg, NJ) for three hours.

2.2 Cytoplasmic and nuclear extract preparation

Cells (either untreated or treated with H_2O_2) were harvested for their cytoplasmic and nuclear fractions using a published protocol (Jagelskà et al., 2002). Total protein concentrations (µg/µl) in the fractions were determined by bincinchoninic acid assay (BCA) (Sigma Chemical, St. Louis, MO) using bovine serum albumin (BSA) as a standard. The p53 (pg/µl) in the two fractions from the cell lines was estimated utilizing the Pantropic p53 ELISA Kit obtained from Calbiochem-EMD (La Jolla, CA).

2.3 Western blots

Following separation of proteins on 10% polyacrylamide gels (BioRad, Hercules, CA) and transfer to nitrocellulose membranes using the iBlot system (Invitrogen, Carlsbad, CA), p53 in the nuclear as well as cytoplasmic extracts was visualized with anti-p53 DO-7 (1:2000 dilution) (Calbiochem-EMD) by incubating the antibody with the nitrocellulose membrane in 5% BSA blocking solution in 1x Tris buffered saline for 3 hours. Actin in cytoplasmic extracts was visualized with anti-β-actin (mouse) (1:1000 dilution) (Sigma Chemicals) by incubating the membrane with antibody for 3 hours. The membranes were then incubated with goat anti-mouse IgG-alkaline phosphatase (AP) (1:1000) secondary antibody (Southern Biotech, Birmingham, AL) in 5% BSA blocking solution in 1x Tris buffered saline for 1 hour and visualized with the colorimetric alkaline phosphatase substrate (KPL, Inc., Gaithersburg, MD) with an exposure time of 3-4 minutes. For p53 phosphoserine detection, p53 pSer15 was visualized with Phosphodetect™ anti-p53 ($pSer^{15}$) (Ab-3) (1:1000 dilution) (Calbiochem-EMD) by incubating the antibody with the membrane for 3 hours. p53 pSer392 was visualized with Phosphodetect™ anti-p53 ($pSer^{392}$) (Ab-4) (1:1000 dilution) (Calbiochem-EMD) by incubating the antibody with the membrane for 18-24 hours. The membrane was then incubated with donkey anti-rabbit IgG(H+L)-AP (1:1000) secondary antibody (Southern Biotech) in 5% BSA blocking solution in 1x Tris buffered saline for 1 hour and visualized with the colorimetric alkaline phosphatase substrate with an exposure time of 10-12 minutes. Signal intensities were observed by means of densitometry and analyzed using Quantity One software by BioRad.

2.4 Streptavidin magnetic bead assay (SA)

This assay based on a published protocol (Chandrachud & Gal 2009) was performed by incubating 50pg of p53 from ARO WRO, and MCF-7 nuclear and cytoplasmic extracts with 20pmoles of biotinylated DNA (30bp) (see Table 1 for sequences) in the other components used previously. Both the 'bound' and 'unbound' fractions along with a pre-bound fraction were separated on 10% SDS-PAGE gels (Bio-Rad), transferred to a PVDF membrane (Millipore, Bedford, MA) and probed for p53 with DO-7 as for the western blots (above) except that PVDF membranes were used and the secondary antibody was conjugated with horse radish peroxidase (HRP) (1:10,000) (Cell Signaling, Danvers, MA). The signal was visualized using a chemiluminescent substrate (Thermofisher Scientific). Signal intensities were quantified by means of densitometry and analyzed using the Quantity One software (Bio-Rad). The percentage of p53 bound to a particular gene regulatory sequence was calculated by adding the intensities in both the 'bound' and 'unbound' fractions and subsequently calculating the percentage in each fraction.

3. Results

We focused our studies on determining the functional status of p53 as a transcription factor and the potential role of phosphorylation as a p53 regulatory mechanism in untreated and H_2O_2 treated ARO and WRO thyroid cancer cells. To accomplish this, we determined the level of p53, its localization in the cell and phosphorylation and the p53 DNA binding specificity for target gene promoter sequences. The thyroid cancer cell lines ARO and WRO have mutations in the p53 within the DNA binding domain at positions 273 (R to H) and 223 (P to L), respectively (Fagin et al., 1993). In some cases, we used the breast cancer cell line, MCF-7 as a comparison for these thyroid cancer cells as it has wild-type p53 (Okumura et al., 2002).

3.1 p53 is predominantly located in the nucleus of ARO and WRO thyroid cancer cells

The level of p53 in nuclear and cytoplasmic fractions from untreated and H_2O_2 treated ARO and WRO thyroid cancer cells was determined using ELISA and compared to the total protein (Table 2). The level of p53 in nuclear and cytoplasmic fractions from untreated ARO and WRO thyroid cancer cells was also determined by western blot analysis (Figure 1). p53 is detected predominantly in the nuclear fraction of all cell extracts with only a minor amount in the ARO cytoplasmic extracts. This latter localization may be an artefact of the extraction procedure or may indicate some retention of p53 in the cytoplasm. p53 was not detected in the cytoplasmic extracts from WRO cells (Figure 1). The relative amounts of p53 in ARO and WRO nuclear extracts are comparable for the same amount of total protein loaded (Figure 1). This observation is not consistent with the p53 quantitation by ELISA showing much lower levels of p53 in the WRO compared to the ARO cells (Table 2). The ELISA kit presumably uses different antibodies than what we used in the western blot analysis which may explain the discrepancy (the identity of the antibodies used in the ELISA kit was not provided by the company when requested).

3.2 Oxidative stress does not result in an increase or change the localization of p53 in ARO and WRO thyroid cancer cell lines

We have determined in our laboratory (Chandrachud & Gal, 2009) that H_2O_2 treatment of MCF-7 breast cancer cells (containing wild-type p53) induces the accumulation of p53 in the nuclear fraction of cell extracts. Using western blot analysis, we determined that the amount of p53 in ARO and WRO nuclear extracts does not change upon H_2O_2 treatment (Figure 2). This is corroborated by the data from the ELISA comparing the levels of p53 with total protein (Table 2). As expected, we observed an increase in the p53 level in MCF-7 breast cancer cells after treatment. H_2O_2 treatment also does not alter the localization of p53 in ARO or WRO thyroid cancer cells (Figure 1 and Table 2).

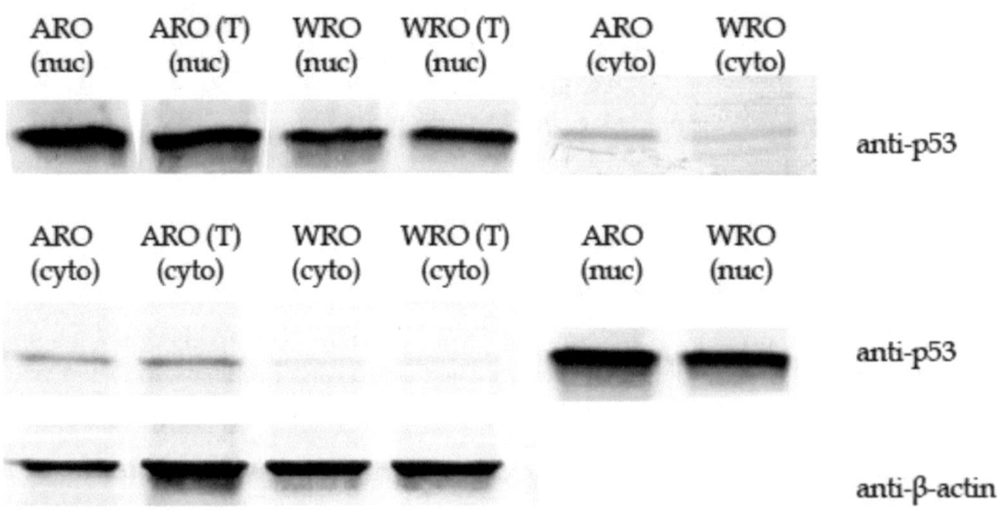

Fig. 1. p53 detection in nuclear and cytoplasmic extracts of ARO and WRO thyroid cancer cells. Western blot analysis shows the distribution of p53 in nuclear (nuc) versus cytoplasmic (cyto) fractions for both ARO and WRO untreated and H_2O_2 treated (T) cells. Total protein amount of 10μg was loaded in each well. β-actin was used as a loading control for cytoplasmic extracts. p53 is predominantly localized in the nuclear fractions from both cell lines.

Extract	ARO	ARO(T)	WRO	WRO(T)	MCF-7	MCF-7(T)
Nuclear p53 (pg/µl)	203	211	43	36	8	18
Cytoplasmic p53(pg/µl)	31	32	9	18	n/a	n/a
Nuc total protein (µg/µl)	7.4	7	8.6	9.2	9	8
Cyto total protein(µg/µl)	8	4.3	4.7	4.4	6	4
Ratio of nuclear p53/total protein	27.3	29.4	5	4	1	2.3

Table 2. Level of p53 and total protein in the nuclear and cytoplasmic extracts of the cell lines. Nuclear and cytoplasmic extracts derived from untreated and cells treated with H_2O_2 for 3 hours (T) were analyzed for p53 by ELISA and for total protein by BCA as described in the Methods section. Two of the cytoplasmic extracts were not analyzed (n/a) for the p53 levels. The level of p53 is higher in the nuclear extracts than in the cytoplasmic extracts and higher in the thyroid cancer cell lines ARO and WRO compared to that in the breast cancer cell line MCF-7 with wild-type p53. Treatment does not increase the level of p53 in the thyroid cancer cells, but does cause an increase in MCF-7 cells as previously published (Chandrachud & Gal, 2009).

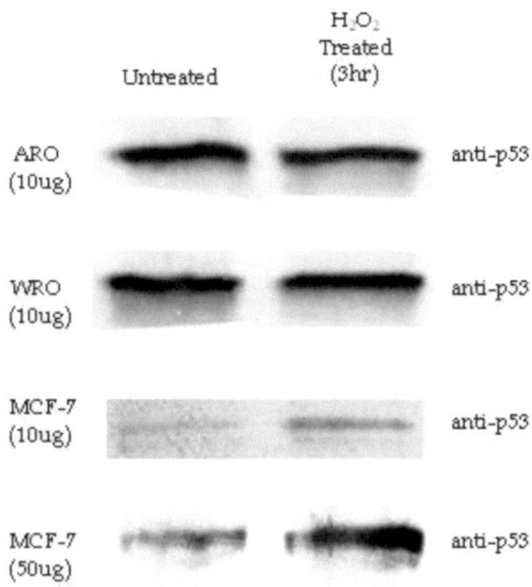

Fig. 2. Levels of p53 in nuclear extracts following H_2O_2 treatment. Western blots were used to monitor the level of p53 in nuclear extracts of ARO, WRO and MCF-7 cells initially (untreated) and following a 3 hour treatment with H_2O_2. Total protein amount of 10µg or 50µg was loaded into each well. The level of p53 does not change in ARO and WRO mutant thyroid cancer cells upon treatment, while the amount of p53 increases in MCF-7 cells after H_2O_2 treatment.

3.3 Phosphorylation of p53 is observed at S15 and S392 in thyroid cancer cells

Phosphorylation of specific residues on p53 has been linked to alterations in the functional status of p53 as a transcription factor (Xu, 2003). p53 is phosphorylated at residues 15 and 392 in extracts from ARO and WRO cells (Figure 3). Phosphorylation of p53 at S15 and S392 is not induced by oxidative stress. Interestingly, H_2O_2 treatment appears to decrease phosphorylation of p53 at residue 392 in ARO and WRO treated cells (Figure 3B). Phosphorylation of p53 at residues 20 and 46 was not detected in the nuclear extracts from the thyroid cancer cells (data not shown).

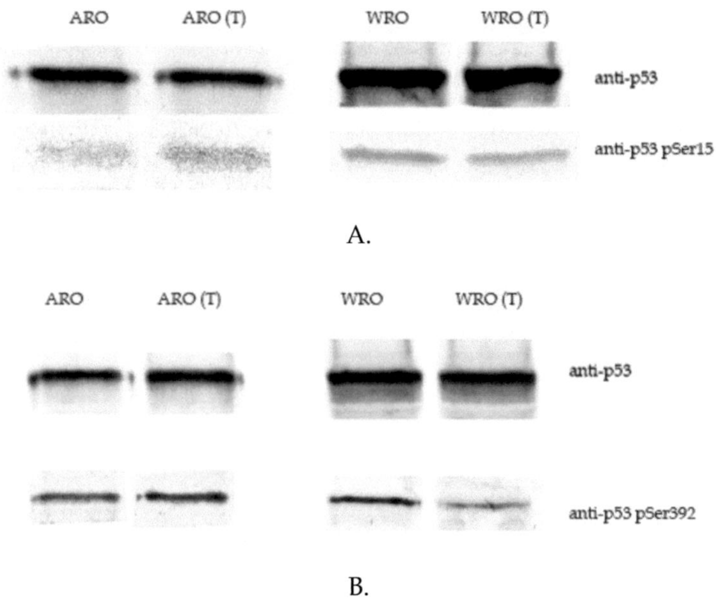

Fig. 3. Western blot analysis of the phosphorylation state of p53 at residues 15 and 392. Nuclear extracts from ARO and WRO thyroid cancer cells containing 300pg of p53 (based on ELISA) were loaded on the gel, and the derived blot probed with antibodies to phosphorylated p53 at S15 (panel A) or at S392 (Panel B) and for total p53 (anti-p53). Phosphorylation of p53 at S15 does not appear to change in response to H_2O_2 treatment, while that modification at S392 appears to decrease after treatment (for WRO cells only).

3.4 DNA binding to some of the sequences by the p53 protein is detected

One measure of the functional status of p53 is the DNA binding and while some work has been done using the DNA consensus sequence with the p53 from these cell lines, we wished to look for differences in binding specificity to several of the more than 100 target sequences recognized by p53. Previously, we have shown that the p53 from these cell lines has somewhat different specificity for the regulatory regions from *p21*, *mdm2* and *cyclin G* (Chandrachud & Gal, 2009). We wanted to extend the sequences analyzed by including 4 other genes, 2 genes regulating the cell cycle and 2 belonging to the apoptotic pathway. Minimal binding was seen to the *cdc25C, bax* and *noxa* regulatory regions by the ARO and WRO nuclear extracts while DNA binding was detected with *p21* and *survivin* gene regulatory regions (Figure 4, Table 3, data not shown). ARO and WRO both bind similarly to *p21* and *survivin* gene regulatory sequences. In a previous publication, the p53 from nuclear extracts from ARO and WRO cells also bound to the *mdm2* and *cyclin G* regulatory gene sequences, both at 10-15% of the p53 bound for ARO and at about 5% bound for the p53 from the WRO cell nuclear extracts using SA (Chandrachud & Gal, 2009). DNA binding

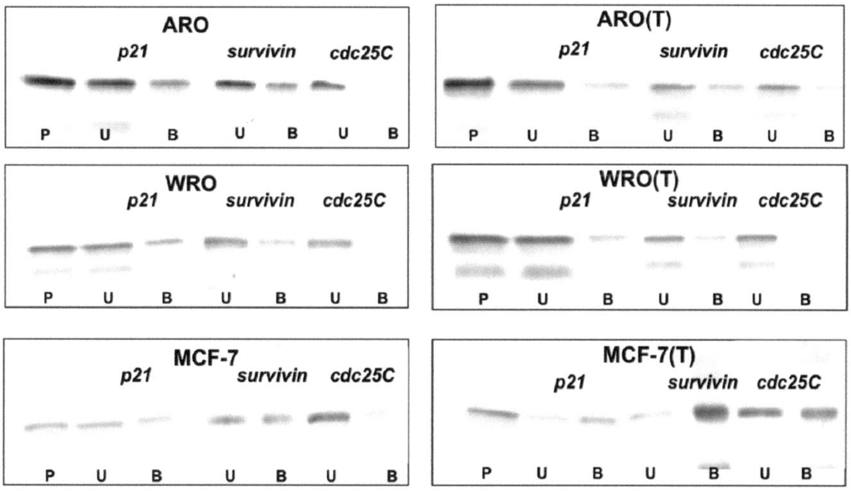

Fig. 4. DNA binding by p53 from nuclear extracts to various DNA sequences. DNA binding by 50pg of p53 to 20pmole biotinylated DNA sequences from the *p21, survivin,* and *cdc25C* promoter regions were performed. The p53 in the DNA bound (B) or unbound (U) fractions and an equivalent aliquot of the protein prior to binding (P) were detected using western blots. Nuclear extracts were derived from ARO, WRO and MCF-7 cells, untreated and following H_2O_2 treatment (T). DNA binding occurs to the *p21* and *survivin* gene promoters while no binding is detected to the *cdc25C* gene by the p53 from the ARO and WRO cells. Binding is detected to all of the sequences by the p53 from the MCF-7 cells, which increases upon treatment with H_2O_2.

Gene	ARO	ARO(T)	WRO	WRO(T)	MCF-7	MCF-7(T)
p21	33	16	32	25	34	83
cdc25C	5.8	5	1.8	2	13	44
bax	1	1.8	0.5	2	11	45.6
noxa	1.5	0.9	0	0	14	56
survivin	33	15.6	32	28	47	76

Table 3. DNA binding specificity of p53 from the nuclear extracts from different cell lines. Nuclear extracts from the different cells untreated or treated with H_2O_2 for 3 hours (T) were prepared and used for the streptavidin DNA binding assay as described for each of the 5 sequences given. The numbers indicate the percent of total p53 in the extract that was bound to the particular sequence using western blots like those shown in Figure 4 as well as data not shown. The experiments using extracts from MCF-7 cells have been repeated at least 3 times, while those with ARO and WRO cell extracts have been repeated twice with the average difference between the replicate values being 1-6%. Binding was detected with the p53 from the ARO, WRO nuclear extracts to the *p21* and *survivin* regulatory regions only and decreased upon treatment with H_2O_2. Binding was detected to all 5 sequences by the p53 from the MCF-7 cells and increased 2-4X upon treatment with H_2O_2.

was also tested with the p53 in the cytoplasmic extracts, but no binding was detected in any of these extracts with the *p21* sequence used here (data not shown). Interestingly, we detected a slightly faster migrating p53 species in some of the extracts, particularly in the cytoplasm of the thyroid cancer cells. This band is not present in the bound fractions using any of the biotinylated gene sequences, consistent with this protein representing a non-DNA binding form of p53. Although the presence of this lower band may be an artefact of the extraction procedure, there are several alternative forms of p53 known (Khoury & Bourdon, 2010). The identity of this faster migrating p53 protein is not known.

3.5 Changes in DNA binding following H_2O_2 treatment

In the previous publication, only the MCF-7 cells had been treated with H_2O_2 to activate p53 (Chandrachud & Gal, 2009). Here, that stress treatment was also applied to the ARO and WRO cells and the nuclear extracts were analyzed for alterations in DNA binding specificity (Figure 4 and Table 3). Insignificant binding is still seen to the *cdc25C, bax* and *noxa* regulatory regions, but for both thyroid cancer cell lines, treatment with H_2O_2 appeared to reduce the level of binding to the *p21* and *survivin* regulatory regions (from the ARO extract by about 50% while that from WRO by between 15 and 25%). In contrast, the binding by the wild-type p53 from the MCF-7 breast cancer cell line was detected for all 5 sequences, and binding to all 5 was enhanced between 2 and 4x after H_2O_2 treatment (Figure 4 and Table 3). This is consistent with previous work showing an increase in binding to the *cyclin G, mdm2* and *p21* regulatory sequences by the p53 from the MCF-7 cells (Chandrachud & Gal, 2009). Thus, there is a different DNA binding specificity of the p53 in MCF-7 cells once the cells are treated with H_2O_2, which is again different from that detected with the mutant p53 from the ARO and WRO cells.

4. Discussion

The functionality of p53 is essential for cells to maintain normal control of the cell cycle and apoptosis. We have looked at the characteristics of p53 from several angles in this chapter and all have provided useful information to better understand this tumor suppressor in the thyroid cancer cell lines, ARO and WRO. As noted above, the p53 in these cells contains a mutation resulting in a different protein from the wild-type protein present in the breast cancer cell line, MCF-7 that we have used for comparison in this work. We have looked at the level of the p53 protein and detected much higher amounts in the thyroid cancer cells compared to the level in the breast cancer cells. We have noted that the protein in ARO and WRO cells is primarily in the nucleus and that it shows phosphorylation at 2 serine residues (15 and 392). The DNA binding by p53 is similar in ARO and WRO cells but shows some significant differences compared to that detected in the MCF-7 cells. We have also compared each of those properties in cells that have been treated to oxidative stress and found that little changes in the p53 from the thyroid cancer cell lines while there is a significant change in the protein from MCF-7 cells. Each of these aspects will be examined further below.

The level of p53 protein observed by ELISA (Table 2) demonstrates a significantly higher level of the p53 present in the thyroid cancer cell lines versus the breast cancer cell line with ARO cell extracts having the most. Western blot analysis of the same extracts loaded at a 10μg total protein (Figure 2) shows a similar level of p53 in both untreated and H_2O_2 treated ARO and WRO cells which is higher than the level of protein observed in MCF-7 cells loaded at both 10μg and 50μg of total protein. We are uncertain of the specificity of the p53 antibody provided in the Pantropic p53 ELISA kit, therefore it is difficult to speculate on the cause of the discrepancy between the ELISA and western blot results observed for the ARO and WRO cell lines (Table 2, Figure 2, respectively). It is evident by densitometry analysis (data not shown) and visual observation of the western blots that both ARO and WRO cell extracts contain very similar levels of the p53 protein. There are several mechanisms to explain the increased level of the p53 observed in the thyroid cancer cells. First, p53 is a transcription factor that is responsible for activating a subset of genes in response to DNA damage, hypoxia and genotoxic agents, such as etoposide and doxorubicin (Vassilev et al., 2004). Both thyroid cancer cell lines express mutations of the p53 protein in the DNA binding domain (ARO, R273H and WRO, P223L) potentially affecting its ability to bind DNA and potentially to induce *mdm2*, which is the primary regulator of p53 (Alarcon-Vargas & Ronai, 2002). Mdm2 binds wild-type p53 with high affinity and acts as a negative modulator of p53 transcriptional activity (Vassilev et. al., 2004). Therefore, the lack of induction of *mdm2* by the mutant p53 may be playing a direct role in the increased stability of p53, resulting in the higher levels of this protein observed in thyroid cancer cells. Another alternative is that the mutant form of p53 is unable to interact with Mdm2 and thus is not targeted for degradation (Prives & White, 2008). Since we do not know the status of Mdm2 (null, wild-type or mutant) in ARO and WRO cells, we can not say definitively whether or not lack of *mdm2* transcription is the causative factor. Research in other cell systems indicates that it is a plausible root cause and could be explored in the future with these thyroid cancer cell lines.

The p53 protein observed in ARO and WRO cells is phosphorylated at serine residues 15 (S15) and 392 (S392) (Figure 3). This is significant because both of these post-translational modifications are known to play important roles in the regulation by Mdm2 by either disrupting interactions between Mdm2 and the N-terminal transactivation domain of p53 (S15) (Xu, 2003) or by blocking ubiquitin-dependent degradation and nuclear export of p53 via the modification in the C-terminal regulatory domain (S392) (Kim et al., 2004). Studies conducted by Kim and colleagues (2004) demonstrate that modification of S392 blocks the binding of the human papilloma virus E6 protein to the p53 and promotes nuclear localization of p53, both of which confer p53 protein stability. We demonstrate that p53 accumulates and is largely retained in the nuclear compartment of thyroid cancer cells in both untreated and H_2O_2 treated cells (Figures 1 and 2). Since the p53 nuclear localization signal (NLS) (residues 316-325) and nuclear export signal (NES) (residues 356-362) are in proximity to the oligomerization domain, Liang and Clarke (2001) have proposed that tetramerization of p53 can inhibit nuclear export by masking the NES and /or NLS required for transport. The observation that the p53 in ARO and WRO thyroid cancer cells is retained in the nucleus and phosphorylated at S15 and S392 indicates that the mutant p53 is likely tetrameric and potentially functional in the cells, although not necessarily able to regulate transcription.

The WRO cells, derived from a follicular carcinoma, are heterozygous for the P223L mutation (Liu et al., 2008). One way in which p53 is regulated in tumor cells is through trans-dominant suppression of wild-type p53 function by a mutant protein. Simultaneous expression of wild-type and mutant p53 has been known to result in hetero-tetramerization of two types of monomers, which could result in a fully intact protein with loss of wild-type protein activity (Chan et al., 2004; Srivastava et al., 1993; Unger et al., 1993). The ARO cells carry the mutation R273H (one of the most common sites altered in all cancers); however, we do not have confirmation as to whether these cells contain a wild-type p53 allele or are homozygous for the mutation. The likelihood for the oligomerization of mixed tetramers would also explain the accumulation of a fully intact, and thus potentially functional protein retained in the nucleus as we demonstrated in this paper.

A variety of treatments are known to stabilize p53 by blocking the Mdm2-mediated degradation of the protein. In this study, we focused on oxidative stress and it's effect on the p53 functionality in the thyroid cancer cell lines as we and others have seen changes in this protein following H_2O_2 treatment of the breast cancer cell line, MCF-7 (Chandrachud & Gal, 2009; Chuang et al., 2002). We did not see significant changes in the level or localization of the mutant p53 protein following H_2O_2 treatment of ARO and WRO cells. This protein is present at a much higher level in these thyroid cancer cells when compared to the level in the MCF-7 cells. It is possible that the protein is already at maximum level and thus can not be further increased. As noted above, the accumulation of p53 could be due to the lack of interaction of the protein with Mdm2 even before oxidative stress treatments, so there may be no change upon treatment. It is also possible there is an alteration in the transducer of the oxidative stress signal (such as the 2-Cys PRX Tpx1 protein) (Veal et al., 2007) in the ARO and WRO cells such that no signal is actually transmitted to cause a change in the accumulation of the p53 protein. One of the upstream regulators of p53 that has been implicated in regulation of p53 activation and stabilization in response to DNA damage is Chk2 (Shieh et al., 2000). Chk2 has been found to induce phosphorylation on Ser 20 of p53 in response to stress which leads to interruption in p53-Mdm2 interaction and a subsequent decrease in p53 ubiquitination (Hirao et al., 2000). We did not observe any phosphorylation at Ser 20 of the p53 from any of the cell lines studied. Phosphorylation of specific serine residues on the p53 protein has been shown following different stress treatments (Hernandez-Vargas et al., 2008). The p53 from ARO and WRO cells has been demonstrated here to be phosphorylated at S15 and S392 in untreated cells (Figure 3). H_2O_2 treatment apparently reduces the level of phosphorylated S392 in WRO cells with no change in the level of this modification in ARO cells. Whether those modifications affect the DNA binding activity of p53 is currently under investigation.

The p53 transcription factor regulates genes in the cell cycle and apoptosis pathways. We monitored DNA binding to 5 genes from these 2 pathways and noted all 5 were recognized by the wild-type p53 from the MCF-7 cells. However, only 2 sequences were recognized by the mutant p53 proteins, those derived from the *survivin* gene which blocks apoptosis and from the *p21* gene regulating the cell cycle. Previous studies link survivin to dedifferentiation in thyroid cancer (Ito et al., 2003), and over-expression of *survivin* has been reported in papillary thyroid carcinomas (Antonaci et al., 2008). Also, it has been reported that increased *survivin* expression is found in the initial stages of colorectal cancer tumor development (Kawasaki et al., 2001). Wild-type p53 binds to the *survivin* regulatory sequence and down-regulates the gene to reduce survival in response to apoptotic stimuli. As mutant p53 also binds to the regulatory element of *survivin*, this gene may be repressed in ARO and WRO cells. The p21 protein blocks cell cycle progression, and its gene is upregulated by wild-type p53 in the event of cellular stress. The mutant p53 proteins from ARO and WRO cells bind the *p21* regulatory element as well, suggesting the p21 protein may also be present in these cells. It is known that some p53 mutants cause growth arrest through upregulation of *p21* (Ludwig et al., 1996). Alternatively, some p53 mutants may have mechanisms of transcriptional activation different from the wild-type protein. In fact, previous work with extracts from WRO cells indicated that the mutant p53 could bind to a DNA sequence, but could not upregulate the gene (Park et al., 1994). It is possible that the binding to the DNA sequences regulating the *p21* and *survivin* genes by mutant p53 may actually prevent binding by wild-type p53 or other transcription factors and in that way disrupt the normal regulation. We did note a modest reduction in the binding to these regulatory sequences by mutant p53 after oxidative stress, while the p53 from the MCF-7 cells had enhanced binding to these DNAs after treatment (Figure 4 and Table 3). This may support the possibility of negative regulation of these genes by the mutant p53. The level of mRNA for these two genes in these cell lines would have to be examined before and after H_2O_2 treatment to test this hypothesis. We observed that the p53 proteins from both ARO and WRO cells do not show any binding to the cell cycle regulatory gene *cdc25C* nor to the regulatory sequences of the pro-apoptotic genes *bax* and *noxa*. Thus, these tumor cells could survive by altering regulation of the cell cycle and the apoptotic pathways. Wild-type p53 down-regulates *cdc25C* to restrict entry into mitosis but upregulates *bax* and *noxa* to promote cell death. Thus, these genes would not be regulated by the mutant p53s resulting in less inhibition of entry into mitosis and a lack of promotion of cell death. The disruption of both pathways would result in growth promotion of the cancer cell lines. These data are in agreement with low apoptotic rates in isolated anaplastic carcinoma cells reported previously (Pavelic et al., 2006).

We have only studied the binding of the p53 proteins here to a small subset of the more than 100 regulatory sequences recognized by the wild-type protein (Menendez, et al., 2009; Riley et al., 2008). The DNA binding recognition of mutant p53 is specific to the sequence of the mutant protein. It is possible with future work in this direction to predict a consensus DNA binding sequence which is exclusively recognized by mutant p53 proteins and thus could explain altered DNA binding and transcriptional activation/ repression of mutant p53 target genes. In many previous publications, only the wild-type consensus DNA sequence has been used to study the p53 DNA binding in different cells and following different treatments. We are aware that DNA binding is not the full picture. For instance, the p53 from both the ARO and WRO cells bound the consensus sequence, but only the ARO cells transactivated the gene regulated by a promoter containing this sequence (Park et al., 1994). Mutant p53 may control transcription of target genes distinct from those regulated by the wild-type protein supporting the concept of a gain-of-function mutation in this master regulator (Deppert et al., 2000, Sigal & Rotter, 2000). Elucidating the molecular mechanisms behind gain-of-function by mutant p53 has proven to be difficult since the observed oncogenic effect often varies with the system under study.

5. Conclusion

The p53 in the ARO and WRO thyroid cancer cells is likely tetrameric as the protein is found in the nucleus and is phosphorylated. This would allow these proteins to affect transcription either directly or via interaction with the wild-type p53 protein. Oxidative stress does not appear to alter the p53 from the thyroid cancer cells in the same way compared to the wild-type protein in breast cancer cells suggesting either altered sensing or already maximal over-produced protein. Our work showing differential DNA binding specificity of mutant and wild-type p53 supports the importance for continuing to study the binding to specific gene regions providing a fuller spectrum of information about the changes in functionality of the p53 protein in cancer cells. Future studies in this direction may identify mutant p53 regulated genes whose action promotes the gain-of-function attribute that makes the thyroid cancers carrying these mutant proteins much more aggressive.

6. Acknowledgment

The authors would like to acknowledge Sanofi Pasteur, Inc. for the use of laboratory facilities and equipment; Amy Fedele for assistance with figures; Dr. Dennis McGee for the use of his tissue culture facilities for part of the work; Diane Messina for assistance with maintenance of tissue culture; Keith Murphy for developing some western blots; Kim Schneider for editorial assistance with the manuscript; and Sally Stem for her assistance with procurement of laboratory reagents. The two first authors both significantly contributed to the experiments described in this work, MTB performing the western blots for level, localization and phosphorylation of p53 while DR performed all the analysis of DNA binding. Both were intimately involved in the writing and revising of the manuscript.

7. References

Alarcon-Vargas, D. & Ronai, Z. (2002). p53-Mdm2--the affair that never ends. *Carcinogenesis,* Vol. 23, pp. 541-547.

Alsner, J.; Jensen, V.; Kyndi, M.; Offersen, B.V.; Vu, P.; Børresen-Dale, A.L. & Overgaard J. (2008). A comparison between p53 accumulation determined by immunohistochemistry and TP53 mutations as prognostic variables in tumours from breast cancer patients. *Acta Oncologica,* Vol. 47, pp. 600-607.

Appella, E. & Anderson, C.W. (2000). Signaling to p53: breaking the posttranslational modification code. *Pathological Biology,*Vol. 48, pp 227–245.

Bai, L. & Zhu, W.G. (2006). P53: Structure, function and therapeutic applications. *Journal of Cancer Molecules,* Vol. 2, pp. 141-153.

Bell, D.; Varley, J.M.; Szydlo, T.E.; Kang, D.H.; Wahrer, D.C.R.; Shannon, K.E.; Lubratovich, M.; Verselis, S.J.; Isselbacher, K.J.; Fraumeni, J.F.; Birch, J.M.; Li, F.P.; Garber, J.E. & Haber, D.A. (1999). Heterozygous germ line hCHK2 mutations in Li-Fraumeni syndrome. *Science,* Vol. 286, pp. 2528-2531.

Blagosklonny, M.V.; Giannakakou, P.; Wojtowicz, M.; Romanova, L.Y.; Ain, K.B.; Bates, S.E. & Fojo, T. (1998). Effects of p53-expressing adenovirus on the chemosensitivity and differentiation of anaplastic thyroid cancer cells. *Journal of Clinical Endocrinology and Metabolism,* Vol. 83, pp. 2516–22.

Chan, W.M.; Siu, W.Y.; Lau, A. & Poon, R.Y. (2004). How many mutant p53 molecules are needed to inactivate a tetramer? *Molecular and Cell Biology,* Vol.24, pp. 3536–3551.

Chandrachud, U. & Gal, S. (2009). Three assays show differences in binding of wild-type and mutant p53 to unique gene sequences. *Technology in Cancer Research and Treatment,* Vol. 8, pp. 445-454.

Chuang, Y.Y.E.; Chen, Y.; Chandramouli, GVR.; Cook, JA.; Coffin, D.; Tsai, MH.; DeGraff, W.; Yan H.; Zhao, S.; Russo, A.; Liu, ET. & Mitchell, J.B. (2002). Gene expression after treatment with hydrogen peroxide, menadione, or t-butyl hydroperoxide in breast cancer cells. *Cancer Research*. Vol. 62, pp. 6246 - 6254.

Collavin, L.; Lunardi, A. & Sal, G. D. (2010). p53-family proteins and their regulators: hubs and spokes in tumor suppression. *Cell Death and Differentiation*, Vol. 17, pp. 901-911.

Deppert, W.; Göhler, T.; Koga, H. & Kim, E. (2000). Mutant p53: "gain of function" through perturbation of nuclear structure and function? *Journal of Cellular Biochemistry*, Vol. 79, pp. 115-122.

Dulic, V.; Kaufmann, W.K.; Wilson, S.J.; Tlsty, T.D.; Lees, E.; Harper, J.W.; Elledge, S.J. & Reed, S.I. (1994). p53-dependent inhibition of cyclin-dependent kinase activities in human fibroblasts during radiation-induced G1 arrest. *Cell*, Vol. 76, pp. 1013-1023.

Fagin, J.A.; Matsuo, K.; Karmakar, A.; Chen, D.L.; Tang, S.H. & Koeffler, H.P. (1993). High prevalence of mutations of the *p53* gene in poorly differentiated human thyroid carcinomas. *Journal of Clinical Investigations*, Vol. 91, pp. 179–184.

Gal, S.; Cook, J. & Howells, L. (2006) Scintillation proximity assay for DNA binding by human p53. *Biotechniques*, Vol. 41, pp. 303-308.

Gamble, S.C.; Cook, M.C.; Riches, A.C.; Herceg, Z.; Bryant, P.E. & Arrand, J.E. (1999). p53 mutations in tumors derived from irradiated human thyroid epithelial cells. *Mutation Research*, Vol. 425 , pp. 231–238.

Gong, B. & Almasan, A. (1999). Differential upregulation of p53-responsive genes by genotoxic stress in hematopoietic cells containing wild-type and mutant p53. *Gene Expression*, Vol. 8, pp. 197-206.

Hernandez -Vargas, H.; Ballestar, E.; Saez, P.C.; Kobbe, C.V.; Rodrıguez, I.B.; Esteller, M.; Bueno, M. & Palacios, J. (2006). Transcriptional profiling of MCF7 breast cancer cells in response to 5-fluorouracil: relationship with cell cycle changes and apoptosis, and identification of novel targets of p53. *International Journal of Cancer*, Vol. 119, pp. 1164-1175.

Hirao, A.; Kong, Y.Y.; Matsuoka, S.; Wakeham, A.; Ruland, J.; Yoshida, H.; Liu, D.; Elledge, S.J. & Mak, T. (2000). DNA damage-induced activation of p53 by the checkpoint kinase Chk2. *Science* , Vol. 287, pp. 1824-1827.

Hoffman, W.H.; Biade, S.; Zilfou, J.T.; Chen, J. & Murphy, M. (2002). Transcriptional repression of the anti-apoptotic survivin gene by wild type p53. *Journal of Biological Chemistry* , Vol. 277, pp. 3247-57.

Horie, S.; Maeta, H.; Endo, K.; Ueta, T.; Takashima, K. & Terada, T. (2001). Overexpression of p53 protein and MDM2 in papillary carcinomas of the thyroid: Correlations with clinicopathologic features. *Pathology International*, Vol. 51, pp. 11–15.

Hunt, J. (2005). Understanding the genotype of follicular thyroid tumors. *Endocrine Pathology*, Vol 16, pp 311–321.

Hussain, S.P. & Harris, C.C. (1998). Molecular epidemiology of human cancer: contribution of mutation spectra studies of tumor suppressor genes. *Cancer Research*, Vol. 58, pp. 4023–4037.

Ito, T.; Seyama, T.; Mizuno, T.; Tsuyama, N.; Hayashi, T.; Hayashi, Y.; Dohi, K.; Nakamura, N. & Akiyama, M. (1992). Unique association of p53 mutations with undifferentiated but not with differentiated carcinomas of the thyroid. *Cancer Research*, Vol. 52, pp. 1369 -1371.

Ito, Y.; Yoshida, H.; Uruno, T.; Nakano, K.; Miya, A.; Kobayashi, K.; Yokozawa, T.; Matsuzuka, F.; Matsuura, N.; Kakudo, K., Kuma, K. & Miyauchi, A. (2003). Survivin expression is significantly linked to the dedifferentiation of thyroid carcinoma. *Oncology Reports*, Vol. 10, pp. 1337-1340.

Jagelská, E.; Brázda, V.; Pospisilová, S.; Vojtesek, B. & Palecek, E. (2002). New ELISA technique for analysis of p53 protein/DNA binding properties. *Journal of Immunological Methods*, Vol. 267, pp. 227-235.

Jeffrey, P.D.; Gorina, S. & Pavletich, N.P. (1995). Crystal structure of the tetramerization domain of the p53 tumor suppressor at 1.7 angstroms. *Science*. Vol. 267, pp. 1498-1502.

Joerger, A.C.; Hwee, C.A. & Fersht, A.R. (2006). Structural basis for understanding oncogenic p53 mutations and designing rescue drugs. *Proceedings of the National Academy of Science* (USA), Vol. 103, pp. 15056-15061.

Jung, E.M., Choi, K.C. & Jeung, E.B. (2011). Expression of calbindin-D28k is inversely correlated with proapoptotic gene expression in hydrogen peroxide-induced cell death in endometrial cancer cells. *International Journal of Oncology*, Vol. 38, pp. 1059-1066.

Kawasaki, H.; Toyoda, M; Shinohara, H.; Okuda, J.; Watanabe, I.; Yamamoto, T.; Tanaka, K.; Tenjo, T. & Tanigawa, N. (2001). Expression of survivin correlates with apoptosis, proliferation and angiogenesis during human colorectal carcinogenesis, *Cancer*, Vol. 91 pp. 2026–2032.

Kern, S.E.; Pietenpol, J.A.; Thiagalingam, S.; Seymour, A., Kinzler, K.W. & Vogelstein, B. (1992). Oncogenic forms of p53 inhibit p53-regulated gene expression. *Science*, Vol. 256, pp. 827–830.

Khoury, M.P. & Bourdon, J.C. (2010). The isoforms of the p53.In: *Cold Spring Harbor Perspectives in Biology 2010*. Levine, A.J. & Lane, D. Vol. 2:a000927, pp. 1-10. Cold Spring Harbor Laboratory Press.

Kim, Y.Y.; Park, B.J.; Kim, D.J.; Kim, W.H.; Kim, S.; Oh, K.S.; Lim, J.Y.; Kim, J.; Park, C. & Park, S.I. (2004). Modification of serine 392 is a critical event in the regulation of p53 nuclear export and stability. *FEBS Letters*, Vol. 572, pp. 92-98.

Kroll, T.G. (2004). Molecular events in follicular thyroid tumors. *Cancer Treatment and Research*, Vol. 122, pp. 85–105.

Kubbutat, M.H.G.; Jones, S. N. & Vousden, K. H. (1997). Regulation of p53 stability by Mdm-2. *Nature*, Vol. 387, pp. 299-303.

Kubbutat, M.H.G.; Ludwig, R.L.; Ashcroft, M. & Vousden, K.H. (1998). Regulation of Mdm2 directed degradation by the C terminus of p53. *Molecular and Cellular Biology*, Vol. 18, pp. 5690-5698.

Lacroix, M.; Toillon, R.-A. & Leclercq, G. (2006) p53 and breast cancer, an update. *Endocrine-Related Cancer*, Vol. 13, pp. 293–325.

Lane, D.P. (1992). p53: Guardian of the genome. *Nature*, Vol. 358, pp. 15-16.

Liang, S.H. & Clarke, M.F. (2001). Regulation of p53 localization. *European Journal of Biochemistry*, Vol. 268, pp. 2779-2783.

Liu, W.; Cheng, S.; Asa, S.L. & Ezzat, S. (2008). The melanoma-associated antigen A3 mediates fibronectin- controlled cancer progression and metastasis. *Cancer Research*, Vol. 68, pp.8104-8112.

Liu, Y & Kulesz-Martin, M. (2001). p53 protein at the hub of cellular DNA damage response pathways through sequence - specific and non-sequence- specific DNA binding. *Carcinogenesis*, Vol. 22, pp. 851-860.

Ludwig, R.L.; Bates, S. & Vousden, K.H. (1996). Differential activation of target cellular promoters by p53 mutants with impaired apoptotic function. *Molecular and Cellular Biology*, Vol. 16, pp. 4952–4960.

Matsuoka, S.; Rotman, G.; Ogawa, A.; Shiloh, Y.; Tamai, K. & Elledge, S.J. (2000). Ataxia telangiectasia-mutated phosphorylates Chk2 in vivo and in vitro. *Proceedings of the National Academy of Sciences USA*, Vol. 97, pp. 10389-10394.

Menendez, D.; Inga, A. & Resnick, MA. (2009). The expanding universe of p53 targets. *Nature Reviews in Cancer*, Vol. 9, pp. 724-737.

Migliorini, D.; Denchi, E.L.; Danovi, D.; Jochemsen, A.; Capillo, M.; Gobbi, A.; Helin, K.; Pelicci, P.G. & Marine, J.C. (2002). MDM4 (MDMx) regulatesp53-induced growth arrest and neuronal cell death during early embryonic mouse development. *Molecular and Cellular Biology*, Vol. 22, pp. 5527–5538.

Milhara, M.; Erster, S.; Zaika, A.; Petrenko, O.; Chittenden, T.; Pancoska, P. & Moll, U. (2003). p53 has direct apoptogenic role at the mitochondria. *Molecular Cell*, Vol. 11, pp. 577-590.

Mirza, A.; McGuirk, M.; Hockenberry, T.N.; Qun, W.; Ashar, H.; Black, S.; Shu F.W.; Luquan, W.; Kirschmeier, P.; Bishop, W.R.; Nielsen, L.L.; Pickett, C.B. & Suxing, L. (2002). Human survivin is negatively regulated by wild-type p53 and participates in p53-dependent apoptotic pathway. *Oncogene*, Vol. 21, pp. 2613- 2622.

Namba, H.; Hara, T.; Tukazaki, T.; et al. (1995). Radiation-induced G1 Arrest Is Selectively Mediated by the p53-WAF1/Cip1 Pathway in Human Thyroid Cells. *Cancer Research*, Vol. 55, pp. 2075-2080.

Nilsson, I. & Hoffmann, I. (2000). Cell cycle regulation by the Cdc25 phosphatase family. *Progress in Cell Cycle Research*, Vol. 4, pp. 107–114.

Okumura, N.; Saji, S.; Eguchi, H.; Hayashi, S.; Saji, S. & Nakashima, S. (2002). Estradiol stabilizes p53 protein in breast cancer cell line, MCF-7. *Japanese Journal of Cancer Research*, Vol. 93, pp. 867-873.

Olivier, M.; Eeles, R.; Hollstein, M.; Khan, M.A.; Harris, C.C. & Hainaut, P. (2002) . The IARC TP53 database: new online mutation analysis and recommendations to users. *Human Mutation*, Vol. 19, pp. 607–614.

Olivier, M.; Hainaut, P. & Børresen-Dale, A.L. (2005). Prognostic and predictive value of TP53 mutations in human cancer, In: *25 Years of p53 research*, Hainaut, P. & Wiman, K.G. pp. 2920–2929, Springer-Verlag, ISBN 1-4020-29220-9, Berlin.

Park, S.; Nakamura, H.; Chumakov, A.; Said, J.; Miller, C.; Chen, D. & Koeffler, H. (1994). Transactivational and DNA binding abilities of endogenous p53 in p53 mutant cell lines. *Oncogene*, Vol. 9, pp. 1899-1906.

Parker, S.B.; Eichele, G.; Zhang, P.; Rawls, A.; Sands, A.T.; Bradley, A.; Olson, E.N.; Harper, J.W. & Elledge, S.J. (1995). p53-independent expression of p21Cip1 in muscle and other terminally differentiating cells. *Science*, Vol. 267, pp. 1024–1027.

Pavelic, K.; Dedivitis, R.A.; Kapitanovic, S.; Cacev, T.; Guirado, C.R.; Danic, D.; Radosevic, S.; Brkic, K.; Pegan, B.; Krizanac, S.; Kusic, Z.; Spaventi, S. & Bura, M. (2006). Molecular genetic alterations of FHIT and p53 genes in benign and malignant thyroid gland lesions. *Mutation Research*, Vol. 599, pp. 45-47.

Pisarchik, A.V.; Ermak, G.; Kartell, N.A. & Figge, J. (2000). Molecular alterations involving p53 codons 167 and 183 in papillary thyroid carcinomas from Chernobyl-contaminated regions of Belarus. *Thyroid*, Vol. 10, pp. 25–30.

Pollina, L.; Pacini, F.; Fontanini, G.; Vignati, S.; Bevilacqua, G. & Basolo, F. (1996). bcl-2, p53 and proliferating cell nuclear antigen expression is related to the degree of differentiation in thyroid carcinomas. *British Journal of Cancer*, Vol. 73, pp.139–43.

Prives, C. & White, E. (2008). Does control of mutant p53 by Mdm2 complicate cancer therapy? *Genes and Development*, Vol. 22, pp. 1259-1264.

Riley, T.; Sontag, E.; Chen, P. & Levine, A. (2008). Transcriptional control of human p53-regulated genes. *Nature Reviews in Molecular and Cell Biology*, Vol. 9, pp. 402-412.

Shahedian, B.; Shi, Y.; Zou, M. & Farid, N.R. (2002). Thyroid carcinoma is characterized by genomic instability: evidence from p53 mutations. *Molecular Genetics and Metabolism*, Vol. 72, pp. 155–163.

Shaulian, E.; Zauberman, A.; Ginsberg, D. & Oren, M. (1992). Identification of minimal transforming domain of p53: negative dominance through abrogation of sequence specific DNA binding. *Molecular and Cellular Biology*, Vol. 12, pp. 5581–5592.

Shieh, S.Y.; Ahn, J.; Tamai, K.; Taya, Y. & Prives, C. (2000). The human homologs of checkpoint kinases Chk1 and Cds1 (Chk2) phosphorylate p53 at multiple DNA damage-inducible sites. *Genes and Development*, Vol. 14, pp. 289-300.

Sigal, A. & Rotter, V. (2000). Oncogenic Mutations of the p53 tumor suppressor: the demons of the guardian of the genome. *Cancer Research*, Vol. 60, pp. 6788-6793.

Soares, P., Cameselle-Teijeiro, J. & Sobrinho-Simoes, M. (1994). Immunohistochemical detection of p53 in differentiated, poorly differentiated and undifferentiated carcinomas of the thyroid, *Histopathology*, Vol. 24, pp. 205–210.

Soussi, T. (2005). The p53 pathway and human cancer. *British Journal of Surgery*, Vol. 92, pp. 1331–1332.

Srivastava, S.; Wang, S.; Tong, Y.O.; Hao, Z.M. & Chang, E. (1993). Dominant negative effect of a germ-line mutant p53: a step fostering tumorigenesis. *Cancer Research*, Vol. 5, pp. 4452–4455.

Unger, T.; Mietz, J.A.; Scheffner, M.; Yee, C.L. & Howley, P.M. (1993). Functional domains of wild-type and mutant p53 proteins involved in transcriptional regulation, transdominant inhibition and transformation suppression. *Molecular and Cellular Biology*, Vol. 1, pp. 5186–5194.

Vassilev, L.T.; Vu, B.T.; Graves, B.; Carvajal, D.; Podlaski, F.; Filipovic, Z.; Kong, N.; Kammlott, U.; Lukacs, C.; Klein, C.; Fotouhi, N. & Liu, E. (2004). In vivo activation of the p53 pathway by small-molecule antagonists of mdm2. *Science*, Vol. 303, pp. 844-848.

Veal, E.A.; Day, A.M. & Morgan, B.A. (2007). Hydrogen peroxide sensing and signaling. *Mol. Cell*, Vol. 26, pp. 1-14.

Vogelstein, B.; Lane, D. & Levine, A.J. (2000). Surfing the p53 network. *Nature*, Vol. 408, pp. 307-310.

Vousden, K.H. & Lu, X. (2002). Live or let die: the cell's response to p53. *Nature Reviews in Cancer*, Vol. 2, pp. 594-604.

Weinberg, R. L.; Veprinstev, D. B. & Fersht, A.R. (2004). Cooperative binding of tetrameric p53 to DNA. *Journal of Molecular Biology*, Vol. 341, pp. 1145-1149.

Weinberg, R. L.; Freund, S.M.V.; Veprinstev, D. B. & Fersht, A.R. (2005). Regulation of DNA binding of p53 by its C-terminal domain. *Journal of Molecular Biology*, Vol. 342, pp. 801-811.

Wu, X.; Webster, S.R. & Chen, J. (2000). Characterization of tumor-associated Chk2 mutations. *Journal of Biological Chemistry*, Vol. 276, pp. 2971-2974.

Xiong, Y.; Hannon, G.J.; Zhang, H.; Casso, D.; Kobayashi, R. & Beach, D. (1999). p21 is a universal inhibitor of cyclin kinases. *Nature*, Vol. 366, pp. 701-704.

Xu, Y. (2003). Regulation of p53 responses by post-translational modifications. *Cell Death and Differentiation*, Vol. 10, pp. 400-403.

Zhou, M.; Gu, L.; Li, F.; Zhu, Y.; Woods, W.G. & Findley, H.W. (2002). DNA Damage Induces a Novel p53-Survivin Signaling Pathway Regulating Cell Cycle and Apoptosis in Acute Lymphoblastic Leukemia Cells. *Journal of Pharmacology and Experimental Therapeutics*, Vol. 303, pp. 124–131.

3

Glycosylation and Glycoproteins in Thyroid Cancer: A Potential Role for Diagnostics

Anna Krześlak, Paweł Jóźwiak and Anna Lipińska
University of Lodz, Poland

1. Introduction

Glycosylation is the most common and the most diverse form of co- and post-translational modifications. An analysis of the Swiss-PROT database has led to the estimation that more than 50% of all proteins are glycosylated. Genes coding proteins involved in all types of oligosaccharides biosynthesis represent 0.5 to 1% of the translated genome (Dennis et al., 1999). Glycoproteins are found ubiquitously in an organism either as soluble (intracellular or extracellular) or as membrane bound molecules. There is a great structural variety of glycoproteins based on the type, length and linkage of a carbohydrate components as well as the degree of saturation of potential glycosylation sites on the protein itself.

Carbohydrates can have a significant influence on the physicochemical properties of glycoproteins, affecting their folding, solubility, aggregation and degradation. Furthermore, glycan chains in glycoproteins play key roles in many biological processes such as embryonic development, immune response and cell-cell interactions in which sugar-sugar or sugar –protein specific recognition is involved (Wei & Li , 2009).

Altered glycosylation is an universal feature of cancer cells, and certain glycan structures and glycoproteins are well-known tumor markers. These include for example glycoproteins such as carcinoembryonic antigen (CEA), commonly used as a marker of colorectal cancer, prostate-specific antigen (PSA) and CA-125 used in the diagnosis of ovarian cancer (Drake et al., 2010). High expression of some glycosyl epitopes for example sialyl Lewis a, sialyl Lewis x, Lewis y, promotes invasion and metastasis. Antibodies against Lewis antigens are used for evaluation of specimens from breast, bladder, colorectal, esophageal and lung carcinomas (Drake et al., 2010). Glycans can regulate different aspects of tumor progression, including proliferation, invasion and metastasis. Cancer-related changes in glycosylation can reflect disease specific alterations in glycan biosynthetic pathways. These include variations in the expression and activity of glycosyltransferases, enzymes that add monosaccharides to acceptors, i.e. proteins or growing carbohydrate chains and glycosidases which catalyze the hydrolysis of the glycosidic linkage to release sugars.

There are three most common categories of protein glycosylation 1) *N*-glycosylation, where glycans are attached to asparagine residues in a consensus sequence N-X-S/T *via* *N*-acetylglucosamine (GlcNAc) residue; 2) *O*-glycosylation, where glycans are attached to serine or threonine *via* *N*-acetylgalactosamine (GalNAc) residue (mucin type glycosylation);

3) *O*-GlcNAcylation, where single *N*-acetylglucosamine residues are attached by *O*-linkage to serine and threonine residues (Fig.1). *N*-oligosaccharides have a common core structure of five sugars and differ in their outer branches. They are divided into three main classes: high mannose, complex and hybrid. High mannose oligosaccharides have additional mannoses linked to the pentasaccharide core and forming the branches. Complex-type oligosaccharides contain characteristic GlcNAc and Gal residues and are often terminated with sialic acid residues. Complex type oligosaccharides can be bi-, tri- or tetraantennary.

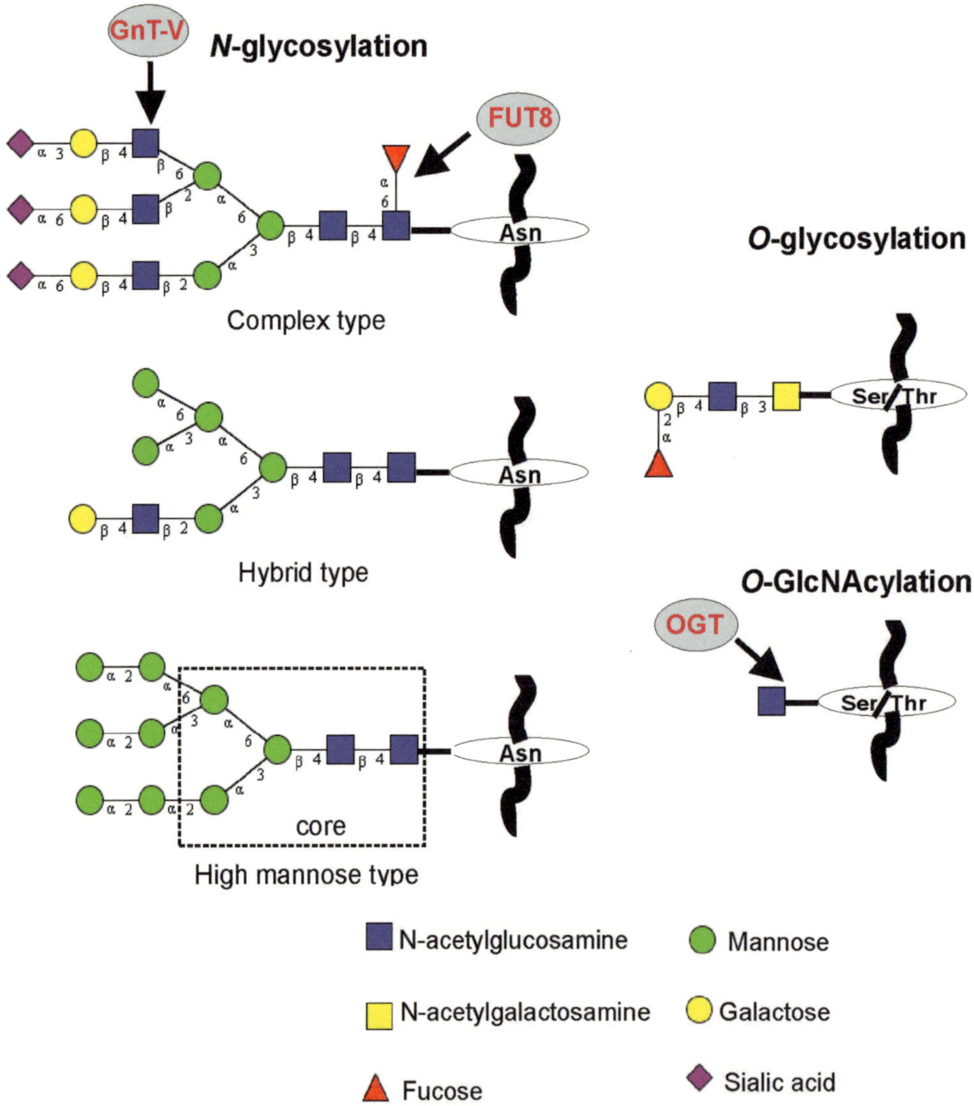

Fig. 1. Examples of carbohydrate structures. Arrows indicate the residues attached by glycosyltransferases the expression of which was studied in thyroid tumors: GnT-V - *N*-acetylglucosaminyltransferase V , FUT8 – α 1,6 –fucosyltransferase, OGT – *O*-GlcNAc transferase

Hybrid oligosaccharides contain one branch that has a complex structure and one or more high-mannose branches (Stanley et al., 2009). The mucin-type *O*-glycan, with *N*-acetylgalactosamine (GalNAc) at the reducing end, is a very common form of *O*-glycosylation in humans (Brockhausen, 1999; Wopereis et al., 2006). In *O*-glycosylated proteins, oligosaccharides range in size from 1 to >20 sugars, displaying considerable structural diversity. In total, 8 mucin-type core structures can be distinguished, depending on the second sugar and its sugar linkage, of which cores 1-6 and core 8 have been described in humans. The *N*-acetylgalactosamine may be extended with sugars such as galactose, *N*-acetylglucosamine, fucose or sialic acid but not mannose, glucose or xylose residues (Brockhausen et al., 2009). The structural variability of glycans is dictated by tissue-specific regulation of glycosyltransferase genes, acceptor and sugar nucleotide donors availability and by competition between enzymes for acceptor intermediates during glycan elongation. Glycosyltransferases catalyze the transfer of a monosaccharide from specific sugar nucleotide donors onto particular position of a monosaccharide in a growing glycan chain in one or two possible anomeric linkages (either α or β) (Dennis et al., 1999). *O*-GlcNAcylation is a specific type of glycosylation since *O*-GlcNAc residues are not elongated and do not form complex structure. This dynamic and inducible modification is more similar to phosphorylation than to classical glycosylation (Hart & Akimoto, 2009).

2. Glycosylation in thyroid cancer

It is known that glycosylation profiles change significantly during oncogenesis (Wei & Li, 2009). Detection of tumor specific alterations could be potentially useful for cancer diagnostics. Lectins are a very good tool for the detection of changes in glycosylation. They are a group of proteins or glycoproteins that have affinity to carbohydrates and can reversibly and specifically interact with certain glycan structural motifs. Some lectins are widely used in cancer diagnostics. For example *Helix pomatia* agglutinin (HPA) which detects αGalNAcβ1-4 Gal, is a part of a panel of markers for histological characterization of gastric cancer specimens. HPA as well as *Ulex europaeus* agglutinin (UEA)(recognize Fucα1-2Galβ) is also used in breast cancer biopsy assessment (Drake et al., 2010).

It has been suggested that lectins might be useful histochemical tools for detecting and analyzing poly-N-acetyllactosamines in thyroid normal and malignant tissues (Ito N et al., 1995,1996). Staining with lectins in combination with endo-beta-galactosidase digestion demonstrated that poly-N-acetyllactosaminyl structures ubiquitously and consistently produced in thyroid papillary carcinomas are highly heterogeneous in their chain length and branching status and quite different from those produced in other thyroid neoplasms (Ito N et al., 1995, 1996). Studies concerning glycosylation of intracellular proteins in benign and malignant thyroid neoplasms showed significant quantitative and qualitative differences in binding of *Erythrina cristagalli* (ECA) and *Ricinus communis* (RCA-120) agglutinins that recognize N-acetyllactosamine or galactose residues (Krześlak et al., 2003). In the majority of carcinoma samples lectin binding to cytosolic proteins was definitely weaker in comparison with adenomas and non-neoplastic specimens which suggests alterations in glycosylation of proteins in thyroid malignant tumors. Also binding patterns of *Sambucus nigra* (SNA) and *Maakia amurensis* (MAA) agglutinins which recognized sialic acids are different in malignant tumors compared with benign thyroid lesions (Krześlak et al., 2007).

Changes in glycosylation are not the random consequence of disordered biology in tumor cells. It is characteristic that of all the possible glycan biosynthetic changes, only a limited subset of changes are correlated with malignant transformation (Varki et al., 2009).

2.1 *N*-acetylglucosaminyltransferase V

The most widely occurring glycosylation change in cancers is enhanced β1,6 GlcNAc side chain branching (see Fig.1.). Increased amounts of β1,6 GlcNAc branched carbohydrates have been linked to tumor invasion and metastasis in case of several human cancers including breast and colon. This carbohydrate structure is a product of increased activity of *N*-acetylglucosaminyltransferase V (GnT-V) (Fernandes et al., 1991; Seelentag et al., 1998; Granovsky et al., 2000).

Ito Y et al. (2006) have studied by immunohistochemistry the expression of GnT-V in thyroid normal and cancer tissues. They found expression of this enzyme in 66 of 68 cases of papillary carcinomas, 10 of 23 - follicular carcinomas, 9 of 13 - follicular adenomas and 6 of 28 - anaplastic carcinomas but the enzyme was not expressed in normal thyroid tissue. It has been shown that matriptase, a tumor-associated type II transmembrane serine protease is a target protein for GnT-V and β 1,6 GlcNAc branching of oligosaccharide on matriptase increases resistance of this protein to proteolytic degradation. Increased expression of matriptase and GnT-V levels were characteristic for papillary carcinoma. Although matriptase is proposed to modulate the metastatic potential of some cancer cells, it is not likely that the matriptase and GnT-V promote invasion and metastasis of papillary thyroid cancers. The levels of expression of both matriptase and GnT-V were significantly high in microcarcinomas. In case of poorly differentaiated and undifferentiated (anaplastic) carcinomas which show local and distant metastasis, expression of these proteins significantly decreased. Thus matriptase and GnT-V probably play a role in early phases of papillary carcinomas growth, but not in their progression (Miyoshi et al., 2010).

2.2 Changes in sialic acid expression

Residues of sialic acid are usually found at the non-reducing terminal position of glycoconjugate sugar chains, α2,3- or α2,6-linked to a galactose (Gal), or α2,6-linked to a *N*-acetylgalactosamine (GalNAc) or *N*-acetylglucosamine (GlcNAc) residues (Harduin-Lepers et al., 2001). Changes in sialic acid expression may be important in cancer progression and metastasis for several reasons. First, sialic acid can prevent cell-cell interactions through charge repulsion effects; second, sialylated structures can be recognized by cell adhesion molecules belonging to selectin or siglec families; third, the addition of sialic acid may mask the underlying sugar structure, thus avoiding recognition by other lectins such as galectins (Dall'Olio & Chiricolo, 2001).

Nozawa et al. (1999) investigated immunohistochemically the reactivity of monoclonal antibody of FB21, which recognizes a sialic acid-dependent carbohydrate epitope with thyroid lesions in order to evaluated the potential diagnostic usefulness of sialic acid expression analysis. The increased FB21 antigen reactivity appeared to be characteristic for follicular and papillary thyroid tumors but not for medullary thyroid carcinoma. FB21 reacted with almost all cases of follicular carcinomas and less than half of cases of papillary carcinomas. A positive reaction was found on the cell surface membranes or apical parts of neoplastic follicles. The normal thyroid follicles, goiters, medullary and anaplastic carcinomas were negative for FB21 reactivity. High frequency of reactivity of follicular carcinoma with FB21 suggested that it may be useful in diagnosis of this histological type of thyroid tumors.

Differences in sialic acid level on luminal surface between thyroid carcinomas and normal thyroid tissue or adenomas and goiters was observed in histochemistry studies using sialic acid binding lectins *Tritrichomonas mobilensis* lectin (TML), *Maackia amurensis* agglutinin (MAA) and *Sambucus nigra* agglutinin (SNA) (Babál et al., 2006). Malignant tumors especially papillary carcinoma had an increased level of sialic acid mainly alpha-2,3-linked and recognized by MAA. These results suggest that increased membrane sialic acid on thyroid gland cells may be an important diagnostic indicator, that could be useful in the distinction of malignant from benign thyroid lesions (Babál et al., 2006).

Cellular sialic acid level is mainly controlled metabolically by sialyltransferases and sialidases. Human sialyltransferases are a family of at least 18 different members that catalyse the transfer of sialic acid residues from their activated form CMP-sialic acid to terminal position of oligosaccharide chains (Harduin-Lepers et al., 2001). Changes in sialyltransferases expression have been observed in cancer tissues and the regulation of their expression is achieved mainly at the transcriptional level (Dall'Olio & Chiricolo, 2001). Sialidases catalyse the removal of sialic acid residues which is an initial step in the degradation of glycoproteins. There are only few studies focusing on sialic acid metabolism in thyroid tissue. Thyroid sialyltransferase 1 (β-galactoside α-2,6-sialyltransferase) and 4 (β-galactoside α-2,3-sialyltransferase) mRNA level and activity are increased in Graves disease (Kiljański et al., 2005). Sialyltransferase 1 showed also a very evident increase of expression in autonomously functioning thyroid nodules (AFTNs) *versus* their surrounding tissues (Eszlinger et al., 2004). Since sialyl Lewis epitopes are more frequently expressed in papillary carcinomas than Lewis a and Lewis b it is speculated that a specific glycosyltransferase, i.e. α2,3 sialyltransferase may be highly activated as compared with α1,4 fucosyltransferase. Moreover, this sialyltransferase seems to be more strongly enhanced in papillary carcinoma than in follicular carcinoma (Kamoshida et al., 2000).

2.3 Fucosylation

Fucosylated glycans are synthesized by fucosyltransferases. Thirteen fucosyltransferase genes have thus far been identified in the human genome. Based on the site of fucose addition fucosyltransferases are classified into α1,2 (FUT1, FUT2), α1,3/4 (FUT 3, 4, 5, 6, 7, 9), α1,6 (FUT8) and *O*-fucosyltransferase (POFUT1) groups (Becker & Lowe, 2003; Ma et al., 2006). Two additional α1,3 fucosyltransferase genes, *FUT10* and *FUT11* and one *O*-fucosyltransferase gene have been identified in the human genome but their protein products have not yet been demonstrated to be enzymatically active although they share primary sequence similarity with active fucosyltransferases. Certain types of fucosylated glycoproteins for example alfa-fetoprotein and several kinds of antibodies, which recognize fucosylated oligosaccharides such as sialyl-Lewis a/x, have been used as tumor markers (Miyoshi et al., 2008). The Lewis blood group antigens are a related set of glycans that carry α1,2/α1,4 fucose residues (Fig.2). Although growing evidence supports the functional significance of fucosylation at various pathophysiological steps of carcinogenesis and tumor progression, the significance of this modification in thyroid cancer has not been widely explored. The results of studies of Vierbuchen et al. (1992) concerning blood group antigens in medullary thyroid carcinoma (MTC) and normal thyroid tissue supported the general concept demonstrated in other carcinomas, that fucosyl- and sialyltransferases might be preferentially activated. The Lewis antigens were absent in normal tissue and present in MTC. Miettinen and Kärkkäinen (1996) analysed immunohistochemically a wide range of thyroid tumors and non-neoplastic tissues by using CD15 antibody, which recognized Lewis x blood group antigen. Nodular goiter and papillary hyperplasia cases either showed no reactivity or were focally positive. Most papillary carcinomas were CD15 positive usually in the majority of tumor cells. However only 50% of follicular carcinomas were positive and anaplastic carcinomas were negative. Similar results were obtained by Fonseca et al. (1996, 1997) who found by using SH1 antibodies that most of papillary and follicular carcinomas were extensively immunoreactive for Lewis x antigen in contrast to the absence of expression of this antigen in normal thyroid.

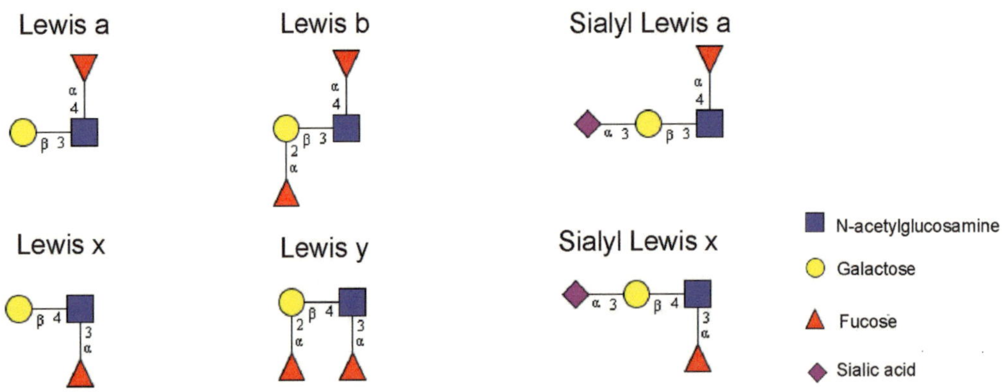

Fig. 2. Lewis antigens.

Ito Y et al. (2003) performed immunohistochemical studies of FUT8 expression in thyroid cancers. FUT8 catalyses the transfer of a fucose residue to the C6 position of the innermost GlcNAc residue of *N*-linked oligosaccharides on glycoproteins to produce core fucosylation (Fig.1.). The expression of FUT8 was very low in normal follicules. A high expression of FUT8 was observed in 33.3% of papillary carcinomas and the incidence was directly linked to tumor size and lymph node metastasis. But the number of cases of follicular carcinomas with high expression of FUT8 was rather low. These results suggest that FUT8 expression may be a key factor in the progression of thyroid papillary carcinomas, but not follicular carcinomas (Ito Y et al., 2003; Miyoshi et al., 2010).

2.4 *O*-GlcNAcylation

O-GlcNAcylation is a post-translational protein modification consisting of *N*-acetylglucosamine moiety attached by *O*-glycosidic linkage to serine and threonine residues (Hart et al., 2007). *O*-GlcNAc is a unique type of glycosylation since it is not elongated to more complex glycan structures and is nearly exclusively on cytoplasmic and nuclear proteins. Furthermore, the addition and removal of *O*-GlcNAc moieties cycles in a very dynamic and inducible manner in response to different stimuli such as hormones, growth factors, and mitogens. That makes *O*-GlcNAcylation more similar to phosphorylation than to classical glycosylation. *O*-GlcNAcylation is one of the most common post-translational modifications. So far, nearly one thousand of cellular proteins have been identified to be *O*-GlcNAcylated (Butkinaree et al., 2010). These proteins belong to diverse functional groups and include nuclear pore proteins, transcription factors, RNA binding proteins, cytoskeletal proteins, chaperones, phosphatases, kinases and other enzymes (Zachara & Hart, 2006). There is growing evidence that *O*-GlcNAc modification is involved in a wide range of biological processes, such as signal transduction, transcription, cell cycle progression and metabolism (Hart et al., 2007). *O*-GlcNAc can modulate protein function by regulating protein activity, protein-protein interaction, localization and protein degradation (Zeidan & Hart, 2010).

There is a relationship between *O*-GlcNAcylation and phosphorylation. All *O*-GlcNAc modified proteins are also phosphoproteins and sometimes *O*-GlcNAc and *O*-phosphate moieties can compete for a binding site or alternatively *O*-GlcNAcylation and phosphorylation can compete *via* steric hindrance when the substrate modification sites are within several aminoacids from each other (Hu et al., 2010). However, unlike phosphorylation, where many kinases and phosphatases regulate the addition and removal of phosphate, *O*-GlcNAcylation is regulated only by two enzymes. The addition of *O*-GlcNAc to proteins is catalyzed by *O*-GlcNAc transferase (OGT) and its removal is catalyzed by *O*-GlcNAc- selective *N*-acetyl-β-D-glucosaminidase (*O*-GlcNAcase, OGA) (Iyer & Hart, 2003). OGT is encoded by a single gene on X chromosome (Lubas & Hanover, 2000; Shafi et al., 2000). Although there is only one *OGT* gene, human OGT has at least three different isoforms because of alternative splicing (Love et al., 2003, Hanover et al., 2003). The main difference between isoforms is the number of tetratricopeptide repeats in N-terminal region. The OGT isoforms differ also in their tissue distribution and probably they may have different functions (Lazarus et al., 2006).

The cloned sequence of *O*-GlcNAcase was found to be identical to that of MGEA5 (meningioma-expressed antigen 5), which was identified genetically in human meningiomas (Heckel et al., 1998; Comtesse et al., 2001). *MGEA5* localizes to chromosome 10q24.1-q24.3 region. *O*-GlcNAcase seems to be a bifunctional enzyme. The N-terminus contains *O*-GlcNAc hydrolase activity and C-terminus bears a putative histone acetyltransferase (HAT) domain (Toleman et. al, 2004). *O*-GlcNAcase is reported both HAT and *O*-GlcNAcase activity *in vitro.*

There is growing evidence that perturbation in *O*-GlcNAc signaling is involved in the pathology of cancers. Overexpression of OGT causes defective cytokinesis increasing polyploidy of cells, a feature common to many cancer cells (Slawson et al., 2005). *O*-GlcNAc is present on many transcription and cell cycle regulatory proteins. The protooncogene c-Myc which regulates transcription of genes involved in cell proliferation, apoptosis and metabolism is modified by *O*-GlcNAc at Thr58 and this potentially stabilizes the protein (Kamemura et al., 2002). The important tumor suppressor p53, which is mutant or dysregulated in many cancers bears *O*-GlcNAc at Ser149. Increased *O*-GlcNAcylation of p53 at Ser149 results in decreased p53 ubiquitination and stabilizes the p53 protein (Yang WH et al., 2006).

Several malignancies have been shown to have increased level of *O*-GlcNAcylation compared to normal tissue (Gu Y et al., 2010; Mi et al., 2011; Caldwell et al., 2010). Elevated

OGT mRNA expression was found in breast cancer cell lines and breast invasive ductal carcinoma compared with normal breast cells and normal breast tissue (Caldwell et. al., 2010; Krześlak et al., 2011a). It has been shown that poorly differentiated breast tumors (grade II and III) had significantly higher OGT expression than grade I tumors and lymph node metastasis is significantly associated with decreased *MGEA5* mRNA expression (Krześlak et al., 2011a). The intracellular *O*-GlcNAcylation has been found to be also associated with the pathogenesis of chronic lymphatic leukemia –CLL (Shi et al., 2010).

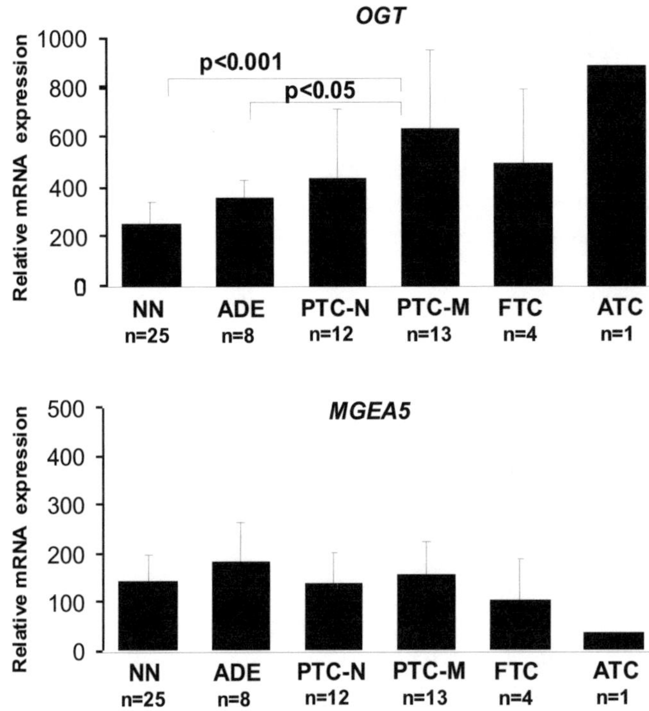

Fig. 3. *OGT* and *MGEA5* expression in thyroid lesions. The expression of *OGT* and *MGEA5* was studied by real time RT-PCR method in series of 25 samples of non-neoplastic lesions - NN (nodular goiters), 8 samples of follicular adenoma - ADE, 25 samples of papillary carcinoma – PTC (12 cases of non-metastatic –N and 13 cases of cancers with lymph node metastasis- M), 4 samples of follicular carcinomas - FTC and 1 sample of anaplastic cancer. TaqMan Gene Expression assays including fluorogenic, FAM labeled probes and sequence specific primers for *MGEA5, OGT* and *GAPDH* were purchased from Applied Biosystems. Assays numbers of OGT, MGEA5 and GAPDH were Hs00201970, Hs00269228 and Hs99999905, respectively. Abundance of *OGT* and *MGEA5* mRNA in samples were quantified by the ΔCt method. ΔCt (Ctgene – CtGAPDH) values were recalculated into relative copy number values (number of *OGT* or *MGEA5* mRNA copies per 1000 copies of GAPDH mRNA). The groups were compared using Mann-Whitney rank sum test. P value < 0.05 was considered statistically significant (non published data).

O-GlcNAcase activity was found to be increased in thyroid papillary, follicular and anplastic cancers in comparison with non-neoplastic lesions and benign tumors. *O*-GlcNAc-modified proteins in thyroid cells had a predominantly nuclear distribution and were more abundant in non-neoplastic lesions than in tumors (Krześlak et al., 2010). However, our preliminary studies concerning *O*-GlcNAc cycling enzymes expression did not show any significant differences in mRNA expression of *MGEA5* between thyroid cancers and non-neoplastic lesions (Fig.3). Contrary, OGT mRNA expression seems to be elevated in cancer samples in comparison to nodular goiters or benign tumors. Moreover, expression of OGT mRNA was higher in papillary carcinoma with lymph node metastasis compared to non-metastatic carcinoma. High expression was also found in case of anaplastic carcinoma. These results might suggest that *O*-GlcNAc transferase is associated with thyroid cancer progression.

Caldwell et al. (2010) have provided evidence that the reduction abnormally elevated OGT and *O*-GlcNAc levels in breast cancer cells inhibits cancer cell growth *in vitro* and *in vivo* and also diminishes breast cancer invasion. Decreasing *O*-GlcNAc levels through knockdown of OGT in cancer cells promotes elevation of the cell-cycle regulator $p27^{kip1}$ and reduces expression of FoxM1 and its transcriptional target matrix metalloproteinase-2. Our studies concerning *O*-GlcNAc role in anaplastic thyroid cancer cells 8305C showed that down-regulation of *O*-GlcNAcase enhanced both basal and IGF-1 stimulated Akt1 activation and cell proliferation (Krześlak et al., 2011b). In cells treated with *O*-GlcNAcase inhibitor - PUGNAc or specific for *O*-GlcNAcase siRNAs phosphorylation of kinase GSK3β and cyclin D1 level were higher than in control cells. These findings suggest that increased proliferation of 8305C cells with down-regulation of *O*-GlcNAcase at least partially depends on IGF-1 - Akt1 - GSK3β - cyclin D_1 pathway.

Although abnormal *O*-GlcNAcylation seems to be a feature of cancer cells its role in tumorigenesis and cancer progression has not been fully elucidated and further investigations in this area are needed. However, it seems that *O*-GlcNAc transferase expression might be a marker for some tumor progression including thyroid. Moreover, regulation of *O*-GlcNAc may be a promissory novel therapeutic strategy for cancer and OGT may be in future a potential drug target.

3. Glycoproteins as thyroid cancer biomarkers

Glycoproteins seem to provide an abounding source for discovering biomarkers for thyroid lesions. Gene expression profiling studies identified some genes coding glycoproteins for example MET, SERPINA1, TIMP1, FN1, CD44, SDC4, DPP4 and PROS1 as important thyroid cancer markers (Griffith et al., 2006). These significantly deregulated genes in thyroid cancer cells may help to develop a panel of markers with sufficient sensitivity and specificity for the diagnostic purpose. Studies of cell surface and secreted protein profiles of human thyroid cancer cell lines (FTC-133, TPC-1, XTC-1, ARO, DRO-1) revealed distinct glycoprotein patterns for each cell line (Arcinas et al., 2009). Of the 333 glycoproteins identified in the five thyroid cancer lines, nearly one third, 105, were found exclusively in a single cell line. FTC-133 and ARO had the fewest (7) and the most (34) uniquely identified glycoproteins, respectively. It is suggested that several glycoproteins have a potential as biomarkers for a specific type of thyroid cancer or as general thyroid cancer biomarkers. For example NCAM-1 is a glycoprotein biomarker candidate for differentiated cancers, syndecan-1 and cadherin-13 for follicular carcinoma, elastin microfibril interfacer-1, hyaluronan and proteoglycan link protein 1, ephrin-B-1 for anaplastic carcinoma, CD157 for Hürthle cell thyroid carcinoma (Arcinas et al., 2009).

Usefulness of some glycoprotein expression analysis for thyroid cancer diagnostics have been already extensively tested.

3.1 Thyroglobulin

Thyroglobulin (Tg) is a large glycoprotein produced by thyroid normal follicular cells and differentiated malignant cells. The production of Tg is low in poorly differentiated cells and absent in anaplastic thyroid cancer (Francis & Schlumberger, 2008). Thyroglobulin provides a matrix for the synthesis of the thyroid hormones, thyroxine (T4) and triiodothyronine (T3), and acts as a storage vehicle for iodine, in the form of iodinated tyrosyl residues (Vali et al., 2000). Tg is a homodimer with molecular weight of 660 kDa and contains 10% of carbohydrate structures. Of the 20 putative N-linked glycosylation sites in the human thyroglobulin polypeptide chain, 16 were shown to be actually glycosylated in the mature protein (Yang SX et al., 1996). Eight of these confirmed glycosylation sites appear to be linked to complex-type oligosaccharide units containing fucose and galactose in addition to mannose and glucosamine. Five sites contain high mannose type units and two sites are linked to oligosaccharide units that may be either hybrid or complex structures (Yang SX et al., 1996). The oligosaccharides of Tg have been shown to affect the structure and function of Tg. They have an impact iodination and hormone synthesis, targeting of Tg to subcellular and extracellular compartments, interactions with a putative membrane receptor and immunoreactivity of Tg (Vali et al., 2000).

Owing to thyroglobulin tissue specificity, its serum level is widely used as a marker for recurrence of thyroid carcinoma following total thyroidectomy. The improved sensitivity of thyroglobulin assays and the adoption of an international calibration standard have made thyroglobulin measurement an essential part of thyroid cancer monitoring (Lin, 2008; Ringel & Ladenson 2004). However, it ought to be remembered that there are some limitations of serum thyroglobulin measurement. The presence of anti-thyroglobulin antibodies interferes with measurements of Tg protein made either by immunometric assay or by radioimmunoassay (Feldt-Rasmussen & Rasmussen, 1985; Mariotti et al, 1995; Spencer, 2004). Due to difficulties with antibody interference, there has been an interest in developing new techniques for thyroid carcinoma monitoring. One of these techniques is the detection of circulating thyroid cells by the measurement of thyroglobulin mRNA (Tg-mRNA) in peripheral blood (Ditkoff et al., 1996). However, there are contradicting results on the usefulness of Tg-mRNA detection in peripheral blood. Some authors suggested the usefulness of this method in the follow-up of thyroid cancer patients (Ringel et al., 1998, 1999; Biscolla et al, 2000; Savagner et al., 2002) but others questioned its reliability (Bojunga et al., 2000; Eszlinger et al., 2002; Span et al., 2003, Elisei et al., 2004). Thyroglobulin mRNA may be expressed in very low concentrations by other cells in the body, including peripheral lymphocytes, through a process known as illegitimate transcription (Verburg et al., 2004).

Since the serum Tg level is increased in the majority of patients with either benign or malignant thyroid nodules, its use is not recommended in the preoperative differentiation between thyroid lesions. However, it is suggested that the carbohydrate structure analysis of thyroglobulin might be useful for thyroid cancer diagnostics. During malignant transformation, epithelial cells modulate the glycosylation profile of their secretion proteins and these post-translational changes may represent specific markers which may be useful diagnostic or prognostic tools. The composition of carbohydrate chains on thyroglobulin from thyroid carcinoma has been reported to differ from that in normal thyroid tissue (Maruyama et al., 1998; Shimizu et al., 2007a). Shimizu et al. (2007b) investigated *Lens culinaris* agglutinin (LCA)-reactive thyroglobulin ratio in serum to evaluate its usefulness for distinguishing between thyroid carcinoma and benign thyroid tumor. Their results were very promising. The *Lens culinaris* agglutinin-reactive thyroglobulin ratio was significantly lower in patients with thyroid carcinoma than in patients with benign thyroid tumor. Moreover, in cases of thyroid carcinoma with lymph node metastasis, *Lens culinaris* agglutinin-reactive Tg ratios were significantly decreased compared to patients with thyroid carcinoma without metastasis. Further studies confirm usefulness of the determination of LCA-reactive Tg ratios using an enzyme-linked immunosorbent assay for distinguishing between benign and malignant lesions (Kanai et al., 2009).

3.2 Fibronectin

Fibronectin (FN) is a high molecular mass adhesive glycoprotein present in the extracellular matrix that plays a significant role in cell adhesion, migration, growth, differentiation and the maintenance of normal cell morphology (Pankov & Yamada, 2002). Although fibronectin is encoded by a single gene it can exist in 20 different isoforms in humans as a results of alternative splicing and post-translational modifications. Fibronectin usually exists as a dimer composed of two ~250 kDa subunits linked by a pair of disulfide bonds near the C-termini. Subunits are composed primarily of three types of repeating module (I, II and III). Sets of modules make up domains for binding to variety of extracellular and cell surface molecules including collagen, glycosaminoglycans, fibrin, integrins and FN itself (Wierzbicka-Patynowski & Schwarzbauer, 2003). FN isoforms can be divided in two groups: soluble plasma FNs which are synthesized predominantly in the liver by hepatocytes and the less-soluble cellular FNs synthesized by other cell types. Heterogenity of fibronectin is also caused by post-translational modification. FN isoforms are glycoproteins that contain 4-9% carbohydrate, depending on the cell type. Glycosylation sites reside predominantly within type III repeats and the collagen-binding domain. The physiological role of the carbohydrates is not certain, but they appear to stabilize FN against hydrolysis and modulate its affinity to some substrates (Pankov & Yamada, 2002). There are seven potential *N*-glycosylation sites in human FN, and these *N*-glycans are largely responsible for the carbohydrate content of this molecule. The *N*-glycan of plasma FN is composed of complex-type biantennary oligosaccharides and is largely sialylated, whereas fibroblast-derived cellular FN contains fucose linked to the innermost *N*-acetylglucosamine (GlcNAc) and is less sialylated (Fukuda et al., 1982, Tajiri et al., 2005). Fetal and neoplastic cells predominantly express a uniquely glycosylated isoform called oncofetal fibronectin (OnfFN). This isoform is characterized by the presence of oncofetal domain situated in the COOH terminal region, which is absent in normal fibronectin. The oncofetal domain of FN is composed of an oligosaccharide linked to a hexapeptide by *O*-glycosylation (Matsuura et al., 1988).

Fibronectin 1 was first reported to be overexpressed in papillary carcinomas (Huang et al., 2001; Wasenius et al., 2003). Prasad et al. (2005) found that FN1 expression was significantly associated with malignancy and highly specific for carcinomas compared to adenomas and non-neoplastic tissues. Immunohistochemical analysis showed that FN1 was expressed in 61 of 67 papillary carcinoma cases, 3 of 6 follicular carcinoma, 4 of 4 anaplastic carcinoma and

6 of 8 Hürthle cells carcinoma cases. Contrary expression of FN1 was observed only in 2 of 29 samples of nodular goiters an 1 of 21 adenoma cases. Coexpression of FN1 with other markers such as galectin-3 or HBME1 was observed only in carcinomas (100% specific) while concurrent absence of FN1 and galectin-3 or HBME1 (Fn_Gal-3_ or FN_HBME1_ immunophenotype) was highly specific (96%) for adenomas (Prasad et al., 2005). Thus, this study suggest that fibronectin 1 is a very useful marker in the diagnosis of thyroid carcinomas. However, some other studies did not confirm high utility of fibronectin 1. Immunohistochemical studies of Nasr et al. (2006) showed that although FN1 was quite specific for papillary carcinomas, a large portion of PTC (31%) were negative. Even those cases that were positive showed weak and focal staining, and there was often significant background staining. The authors suggested that low sensitivity, focal staining and high background positivity significantly impair the utility of FN1 in diagnostics.

Using the reverse transcription-PCR technique, Takano et al. (1998, 1999) have suggested that oncofetal fibronectin (onfFN) may be an accurate molecular preoperative diagnostic marker for papillary thyroid carcinoma. They analyzed the expression of onfFN in fine-needle aspiration biopsies. The sensitivity and specificity of this method were 96% and 100%, respectively. They also showed high onfFN expression in anaplastic cancer tissues and cell lines (Takano et al., 2007). It has been suggested that oncofetal fibronectin may be a better tumor-specific marker in detecting minimal residual disease in differentiated thyroid carcinoma than thyroglobulin (Hesse et al., 2005). Thyroglobulin mRNA was thought to originate from circulating thyrocytes, but other studies demonstrated that physiological blood cells such as leukocytes are capable of ectopic Tg mRNA transcription (Verburg et al., 2004) In order to monitor patients with DTC for minimal residual disease by blood assays, Hesse et al. (2005) developed and optimized a specific, sensitive real-time RT-PCR assay using FRET technology to quantify absolute amounts of onfFN templates. High expression rate of onfFN transcripts in DTCs was demonstrated, while onfFN mRNA was not found to be illegitimately transcribed by peripheral blood cells. The authors suggested that onfFN mRNA analysis may be a specific tool for monitoring micrometastases in the context of minimal residual disease or for assessing tumor response to therapy. Continuing their studies they performed the analysis of mRNA level in peripheral blood of PTC patients who were previously treated by thyreoidectomy and treated by levothyroxine to determine if onfFN levels are correlated with the status of the disease or with thyroid-stimulating hormone (TSH) serum concentrations (Wehmeier et al 2010). The mean value of onfFN mRNA in bloods from healthy subjects was used as control. OnfFN transcripts were highly abundant in the peripheral blood of the patients, but the levels of onfFN mRNA did not differ significantly among the patients who were free of the disease, had local residual disease or metastatic disease. However, there was a trend towards higher expression rates of onfFN mRNA in patients with metastases than those free of disease. Discrimination between the disease states was better without TSH stimulation. The authors suggest that circulating onfFN mRNA, may be a useful tool to detect circulating thyroid cancer cells.

3.3 CD44

The CD44 glycoprotein is an acidic molecule whose charge is largely determined by sialic acid. CD44 plays a critical role in a variety of cellular behaviors, including adhesion, migration, invasion, and survival. The main ligand for CD44 is a hyaluronan but CD44 has an afifinity to other extracellular matrix constituents such as osteopontin, collagens, and matrix metalloproteinases (MMPs) (Cichy & Puré, 2003). The gene for CD44 contains 20 exons, 12 of which are expressed by the most common form of CD44, referred to as standard CD44 (CD44s). Isoforms of CD44 are generated by the insertion of alternative exons (V1–V11) at a single site within the membrane-proximal portion of the extracellular domain (Ponta et al., 2003). Molecules containing the variable exons or their peptide products are designated CD44v. The most abundant standard protein consists of three regions, a 72 amino acid (aa) C-terminal cytoplasmic domain, a 21 aa transmembrane domain, and a 270 aa extracellular domain (Goodison et al., 1999). The degree of glycosylation can affect the ligand binding characteristics of the protein and therefore alter its function. The regulation of the amount and the type of post-translational modification can add further diversity to the range of potential functions of CD44 isoforms. Expression of multiple CD44 isoforms is frequently upregulated during neoplastic transformation. CD44, particularly its variants, may be useful as a diagnostic or prognostic marker of malignancy (Goodison et al., 1999).

Expression of CD44 both on mRNA and protein levels was intensively studied in thyroid pathological lesions in order to evaluate its utility in distinguishing benign and malignant tumors. Immunohistochemical and immunocytochemical analyses showed that CD44 molecule was preferentially expressed in papillary thyroid carcinoma compared with other thyroid neoplasms and non-neoplastic lesions (Figge et al., 1994; Böhm et al., 2000; Kim et al., 2002). Variant isoforms of CD44 (CD44v3 and CD44v6) were detected in follicular and papillary carcinomas as well as in follicular adenomas but not in non-neoplastic lesions (Gu et al., 1998). The frequency of both variants expression was significantly higher in PTC with node metastasis than in PTC without metastasis (Gu et al., 1998). Since CD44v6 is not expressed by normal thyrocytes and is variably detected in benign and malignant lesions Gasbarri et al. (1999) suggested that it could be a preoperative marker to identify malignant lesions. Its immunodetection in cytologic specimens obtained by fine-needle aspiration biopsy could be useful for selecting those nodular lesions of the thyroid gland that need to be surgically resected (Gasbarri et al., 1999). Böhm et al. (2000) found that reduced level of CD44s in differentiated thyroid cancer patients seemed to be an independent prognostic factor for unfavorable disease outcome. Age older than 60 years, distant metastases and advanced pTNM stage were related to the loss of CD44s expression.

The main problem in preoperative diagnostics of thyroid neoplastic lesions is distinguishing between follicular carcinomas and follicular adenomas. Nasir et al. (2004) tested usefulness of CD44v6 among other markers in differentiating benign and malignant follicular neoplasms. They found membranous CD44v6 staining in 81% of FTC but in only 20% of follicular adenomas and suggested that its immunohistochemical detection may be useful for follicular neoplasm diagnostics. Maruta et al. (2004) analysed CD44v6 immunostaining in fine-needle aspiration cytology of 35 follicular carcinoma specimens and 44 cases of follicular adenomas and observed positive reaction in 74% of carcinoma cases and 30% of adenomas. There was no correlation between the expression of CD44v6 in follicular carcinomas and characteristics such as capsular invasion, vascular invasion, metastasis, or tumor size (Maruta et al., 2004).

Since CD44 is often detected in benign lesions its diagnostic importance is questioned by some authors (Nikiel et al., 2006). Matesa et al. (2007) analyzed CD44v6 mRNA expression in order to answer whether the presence of macrophages and Hürthle cells are responsible for positive expression detected in benign lesions. They found a statistically significant relationship between presence of Hürthle cells and positive expression of CD44v6 in nodular goiter cytological samples.

3.4 Osteopontin

Osteopontin (OPN) is an acidic hydrophilic glycophosphoprotein rich in aspartic acid, glutamic acid and serine and contains ~30 monosaccharides, including 10 residues of sialic acid. One carbohydrate chain is attached by *N*-glycosyl bond to protein and 5-6 chains are linked by *O*-glycosyl bond (Rangaswami et al., 2006). OPN is a member of a small integrin binding ligand *N*-linked glycoprotein (SIBLING) family of proteins which include bone sialoprotein (BSP), dentin matrix protein 1 (DMP1), dentin sialoprotein (DSPP), and matrix extracellular phoshoglycoprotein (MEPE) (Wai & Kuo, 2008). OPN functions by mediating cell-matrix interactions and cellular signaling through binding with integrin and CD44 receptors. Many studies have indicated that OPN is highly expressed in several malignancies. OPN expression is associated with tumor invasion, progression or metastasis in breast, stomach, lung, prostate, liver and colon cancers (for a review see Wai & Kuo, 2008; Rangaswami et al., 2006).

Castellone et al. (2004) showed that osteopontin was a major RET/PTC - induced transcriptional target in PC Cl3 thyroid follicular cells. RET/PTC also induced a strong overexpression of CD44 which is a cell surface signaling receptor for OPN. These results prompt further studies to ascertain whether OPN could be a useful PTC tumor marker. OPN expression was studied by immunohistochemistry in 117 samples of thyroid papillary cancer, benign lesions and normal tissues (Guarino et al., 2005). OPN was found to be overexpressed in PTCs compared with normal thyroid tissue, follicular adenomas and multinodular goiters. Moreover, OPN up-regulation was correlated with aggressive clinicopathological features of PTC. The prevalence and intensity of OPN staining were significantly correlated with the presence of lymph node metastases and tumor size. However, follicular variant of PTC had lower prevalance of OPN expression compared to classical type. Studies of Briese et al. (2010) on a large number of thyroid samples showed that normal thyroid was negative for OPN, thyroid adenomas were weakly OPN positive, whereas many carcinomas were strongly positive. However, there was no association between OPN expression and tumor size and metastasis status.

mRNA level of *SPP1* (osteopontin gene) was validated in a panel of 57 thyroid tumors using quantitative PCR (qPCR) (Oler et al., 2008). SPP1 was overexpressed in PTCs but the difference was not considered significant. However, *SPP1* expression was associated with the presence of lymph node metastasis for tumors >1 cm. The expression levels of *SPP1* in follicular variant of PTC and follicular carcinoma were lower than in classical type of PTC.

Recently Wang et al. (2010) found that osteopontin expression is positively correlated in thyroid papillary carcinoma with phosphorylated c-Jun kinase (p-JNK). Activation of the JNK signaling pathway appears to be an important event in thyroid tumorigenesis and, perhaps, in tumor progression making p-JNK a possible target in cancer treatment. Coordinated expression of p-JNK and OPN immunoreaction suggest an involvement of both genes in the same molecular pathway in thyroid lesions (Wang et al., 2010).

3.5 NCAM

Neuronal cell adhesion molecule (NCAM, CD56) mediates homotypic and heterotypic cell-cell adhesion (Crossin & Krushel, 2000). NCAM structurally belongs to the immunoglobulin superfamily. The extracellular part of NCAM consists of five Ig-like domains and two fibronectin type III-like domains. Alternative mRNA splicing results in three major isoforms: a 120 kDa isoform which is predominantly expressed in normal and well differentiated tissues and a 140 and 180 kDa isoforms that are found predominantly in less differentiated or malignant cell types (Jensen & Berthold, 2007). NCAM is unique among adhesion molecules because it carries a large amount of the negatively charged sugar, polysialic acid (PSA) (Crossin & Krushel, 2000). The presence of PSA can affect the strength or stability of adhesion systems in which NCAM is involved.

NCAM is present on follicular epithelial cells of the normal thyroid but its expression is reduced by malignant transformation and may affect the migratory capability of tumor cells (Zeromski et al., 1998, 1999; Satoh et al., 2001). Scarpino et al. (2007) analyzed NCAM expression in tissue sections of 61 cases of papillary thyroid carcinoma (PTC) using immunohistochemistry and quantitative real-time PCR. Reduced NCAM protein expression was observed by immunohistochemistry in all histological variants of PTC and also in lymph node metastases. Reduced expression of NCAM protein was associated with a significant reduction of NCAM mRNA in the tumor tissue compared with the paired normal thyroid tissue. Other studies showed NCAM to be extremely useful in the distinction between PTC and follicular benign or malignant lesions (El Demellawy et al., 2008, 2009; Ozolins et al., 2010). El Demellawy et al. (2009) evaluated the diagnostic value of protein expression using antibodies against NCAM in normal follicular thyroid epithelium, benign thyroid lesions, and thyroid carcinomas. Their aim was to study the applicability of difference in NCAM expression as a marker that distinguishes PTC, including the follicular variant from other follicular thyroid lesions and follicular thyroid carcinoma. They found that NCAM is of value in distinguishing PTC from other thyroid follicular pathology with a sensitivity of 100% and a specificity of 100%.

The potential role of NCAM in tumor cell biology was investigated by silencing the *NCAM* gene in the TPC1 thyroid papillary carcinoma cell line (Scarpino et al., 2007). The results confirm that modifications of NCAM expression cause profound alterations in the adhesive and migratory properties. However, contrary to the observation that loss of NCAM is usually associated with increased tumor invasiveness *in vivo,* NCAM-silenced TPC-1 cells were more adhesive to different extracellular matrix components, and were less efficient in cell migration and invasiveness. This discrepancy requires further investigations.

3.6 TIMPs

Tissue inhibitors of metalloproteinases (TIMPs) have a dual role in the process of tumor progression with both pro- and anti-tumorigenic activities. Although originally characterized by their ability to inhibit matrix metalloproteinases (MMPs) activity, TIMPs have additional biological activities and have been shown to regulate a number of cellular processes including cell growth, migration, and apoptosis (Stetler-Stevenson, 2008). Four TIMPs have been currently characterized in human and designated as TIMP-1, -2, -3 and -4. They are expressed by a variety of cell types and are present in most tissues and body fluids.

TIMP-1 gene differs from the other members of the family in having a short exon 1 that is transcribed but not translated. The function of exon 1 appears to be related to the control of the specificity of tissue expression and may contain tissue-specific repressor elements. TIMP-1 is a glycosylated protein and the *N*-linked oligosaccharides are composed of sialic acid, mannose, galactose and *N*-acetylglucosamine. The TIMP-1 glycosylation seems to play a role in various functions including correct folding of the nascent protein, transport of the molecule to cell surface and enhanced stability of the protein (Lambert et al., 2004). TIMP-3 has also one glycosylation site.

TIMP-1 mRNA or protein overexpression was found in thyroid papillary cancers compared to normal tissue or goiters (Hawthorn et al., 2004; Maeta et al., 2001). Shi et al. (1999) investigated TIMP-1 gene expression in 39 primary thyroid tumors to see whether there is a correlation between TIMP-1 expression and the aggressiveness of the disease. They also transfected human TIMP-1 cDNA into a papillary thyroid carcinoma cell line (NPA) to study the effect of TIMP-1 expression on its invasive potential using an *in vitro* tumor invasion assay. The results showed that TIMP-1 mRNA level correlated directly with tumor aggressiveness: the highest number of TIMP-1 transcripts was found in stages III and IV *versus* benign goitres. However, overexpression of TIMP-1 by gene transfer resulted in a significant suppression of the malignant phenotype of NPA cells which suggests that TIMP-1 may function as a thyroid tumor invasion/metastasis suppressor. To explain these discrepancies, the authors suggested that the increased levels of TIMP-1 transcripts observed in cancer samples came from stroma cells to counteract tumor invasion and metastasis.

Kebebew et al. (2006) performed a real-time quantitative reverse-transcriptase polymerase chain reaction (RT-PCR) assay of several candidate diagnostic markers to distinguish benign from malignant thyroid neoplasms, and to predict the extent of the disease. TIMP-1 mRNA expression level as well as ECM1 (extracellular matrix protein 1), TMPRSS4 (transmembrane protease, serine 4) and ANGPT2 (angiopoietin 2) mRNA levels were found to be independent diagnostic markers of malignant thyroid neoplasms. The AUC (the area under the receiver operating characteristic (ROC) curve) for 4 diagnostic genes in combination was 0.993 with sensitivity of 100%, specificity of 94.6%, positive predictive value of 96.5%, and negative predictive value of 100%. Thus the RT-PCR multigene assay involving TIMP1 is an excellent diagnostic marker for differentiated thyroid cancer and it will be a helpful adjunct to FNA biopsy of thyroid nodules.

The plasma concentration of MMP-1, 2, 3, 8 and 9 as well TIMP-1 and 2 was evaluated by enzyme-linked immunosorbent assay (ELISA) in patients with thyroid cancers (papillary, anaplastic and medullary) and in healthy subjects. The author suggests that, predominance of MMP-2 over TIMP-2 and TIMP-1 over MMP-1 is a common feature in patients with thyroid cancer (Komorowski et al., 2002).

Recently Nam et al. (2011) have studied the expression of matrix metalloproteinase-13 (MMP-13) and tissue inhibitor of metalloproteinase-13 (TIMP-3) in thyroid cancer by RT-PCR. They found that MMP-13 and TIMP-3 expression levels were significantly decreased in PTC samples compared with normal thyroid tissues.

3.7 Dipeptidyl peptidase IV

Dipeptidyl peptidase IV (DPPIV), assigned to the CD26 cluster, is a multifunctional protein expressed on epithelial cells and lymphocytes. DPPIV is a type II transmembrane glycoprotein which consists of a large extracellular domain (C-terminus) connected by a flexible stalk region to a hydrophobic transmembrane domain and short intarcellular tail (N-terminus) (Kotacková et al., 2009). It preferentially cleaves N-terminal dipeptides from polypeptides with proline or alanine in the penultimate position and regulates the activities of a number of hormones, neuropeptides, cytokines and chemokines (Havre et al., 2008; Kotacková et al., 2009). DPPIV palys an important role in immune regulation, signal transduction, chemotaxis, cell adhesion and apoptosis. It is suggested that DPPIV is also involved in the neoplastic transformation and tumor progression (Pro & Dang, 2004; Kotacková et al., 2009).

Numerous early studies showed that DPPIV is abnormally expressed in thyroid carcinomas and may be useful for the diagnosis of thyroid tumors (Aratake et al., 1991; Kotani et al., 1992; Tanaka et al., 1995; Umeki et al., 1996; Tang et al., 1996; Hirai et al., 1999). DPPIV-like enzymatic activity and DPPIV protein expression were up-regulated in thyroid cancers. However, DPPIV positivity is limited to the group of well-differentiated carcinomas, particularly papillary carcinoma (Kholová et al., 2003; de Micco et al., 2008). DPPIV sensitivity to malignant follicular tumors including the follicular variant of PTC was low with a misdiagnosis rate of 20–30%, especially with tumors presenting Hürthle or tall-cell features. Although, the use of DPPIV can increase specificity and positive predictive value of the cytological diagnosis, the value of the marker in the individual cases is very limited (Kholová et al., 2003). The analysis of DPPIV mRNA level in 102 PTCs and 77 normal thyroid fragments with the use of Q-PCR reaction confirmed the increase of DPPIV expression in papillary thyroid carcinoma. However, the ROC analysis revealed that the diagnostic efficiency of DPPIV estimation is limited. Thus diagnostic usefulness of DPPIV as a single PTC marker is also doubtful (Ożóg et al. 2006).

3.8 E-cadherin and dysadherin

Cadherins are members of a large family of transmembrane glycoproteins, many of which participate in Ca^{2+}-dependent homophilic cell-cell adhesion and play an important role in the formation of tissue architecture (Shapiro & Weis, 2009). E-cadherin is necessary for normal epithelial function. Dysadherin is a cancer-associated cell membrane glycoprotein. It inactivates E-cadherin function in a post-transcriptional manner, has an anti-cell-cell adhesion function and plays an important role in tumor progression and metastasis (Ino et al., 2002).

Several authors have investigated the expression of E-cadherin in thyroid cancers (Scheumman et al., 1995; Serini et al., 1996; von Wasielewski et al., 1997; Kapran et al., 2002; Rocha et al., 2003; Kato et al., 2002; Choi et al. 2005; Brecelj et al., 2005). In general, it appears that E-cadherin expression is retained in follicular neoplasms but it is reduced in papillary carcinomas and lost in anaplastic and poorly differentiated carcinomas. Reduction or loss of E-cadherin has been correlated with widely invasive growth and lymph node metastases (Naito et al., 2001). E-cadherin reactivity is reported to be an important prognostic factor in papillary thyroid carcinomas (Scheumman et al., 1995; Rocha et al., 2003). Lack of E-cadherin expression has been considered as an adverse prognostic factor for survival.

Dysadherin expression in thyroid cancer was reported by two studies. Sato et al. (2003) analyzed by immunohistochemistry dysadherin and E-cadherin expression in 92 thyroid carcinomas. Dysadherin was detected in 39 of 51 papillary carcinomas and in all 31 undifferentiated carcinomas but not in follicular carcinomas or normal thyroid tissue controls. Dysadherin expression correlated significantly with tumor size, regional lymph node metastasis, and distant metastasis of the primary carcinoma. A significant association was also observed between dysadherin expression and death from thyroid carcinoma. Dysadherin expression showed a significant negative correlation with E-cadherin expression (Sato et al., 2003).

Batistatou et al. (2008) compared the dysadherin expression in papillary carcinomas and papillary microcarcinomas (PMC) to find out whether there are any differences in the cell–cell adhesion system between these two malignancies that have different biological behavior. PMC has been defined as a papillary neoplasm measuring 1cm or less in diameter and usually remains clinically silent and is often identified incidentally in surgically removed thyroid glands for other reasons (e.g. nodular hyperplasia, thyroiditis). A statistically significant difference in dysadherin and E-cadherin expression between PC and PMC and a negative correlation between E-cadherin and dysadherin expression regardless of tumor size were noted (Batistatou et al., 2008).

3.9 Mucins

Mucins are defined as high molecular weight glycoproteins that contain tandem repeat structures extensively glycosylated through GalNAc *O*-linkages at the threonine and serine residues. To date, twenty one members of human mucin (MUC) family have been reported and they are designed chronologically in order of discovery. On the basis of their structural and physiologic characteristics, mucins have been divided into three sub-classes: the secreted/gel-forming mucins, the soluble mucins, and the membrane- associated mucins (Kufe, 2009; Ohashi et al., 2006).

Mucins are multifaceted glycoproteins that play a crucial role in maintaining homeostasis and promoting cell survival. They form a physical barrier, which separates an apical surface of epithelial cells from the external environment and protects against infection and proteolytic degradation. The membrane-associated mucins are anchored to the surface of the cell by a transmembrane domain and then have short cytoplasmic tail that interacts with cytoskeletal elements and cytosolic adaptor proteins. Therefore, they can act as putative receptors that engage diverse signaling pathway linked to differentiation, proliferation and apoptosis. Several reports indicate that aberrant upregulations of mucins especially transmembrane forms may promote the malignant phenotype of human carcinomas. In many types of tumor overexpression of transmembrane mucins contribute to the oncogenesis by disrupting epithelial polarity and cell-cell interactions, to constitutive activation of growth and survival pathways and to blocking stress-induced apoptosis and necrosis (Bafna et al., 2010; Kufe, 2009; Carraway et al., 2003).

The production of mucins has been relatively frequently observed in thyroid carcinomas. In a study of 142 cases of thyroid neoplasms, Mlynek et al. (1985) found mucinous substances, which occurred in about 50% of the papillary and medullary carcinomas, 35% of the follicular carcinomas and 21% of the anaplastic varieties. The most widely studied mucin, associated with thyroid malignancies is MUC1, encoded by gene located on the chromosome 1q21-24. Wreesmann et al. (2004) suggested that up-regulation of MUC1 expression in papillary thyroid carcinoma correlates with 1q21 amplifications and aggressive behavior. The MUC1 gene overexpression was present in 97,5% of tall-cell variant of PTCs (TCV) as compared with only 35% of conventional PTCs. These results are in contrast to the previous analysis of Bièche et al. (1997) who detected no MUC1 gene amplification in 14 tumor samples (6 adenomas and 8 PTC) informative for the MUC1 gene. However, these studies showed higher MUC1 expression level in 6 out of 11 papillary carcinoma cases in comparison with 10 macrofollicular adenoma cases and normal thyroid tissue. Moreover, the authors observed that intracytoplasmic MUC1 staining occurred in 75% (3/4) of "high-risk" papillary thyroid carcinomas and in only 28,5% (2/7) of the "low-risk" PTC without extrathyroidal invasion or lymph node involvement, suggesting that MUC1 can be associated with more aggressive tumors. Indeed, comparing human thyroid cancer cell lines, Patel et al. (2005) found increased MUC1 expression in aggressive thyroid cancer cell lines (8305C, KAT4, ARO, BHP2-7, BHP10-3, BHP7-13, BHP18-21) but not in other papillary and follicular thyroid cancer cell lines (KAT5, KAT10, NPA, WRO, FRO). In addition, they demonstrated that targeting MUC1 with monoclonal antibody selectively affects cell viability and confirmed that MUC1 plays a crucial role in the thyroid behavior. Furthermore, a relationship was observed between cytoplasmic MUC1 and cyclin D1 immunostaining in the conventional PTCs and in papillary microcarcinomas (PMCs), implying that MUC1 may be involved in the regulation of Wnt pathway and has a role in B-catenin/cyclin D1 signaling. However, due to a very broad MUC1 expression in different histological variants, the authors were not able to determinate its prognostic utility (Abrosimov et al., 2007). Magro et al. (2003) found that MUC1 may co-exist in variety of glycosylated forms in different cellular compartments. They supposed that post-translational modification of mucins, rather than alterations in expression levels, may be stronger associated with tumor progression and specific glycosylation traits of MUC1 and could be an ancillary tool in histopathological diagnosis. Other investigators found MUC1 mRNA overexpression in 15 cases of PTC in contrast to 22-follicular adenomas and 22-normal thyroid tissues (Baek et al., 2007). More recently, Morari et al. (2010) basing on the study of 410 patients reported that MUC1 expression distinguished benign from malignant thyroid tissue with sensitivity of 89%; specificity of 52%; predictive positive value=75%; predictive negative value=74%. In conclusion, they suggested that MUC1 is not a reliable prognostic marker but may be useful in characterization of thyroid carcinomas, especially the follicular patterned thyroid lesions. The expression of other mucins in thyroid neoplasms has been poorly investigated. Nam et al. (2011) have suggested that MUC4 and MUC15 are the other important mucins associated with thyroid transformation. They showed significantly increased MUC4 and MUC15 mRNA level and positive immunoreactivities in PTC compared with normal tissue. High MUC4 expression correlated with small tumor size and papillary thyroid microcarcinoma subtype whereas overexpression of MUC15 was associated with age, the presence of multifocality and distant metastasis. The results of this study suggest, that MUC4 and MUC15 may play a crucial role in thyroid malignancy, especially the MUC15 may be a new prognostic marker and potential therapeutic target. However, there are some discrepancies between the previously published reports that indicated weakly positive or negative MUC4 staining of both benign and malignant thyroid carcinomas (Baek et al., 2007; Magro et al., 2003). The expression of MUC2, MUC3, MUC5AC, MUC5B and MUC6 in thyroid neoplasms has been tested, though none of these glycoproteins was associated with clinicopathological features of thyroid carcinomas (Magro et al., 2003; Alves et al., 1999). The clinical and prognostic significance of mucins in thyroid tumors is still an open question.

4. Galectins

Galectins are endogenous lectins defined by shared consensus amino acid sequences and an affinity for β-galactose containing oligosaccharides. Fifteen members of galectin family have been identified and classified into three subgroups based on their structure: prototype (galectin-1, 2, 5, 10, 11, 13, 14, 15), tandem repeat type (galectin-6, 8, 9, 12) and chimera type (galectin-3). The presence of at least one carbohydrate recognition domain (CRD) is a common characteristic of galectins (Krześlak & Lipińska, 2004; Elola et al., 2007; Boscher et al., 2011). Galectins have both intra- and extracellular localization. Galectins can be secreted by non-classical pathway and depending on the cell type or differentiation state, they are found in the cytoplasm and the nucleus, on the cell surface and in the extracellular matrix (Hughes, 2001; Haudek et al., 2010; Garner & Baum, 2008). Galectins have been shown to play roles in diverse biological processes, such as embryogenesis, adhesion and proliferation of cells, apoptosis, mRNA splicing and modulation of immune response (Krześlak & Lipińska, 2004; Elola et al., 2007; Boscher et al., 2011).

Among various galectins, galectin-1, 3 and 7 have gained attention as potential markers of thyroid malignancy. However, the data concerning galectin -1 and 7 expression in thyroid are very limited. Chiariotti et al. (1995) analyzed mRNA and protein levels of galectin-1 in 74 human thyroid specimens of neoplastic, hyperproliferative and normal tissues. Galectin-1 mRNA levels was increased in 28 of 40 papillary carcinomas and in 6 of 7 anaplastic carcinomas compared with normal or hyperplastic thyroid. Immunohistochemical analysis of normal thyroid and papillary carcinoma sections revealed a higher content of galectin-1 protein in neoplastic cells than in normal cells. Similarly Xu et al. (1995) showed that all studied by them thyroid malignancies of epithelial origin (i.e., papillary and follicular carcinomas) and metastatic lymph node from a papillary carcinoma expressed high levels of galectin-1. In contrast neither benign thyroid adenomas nor adjacent normal thyroid tissue expressed galectin-1. There are only two studies concerning galectin-7 expression in thyroid cancers (Rorive et al., 2002; Than et al., 2008). The profile of galectin-7 expression is different from that of galectin-1 and 3. The results of immunohistochemical analysis revealed that this galectin is markedly down-regulated in adenomas compared with multinodular goiters and carcinomas (Rorive et al., 2002). Than et al. (2008) did not show any diagnostic value of galectin-7 in thyroid malignancy, even for a simple differentiation between obvious benign and malignant thyroid lesions .

In contrast to galectin-1 and 7, galectin-3 is one of the best studied molecular markers for thyroid diagnosis (for rewiew see Sanabria et al., 2007; Chiu et al., 2010) . The expression of this protein was widely studied both in cancer tissues and in cytological specimens. Numerous studies have reported that galectin-3 is a very sensitive and reliable diagnostic marker for identification of thyroid carcinomas with high sensitivity and specificity (Orlandi et al., 1998; Gasbarri et al., 1999; Inohara et al., 1999; Bartolazzi et al., 2001; Saggiorato et al., 2001,2004; Pisani et al., 2004). However there are studies which did not confirm this diagnostic utility of galectin-3 (Niedziela et al., 2002, Mehrotra et al., 2004, Mills et al., 2005) The discrepancies observed in these reports could have resulted from different methods used for galectin-3 expression analysis. These methods differ in sample preparation details, the used antibody, dilution of antibodies, assessement of positive results (percentage of marked cells and intensity of staining). Moreover, in the thyroid gland, oxyphilic cells are rich in endogenous biotin and galectin-3 immunocytochemistry may provide false-positive results in oxyphilic cell lesions due to biotin-based detection systems (Volante et al., 2004).

Recently, the diagnostic utility of galectin-3 in distinguishing benign from malignant follicular thyroid nodules was evaluated in a multicenter trial comprised a large cohort of patients (Bartolazzi et al., 2008). Galectin-3 expression analysis was applied preoperatively on 465 follicular thyroid FNAB samples and diagnostic accuracy was compared with final histology. Galectin-3 expression had an overall reported sensitivity of 78%, specificity of 93% and accuracy of 88% for distinguishing benign and malignant thyroid tumors. Similar results were obtained in two center trial reported by Franco et al. (2009). They compared galectin-3 staining results in suspicious or indeterminate FNABs samples with the histologic diagnosis of the thyroidectomy specimens. Galectin-3 expression was found to have sensitivity of 83%, specificity of 81%, positive predictive value of 84%, and negative predictive value of 80%.

Few studies have evaluated the correlation between galectin-3 expression and clinicopathological parameters of thyroid cancers such as tumor size and grade, capsular invasion or lymph node metastasis status. The galectin-3 expression level in follicular carcinoma was significantly increased with the degree of vascular or capsular invasion (Ito Y et al. 2005). High galectin-3 expression was also associated with lymph node metastasis in MTC (Faggiano et al., 2002; Cvejic et al., 2005). Contrary, Kawachi et al. (2000) reported significantly higher galectin-3 expression in the primary foci of the thyroid tumors with lymph node metastases, but they found lower levels of galectin-3 in their metasatsis offspring. Recently, Türköz et al. (2008) suggested that galectin-3 overexpression is more profound in early stages of papillary carcinoma, and its expression intensity decreases during tumor progression.

Two studies have analyzed the serum level of galecin-3 in thyroid cancer patients (Inohara et al. 2008; Saussez et al., 2008). They measured serum level of galectin-3 by ELISA method and compared with histological diagnosis after thyroidectomy. Although Sauessez et al. (2008) showed that higher serum level of galectin 3 was associated with thyroid disease there were no significant differences between benign and malignant thyroid tissues. Inohara et al. (2008) showed that serum galectin concentration in patients with papillary carcinomas did not differ significantly from that in patients with follicular carcinoma or adenoma and in healthy individuals.

Studies of Bartolazzi et al. (2008) and Franco et al. (2009) suggest that galectin-3 expression analysis may represent useful diagnostic method for those follicular nodules that remain indeterminate by cytological diagnosis and may improve the selection of patients for surgery. However before it can be used in clinical practice there is an urgent need for validation of methods of galectin-3 expression analysis. Some other studies suggest that diagnostic usefulness of galectin-3 may be significantly increased by combining with other potential thyroid cancer markers such as HBME1, cytokeratin-19, DPPIV, CD44v6, thyroid peroxidase (Aratake et al., 2002; Weber et al., 2004; Maruta et al. 2004; de Matos et al., 2005; Prasad et al., 2005; Papotti et al., 2005; Liu et al., 2008; Barut et al., 2010).

5. Conclusion

Fine needle aspiration biopsy (FNAB) is a practical and the most effective diagnostic technique for the preoperative detection of malignant nodule. However, the important limitation of FNAB is the lack of sensitivity in the evaluation of follicular neoplasms due to its inability to differentiate benign follicular lesions from their malignant counterparts. Moreover, for definite diagnosis of malignancy a complete excision with unequivocal evidence of capsular or vascular invasion is required. Therefore, new markers that may allow for accurate diagnosis of thyroid malignancy and eliminate potentially unnecessary surgery are needed. Glycosylation changes and the analyses of expression of some glycoproteins or galectins can provide a novel strategy for improvement of thyroid cancer diagnostics. So far, the most promising results have been obtained in the case of galectin-3 expression. Currently an improved galectin-3 immunodetection method represents a new methodological approach that can be used to optimize the preoperative selection of thyroid nodules. Further studies concerning alterations of glycosylation and glycoprotein patterns in thyroid pathological specimens may potentially lead to the discovery of novel biomarkers.

6. Acknowledgment

This work was supported by the statutory fund for Department of Cytobiochemistry, University of Lodz.

7. References

Abrosimov, A.; Saenko, V.; Meirmanov, S.; Nakashima, M.; Rogounovitch, T.; Shkurko, O.; Lushnikov, E.; Mitsutake, N.; Namba, H. & Yamashita, S. (2007). The cytoplasmic expression of MUC1 in papillary thyroid carcinoma of different histological variants and its correlation with cyclin D1 overexpression. *Endocrine Pathology*, Vol.18, No.2, (Summer 2007), pp. 68-75, ISSN 1046-3976

Alves, P.; Soares, P.; Fonseca, E. & Sobrinho-Simões M. (1999). Papillary thyroid carcinoma overexpresses fully and underglycosylated mucins together with native and sialylated simple mucin antigens and histo-blood group antigens. *Endocrine Pathology*, Vol.10, No.4, (Winter 1999), pp. 315-324, ISSN 1046-3976

Aratake, Y.; Kotani, T.; Tamura, K.; Araki, Y.; Kuribayashi, T.; Konoe, K.& Ohtaki, S. (1991) Dipeptidyl aminopeptidase IV staining of cytologic preparations to distinguish benign from malignant thyroid diseases. *American Journal of Clinical Pathology*, Vol.96, No.3, (September 1991), pp. 306-310, ISSN 0002-9173

Aratake, Y.; Umeki, K.; Kiyoyama, K.; Hinoura, Y.; Sato, S.; Ohno, A.; Kuribayashi, T.; Hirai, K.; Nabeshima, K. & Kotani, T. (2002) Diagnostic utility of galectin-3 and CD26/DPPIV as preoperative diagnostic markers for thyroid nodules. *Diagnostic Cytopathol*ogy,Vol.26, No.6, (June 2002), pp.366-372, ISSN 1097-0339

Arcinas, A.; Yen, T.Y.; Kebebew, E. &Macher, B.A. (2009) Cell surface and secreted protein profiles of human thyroid cancer cell lines reveal distinct glycoprotein patterns. *Journal of Proteome Research*, Vol.8, No.8, (August 2009),pp. 3958-3968, ISSN 1535-3893

Babál, P.; Janega, P.; Cerná, A.; Kholová, I. & Brabencová, E. (2006) Neoplastic transformation of the thyroid gland is accompanied by changes in cellular sialylation. *Acta Histochemica,* Vol. 108, No.2, (May 2006), pp. 133-140, ISSN 0065-1281

Baek, S.K.; Woo, J.S.; Kwon, S.Y.; Lee, S.H.; Chae, Y.S. & Jung K.Y. (2007). Prognostic significance of the Muc1 and Muc4 expressions in thyroid papillary carcinoma. *The Laryngoscope,* Vol.117, No.5, (May 2007), pp. 911-916, ISSN 0023-852X

Bafna, S.; Kaur, S. & Batra, S.K. (2010). Membrane-bound mucins: the mechanistic basis for alterations in the growth and survival of cancer cells. *Oncogene,* Vol.29, No.20, (May 2010), pp. 2893-2904, ISSN 0950-9232

Bartolazzi, A.; Gasbarri, A.; Papotti, M.; Bussolati, G.; Lucante, T.; Khan, A.; Inohara, H.; Marandino, F.; Orlandi, F.; Nardi, F.; Vecchione, A.; Tecce, R. & Larsson, O. (2001). Thyroid Cancer Study Group. Application of an immunodiagnostic method for improving preoperative diagnosis of nodular thyroid lesions. *The Lancet,*Vol.357, No.9269, (May 2001), pp. 1644-1650, ISSN 0140-6736

Bartolazzi, A.; Orlandi, F.; Saggiorato, E.; Volante, M.; Arecco, F.; Rossetto, R.; Palestini, N.; Ghigo, E.; Papotti, M.; Bussolati, G.; Martegani, M.P.; Pantellini, F.; Carpi, A.; Giovagnoli, M.R.; Monti, S.; Toscano, V.; Sciacchitano, S.; Pennelli, G.M.; Mian, C. ;Pelizzo, M.R.; Rugge, M.; Troncone, G.; Palombini, L.; Chiappetta, G.; Botti, G.; Vecchione, A.& Bellocco, R. (2008) Italian Thyroid Cancer Study Group (ITCSG). Galectin-3-expression analysis in the surgical selection of follicular thyroid nodules with indeterminate fine-needle aspiration cytology: a prospective multicentre study. *The Lancet Oncolgy,* Vol. 9, No. 6, (June 2008),pp. 543-549, ISSN 1470-2045

Barut, F.; Onak, Kandemir, N., Bektas, S.; Bahadir B., Keser, S. & Ozdamar, S.O. (2010) Universal markers of thyroid malignancies: galectin-3, HBME-1, and cytokeratin-19. *Endocrine Pathology,* Vol. 21, No.2, (June 2010), pp. 80-89, ISSN 1046-3976

Batistatou, A.; Charalabopoulos, K.; Nakanishi, Y.; Vagianos, C.; Hirohashi, S.; Agnantis, N.J.& Scopa, C.D. (2008) Differential expression of dysadherin in papillary thyroid carcinoma and microcarcinoma: correlation with E-cadherin. *Endocrine Pathology,* Vol. 19, No.3 (Fall 2008), pp. 197-202, ISSN 1046-3976

Becker, D.J. & Lowe, J.B. (2003) Fucose: biosynthesis and biological function in mammals. *Glycobiology,* Vol. 13, No.7, (July 2003), pp. 41R-53R, ISSN 0959-6658

Bièche, I.; Ruffet, E.; Zweibaum, A.; Vildé, F.; Lidereau, R.; & Franc, B. (1997). Muc1 mucin gene, transcripts, and protein in adenomas and papillary carcinomas of the thyroid. *Thyroid,* Vol.7, No.5, (October 1997), pp. 725-731, ISSN 1050-7256

Biscolla, R.P.M.; Cerutti, J.M. & Maciel, R.M.B. (2000) Detection of recurrent thyroid cancer by sensitive nested reverse transcription–polymerase chain reaction of thyroglobulin and sodium/iodide symporter messenger ribonucleic acid transcripts in peripheral blood. *Journal of Clinical Endocrinology & Metabolism,* Vol. 85,(October 2000), pp. 3623–3627, ISSN 0021-972X

Böhm, J.P; Niskanen, L.K.; Pirinen, R.T.; Kiraly, K.; Kellokoski, J.K.; Moisio, K.I.; Eskelinen, M.J.; Tulla, H.E.; Hollmen, S. Alhava, E.M. & Kosma, V.M. (2000) Reduced CD44 standard expression is associated with tumour recurrence and unfavourable outcome in differentiated thyroid carcinoma. *The Journal of Pathology.* Vol. 192, No. 3, (November 2000), pp. 321-327, ISSN 1096-9896

Bojunga, J.; Roddiger, S.; Stanisch, M.; Kusterer, K.; Kurek, R.; Renneberg, H.; Adams, S.; Lindhorst, E.; Usadel, K.H. & Schumm-Draeger, P.M. (2000) Molecular detection of thyroglobulin mRNA transcripts in peripheral blood of patients with thyroid disease by RT–PCR. *British Journal of Cancer,* Vol. 82, No. 10, (May 2000), pp. 1650–1655, ISSN 0007-0920

Boscher, C.; Dennis, J.W. & Nabi, I.R. (2011) Glycosylation, galectins and cellular signaling. *Current Opinions in Cell Biology*. doi:10.1016/j.ceb.2011.05.001, ISSN 0955-0674

Brecelj, E.; Frković, Grazio, S.; Auersperg, M. &Bracko, M. (2005) Prognostic value of E-cadherin expression in thyroid follicular carcinoma. *European Journal of Surgical Oncology*, Vol. 31, No. 5, (June 2005), pp. 544-548. ISSN 0748-7983

Briese, J.; Cheng, S.; Ezzat, S.; Liu, W.; Winer, D.; Wagener, C.; Bamberger, A.M& Asa, S.L. (2010). Osteopontin (OPN) expression in thyroid carcinoma. *Anticancer Research*, Vol. 30, No. 5, (May 2010), pp.1681-1688, ISSN 0250-7005

Brockhausen, I. (1999) Pathways of *O*-glycan biosynthesis in cancer cells. *Biochimica et Biophysica Acta* , Vol. 1473, No.1, (December 1999) pp. 67–95, ISSN 0304-4165

Brockhausen, I.; Schachter, H.& Stanley P. (2009). O-GalNAc Glycans. In: *Essentials of Glycobiology*, Varki, A.; Cummings, R.D.; Esko, J.D.; Freeze, H.H.; Stanley, P., Bertozzi, C.R.; Hart, G.W. & Etzler, M.E.,: Cold Spring Harbor Laboratory Press; 2009, ISBN-13: 9780879697709, Cold Spring Harbor (NY)

Butkinaree, C.; Park, K. & Hart, G.W. (2010). O-linked beta-N-acetylglucosamine (O-GlcNAc): Extensive crosstalk with phosphorylation to regulate signaling and transcription in response to nutrients and stress. *Biochimica et Biophysica Acta*, Vol. 1800, No. 2, (February 2010), pp. 96-106, ISSN 0304-4165

Caldwell, S.A.; Jackson, S.R.; Shahriari, K.S.; Lynch, T.P.; Sethi, G.; Walker, S.; Vosseller, K. & Reginato, M.J. (2010). Nutrient sensor O-GlcNAc transferase regulates breast cancer tumorigenesis through targeting of the oncogenic transcription factor FoxM1. *Oncogene*, Vol. 29, No.19 (May 2010), pp. 2831-2842 , ISSN 0950-9232

Carraway, K.L.; Ramsauer, V.P.; Haq, B. & Carothers Carraway, C.A. (2003). Cell signaling through membrane mucins. *BioEssays*, Vol.25, No.1, (January 2003), pp. 66-71, ISSN 0265-9247

Castellone, M.D.; Celetti, A.; Guarino, V.; Cirafici, A.M.; Basolo, F.; Giannini, R.; Medico, E.; Kruhoffer, M.; Orntoft, T.F.; Curcio, F.; Fusco, A.; Melillo, R.M. & Santoro, M. (2004). Autocrine stimulation by osteopontin plays a pivotal role in the expression of the mitogenic and invasive phenotype of RET/PTC-transformed thyroid cells. *Oncogene*, Vol. 23, No. 12., (March 2004), pp. 2188-2196, ISSN 0950-9232

Chiariotti, L.; Berlingieri, M.T.; Battaglia, C.; Benvenuto, G.; Martelli, M.L.; Salvatore, P.; Chiappetta, G.; Bruni, C.B. & Fusco, A. (1995). Expression of galectin-1 in normal human thyroid gland and in differentiated and poorly differentiated thyroid tumors. *International Journal of Cancer*, Vol. 64, No. 3, (June 1995), pp. 171-175, ISSN 1097-0215

Chiu, C.G.; Strugnell, S.S.; Griffith, O.L.; Jones, S.J.; Gown, A.M.; Walker, B.; Nabi, I.R. & Wiseman, S.M. (2010). Diagnostic utility of galectin-3 in thyroid cancer. *American Journal of Pathology*, Vol. 176, No. 5, (May 2010), pp. 2067-2081, ISSN 0002-9440

Choi, Y.L.; Kim, M.K.; Suh, J.W.; Han, J.; Kim, J.H.; Yang, J.H. & Nam, S.J. (2005). Immunoexpression of HBME-1, high molecular weight cytokeratin, cytokeratin 19, thyroid transcription factor-1, and E-cadherin in thyroid carcinomas. *Journal of Korean Medical Science*, Vol. 20, No. 5, (October 2005), pp.853-859, ISSN 1011-8934.

Cichy, J. & Puré, E. (2003). The liberation of CD44. *The Journal of Cell Biology*, Vol. 161, No. 5, (June 2003), pp. 839-843, ISSN 0021-9525

Comtesse, N.; Maldener, E. & Meese, E. (2001). Identification of a nuclear variant of MGEA5, a cytoplasmic hyaluronidase and a beta-N-acetylglucosaminidase. *Biochemical and Biophysical Research Communications*, Vol.283, No.3, (May 2001), pp. 634-640, ISSN 0006-291X

Crossin, K.L. & Krushel, L.A. (2000). Cellular signalling by neural cell adhesion molecules of the immunoglobulin superfamily. *Developmental Dynamics*, Vol. 218, No. 2, (June 2000), pp. 260–279, ISSN 1097-0177

Cvejic, D.S.; Savin, S.B.; Petrovic, I.M.; Paunovic, I.R.; Tatic, S.B. & Havelka, M.J. (2005). Galectin-3 expression in papillary thyroid carcinoma: relation to histomorphologic growth pattern, lymph node metastasis, extrathyroid invasion, and tumor size. *Head & Neck*, Vol. 27, No. 12, (December 2005), pp. 1049-1055, ISSN 1097-0347

Dall'Olio, F. & Chiricolo, M. (2001). Sialyltransferases in cancer. *Glycoconjugate Journal*, Vol. 18, No. 11-12, (November 2001), pp. 841-850, ISSN 0282-0080

de Matos, P.S.; Ferreira, A.P.; de Oliveira Facuri, F.; Assumpção, L.V.; Metze, K. & Ward, L.S. (2005). Usefulness of HBME-1, cytokeratin 19 and galectin-3 immunostaining in the diagnosis of thyroid malignancy. *Histopathology*, Vol. 47, No. 4, (October 2005), pp. 391-401, ISSN 1365-2559

de Micco, C.; Savchenko, V.; Giorgi, R.; Sebag, F. & Henry, J.F. (2008). Utility of malignancy markers in fine-needle aspiration cytology of thyroid nodules: comparison of Hector Battifora mesothelial antigen-1, thyroid peroxidase and dipeptidyl aminopeptidase IV. *British Journal of Cancer*, Vol. 98, No. 4, (February 2008), pp. 818-823, ISSN 0007-0920

Dennis, J.W.; Granovsky, M., & Warren, C.E. (1999). Protein glycosylation in development and disease. *Bioessays*. Vol. 21, No. 5, (May 1999), pp. 412-421, ISSN 1521-1878

Ditkoff, B.A.; Marvin, M.R.; Yemul, S.; Shi, Y.J.; Chabot, J.; Feind, C. & Lo Gerfo, P.L. (1996). Detection of circulating thyroid cells in peripheral blood. *Surgery*, Vol.120, No.6, (December 1996), pp. 959–964, ISSN 0039-6060

Drake, P.M.; Cho, W.; Li, B.; Prakobphol, A.; Johansen, E.; Anderson, N.L.; Regnier, F.E.; Gibson, B.W. & Fisher, S.J. (2010). Sweetening the pot: adding glycosylation to the biomarker discovery equation. *Clinical Chemistry*, Vol.56, No.2, (February 2010), pp. 223-236, ISSN 0009-9147

El Demellawy, D.; Nasr, A. & Alowami, S. (2008). Application of CD56, P63 and CK19 immunohistochemistry in the diagnosis of papillary carcinoma of the thyroid. *Diagnostic Pathology*, Vol.3, (February 2008), pp. 5, ISSN 1746-1596

El Demellawy, D.; Nasr, A.L.; Babay, S. &Alowami S. (2009). Diagnostic utility of CD56 immunohistochemistry in papillary carcinoma of the thyroid. *Pathology Research & Practice*, Vol. 205, No. 5(January 2009), pp. 303-309. ISSN 0344-0338

Elisei, R.; Vivaldi, A.; Agate, L.; Molinaro, E.; Nencetti, C.; Grasso, L.; Pinchera, A. &Pacini, F. (2004). Low specificity of blood thyroglobulin messenger ribonucleic acid assay prevents its use in the follow-up of differentiated thyroid cancer patients. *The Journal of Clinical and Endocrinology & Metabolism*. Vol.89, No.1, (January 2004), pp. 33-39, ISSN 0021-972X

Elola, M.T.; Wolfenstein-Todel, C.; Troncoso, M.F.; Vasta, G.R. & Rabinovich, G.A. (2007). Galectins: matricellular glycan-binding proteins linking cell adhesion, migration, and survival. *Cellular and Molecular Life Science*, Vol.64, No.13, (July 2007), pp. 1679-700, ISSN 1420-682X

Eszlinger, M.; Krohn, K.; Frenzel, R.; Kropf, S.; Tönjes, A. & Paschke, R. (2004). Gene expression analysis reveals evidence for inactivation of the TGF-beta signaling cascade in autonomously functioning thyroid nodules. *Oncogene*, Vol.23, No.3, (January 2004), pp. 795-804, ISSN 0950-9232

Eszlinger, M.; Neumann, S.; Otto, L. & Paschke, R. (2002). Thyroglobulin mRNA quantification in the peripheral blood is not a reliable marker for the follow-up of patients with differentiated thyroid cancer. *European Journal of Endocrinology,* Vol.147, No.5 (November 2004), pp. 575–582, ISSN 0804-4643

Faggiano, A.; Talbot, M.; Lacroix, L.; Bidart, J.M.; Baudin, E.; Schlumberger, M. & Caillou B. (2002). Differential expression of galectin-3 in medullary thyroid carcinoma and C-cell hyperplasia. *Clinical Endocrinology,* Vol.57, No.6, (December 2002), pp. 813-819, ISSN 1365-2265

Feldt-Rasmussen, U. & Rasmussen, A.K. (1985). Serum thyroglobulin (Tg) in presence of thyroglobulin autoantibodies (TgAb). Clinical and methodological relevance of the interaction between Tg and TgAb in vitro and in vivo. *Journal of Endocrinooglical Investigation,* Vol.8, No.6, (December 1985), pp. 571–576, ISSN 0391-4097

Fernandes, B.; Sagman, U.; Auger, M.; Demetrio, M. & Dennis, J.W. (1991). Beta 1-6 branched oligosaccharides as a marker of tumor progression in human breast and colon neoplasia. *Cancer Research,* Vol.51, No.2, (January 1991), pp. 718-723, ISSN 0008-5472

Figge, J.; del Rosario, A.D.; Gerasimov, G.; Dedov, I.; Bronstein, M., Troshina, K.; Alexandrova, G.; Kallakury, B.V.; Bui, H.X.; Bratslavsky, G. & Ross, J.S. (1994). Preferential expression of the cell adhesion molecule CD44 in papillary thyroid carcinoma. *Experimental and Molecular Pathology,* Vol.61, No.3, (December 1994), pp. 203-211, ISSN 0014-4800

Fonseca, E.; Castanhas, S. & Sobrinho-Simoes M. (1996). Expression of simple mucin type antigens and Lewis type 1 and type 2 chain antigens in the thyroid gland: an immunohistochemical study of normal thyroid tissues, benign lesions, and malignant tumors. *Endocrine Pathology,* Vol.7, No.4, (Winter 1996), pp. 291-301, ISSN 1046-3976

Fonseca, E.; Castanhas, S. & Sobrinho-Simoes, M. (1997). Carbohydrate antigens as oncofetal antigens in papillary carcinoma of the thyroid gland. *Endocrine Pathology,* Vol.8, No.4, (Winter 1997), pp. 301-303, ISSN 1046-3976

Francis, Z. & Schlumberger, M. (2008). Serum thyroglobulin determination in thyroid cancer patients. *Best Practice & Research Clinical Endocrinology & Metabolism,* Vol.22, No.6, (December 2008), pp. 1039-1046, ISSN 1521-690x

Franco, C.; Martínez, V.; Allamand, J.P.; Medina, F.; Glasinovic, A.; Osorio, M. & Schachter, D. (2009). Molecular markers in thyroid fine-needle aspiration biopsy: a prospective study. *Applied Immunohistochemistry and Molecular Morphology,* Vol.17, No.3, (May 2009), pp. 211-215, ISSN 1533-4058

Fukuda, M.; Levery, S.B. & Hakomori S. (1982). Carbohydrate structure of hamster plasma fibronectin. Evidence for chemical diversity between cellular and plasma fibronectin. *Journal of Biological Chemistry,* Vol.257, No.12, (April 1982), pp. 6856–6860, ISSN 0021-9258

Garner, O.B. & Baum, L.G. (2008). Galectin-glycan lattices regulate cell-surface glycoprotein organization and signalling. *Biochemical Society Transactions,* Vol.36, No.6, (December 2008), pp. 1472-1477, ISSN 0300-5127

Gasbarri, A.; Martegani, M.P.; Del Prete, F.; Lucante, T.; Natali, P.G. & Bartolazzi A. (1999). Galectin-3 and CD44v6 isoforms in the preoperative evaluation of thyroid nodules. *Journal of Clinical Oncology,* Vol.17, No.11, (November 1999), pp. 3494-3502, ISSN 0732-183X

Goodison, S.; Urquidi, V. & Tarin, D. (1999). CD44 cell adhesion molecules. *Molecular Pathology,* Vol.52, No.4, (August 1999), pp. 189-196, ISSN 1472-4154

Granovsky, M.; Fata, J.; Pawling, J.; Muller, W.J.; Khokha, R. & Dennis, J.W. (2000). Suppression of tumor growth and metastasis in Mgat5-deficient mice. *Nature Medicine,* Vol.6, No.3, (March 2000), pp. 306-312, ISSN 1078-8956

Griffith, O.L.; Melck, A.; Jones, S.J. & Wiseman, S,M. (2006). Meta-analysis and meta-review of thyroid cancer gene expression profiling studies identifies important diagnostic biomarkers. *Journal of Clinical Oncology,* Vol.24, No.31, (November 2006), pp. 5043-5051, ISSN 0732-183X

Gu, J.; Daa, T.; Kashima, K.; Yokoyama, S.; Nakayama, I. & Noguchi, S. (1998). Expression of splice variants of CD44 in thyroid neoplasms derived from follicular cells. *Pathology International,* Vol.48, No.3, (March 1998), pp. 184-190, ISSN 1320-5463

Gu, Y.; Mi, W.; Ge Y.; Liu, H.; Fan, Q.; Yang, J.& Han, F. (2010). GlcNAcylation plays an essentials role in breast cancer metastasis. *Cancer Research,* Vol.70, No.15 (August 2010), pp. 6344- 6351, ISSN 0008-5472

Guarino, V.; Faviana, P.; Salvatore, G.; Castellone, M.D.; Cirafici, A.M.; De Falco, V.; Celetti, A.; Giannini, R.; Basolo, F.; Melillo, R.M. & Santoro, M. (2005). Osteopontin is overexpressed in human papillary thyroid carcinomas and enhances thyroid carcinoma cell invasiveness. *The Journal of Clinical and Endocrinology & Metabolism,* Vol.90, No.9, (September 2005), pp. 5270-5278, ISSN 0021-972X

Hanover, J.A.; Yu, S.; Lubas, W.B.; Shin, S.H.; Ragano-Caracciola, M.; Kochran, J. & Love, D.C. (2003). Mitochondrial and nucleocytoplasmic isoforms of O-linked GlcNAc transferase encoded by a single mammalian gene. *Archives of Biochemistry and Biophysics,* Vol.409, No.2, (January 2003), pp. 287-297, ISSN 0003-9861

Harduin-Lepers, A.; Vallejo-Ruiz, V.; Krzewinski-Recchi, M.A.; Samyn-Petit, B.; Julien, S. & Delannoy, P. (2001). The human sialyltransferase family. *Biochimie,* Vol.83, No.8, (August 2001), pp. 727-737, ISSN 0300-9084

Hart, G.W.& Akimoto, Y. (2009) The O-GlcNAc Modification. In: *Essentials of Glycobiology,* Varki, A.; Cummings, R.D.; Esko, J.D.; Freeze, H.H.; Stanley, P., Bertozzi, C.R.; Hart, G.W. & Etzler, M.E.,: Cold Spring Harbor Laboratory Press; 2009, ISBN-13: 9780879697709, Cold Spring Harbor (NY)

Hart, G.W.; Housley, M.P. & Slawson, C. (2007). Cycling of O-linked β-N-acetylglucosamine on nucleocytoplasmic proteins. *Nature,* Vol.446, No.7139, (April 2007), pp. 1017-1022, ISSN 0028-0836

Haudek, K.C.; Spronk, K.J.; Voss, P.G.; Patterson, R.J.; Wang, J.L. & Arnoys, E.J. (2010). Dynamics of galectin-3 in the nucleus and cytoplasm. *Biochimica et Biophysica Acta,* Vol.1800, No.2, (February 2010), pp. 181-189, ISSN 0304-4165

Havre, P.A.; Abe, M.; Urasaki, Y.; Ohnuma, K.; Morimoto, C. & Dang, N.H. (2008). The role of CD26/dipeptidyl peptidase IV in cancer. *Frontiers in Bioscience,* Vol.13, (January 2008), pp. 1634-1645, ISSN 1093-9946.

Hawthorn, L.; Stein, L.; Varma, R.; Wiseman, S.; Loree, T. & Tan, D. (2004). TIMP1 and SERPIN-A overexpression and TFF3 and CRABP1 underexpression as biomarkers for papillary thyroid carcinoma. *Head & Neck,* Vol.26, No.12, (December 2004), pp. 1069-1083, ISSN 1097-0347

Heckel, D.; Comtesse, N.; Brass, N.; Blin, N.; Zang, K.D. & Meese, E. (1998). Novel immunogenic antigen homologous to hyaluronidase in meningioma. *Human Molecular Genetics,* Vol.7, No.12, (November 1998), pp. 859-1872, ISSN 0964-6906

Hesse, E.; Musholt, P.B.; Potter, E.; Petrich, T.; Wehmeier, M.; von Wasielewski, R.; Lichtinghagen, R. & Musholt, T.J. (2005) Oncofoetal fibronectin–a tumour-specific marker in detecting minimal residual disease in differentiated thyroid carcinoma.

The British Journal of Cancer, Vol.93, No.5, (September 2005), pp. 565-570. ISSN 0007-0920

Hirai, K.; Kotani, T.; Aratake, Y.; Ohtaki, S. & Kuma, K. (1999). Dipeptidyl peptidase IV (DPP IV/CD26) staining predicts distant metastasis of 'benign' thyroid tumor. *Pathology International*, Vol.49, No.3, (March 1999), pp. 264-275, ISSN 1320-5463

Hu, P.; Shimoji, S. & Hart, G.W. (2010). Site-specific interplay between O-GlcNAcylation and phosphorylation in cellular regulation. *FEBS Letters*, Vol.584, No.12, (June 2010), pp. 2526-2538, ISSN 0014-5793

Huang, Y.; Prasad, M.; Lemon, W.J.; Hampel, H.; Wright, F.A.; Kornacker, K.; LiVolsi, V.; Frankel, W.; Kloos, R.T.; Eng, C.; Pellegata, N.S. & de la Chapelle, A. (2001). Gene expression in papillary thyroid carcinoma reveals highly consistent profiles. *Proceedings of the National Academy of Science of the United States of America*, Vol. 98, No.26 (December 2001), pp. 15044–15049, ISSN 1091-6490

Hughes, R.C. (2001). Galectins as modulators of cell adhesion. *Biochimie*, Vol.83, No.7, (July 2001), pp. 667-676, ISSN 0300-9084

Ino, Y.; Gotoh, M.; Sakamoto, M.; Tsukagoshi, K. & Hirohashi, S. (2002). Dysadherin, a cancer-associated cell membrane glycoprotein, down-regulates E-caherin and promotes metastasis. *Proceedings of the National Academy of Science of the United States of America*, Vol.99, No.1, (January 2002), pp. 365-370, ISSN 1091-6490

Inohara, H.; Honjo, Y.; Yoshii, T.; Akahani, S.; Yoshida, J.; Hattori, K.; Okamoto, S.; Sawada, T.; Raz, A. & Kubo, T. (1999) Expression of galectin-3 in fine-needle aspirates as a diagnostic marker differentiating benign from malignant thyroid neoplasms. *Cancer*, Vol.85, No.11, (June 1999), pp. 2475-2484, ISSN 1528-9117

Inohara, H.; Segawa, T.; Miyauchi, A.; Yoshii, T.; Nakahara, S.; Raz, A.; Maeda, M.; Miyoshi, E.; Kinoshita, N.; Yoshida, H.; Furukawa, M.; Takenaka, Y.; Takamura, Y.; Ito, Y. & Taniguchi N. (2008). Cytoplasmic and serum galectin-3 in diagnosis of thyroid malignancies. *Biochemical and Biophysical Research Communications*, Vol.376, No.3, (November 2008), pp. 605-610, ISSN 0006-291X

Ito, N.; Yokota, M.; Kawahara, S.; Nagaike, C,; Morimura, Y.; Hirota, T. & Matsunaga, T. (1995). Histochemical demonstration of different types of poly-N-acetyllactosamine structures in human thyroid neoplasms using lectins and endo-beta-galactosidase digestion. *The Histochemical Journal*, Vol.27, No.8, (August 1995), pp. 620-629, ISSN 0018-2214

Ito, N.; Yokota, M.; Nagaike, C.; Morimura, Y.; Hatake, K. & Matsunaga, T. (1996). Histochemical demonstration and analysis of poly-N-acetyllactosamine structures in normal and malignant human tissues. *Histology and Histopathology*, Vol.11, No.1, (January 1996), pp. 203-214, ISSN 0213-3911

Ito, Y.; Akinaga, A.; Yamanaka, K.; Nakagawa, T.; Kondo, A.; Dickson, R.B.; Lin, C.Y.; Miyauchi, A.; Taniguchi, N. & Miyoshi, E. (2006). Co-expression of matriptase and N-acetylglucosaminyltransferase V in thyroid cancer tissues-its possible role in prolonged stability in vivo by aberrant glycosylation. *Glycobiology*, Vol.16, No.5, (May 2006), pp.368-374, ISSN 0959-6658

Ito, Y.; Miyauchi, A.; Yoshida, H.; Uruno, T.; Nakano, K.; Takamura, Y.; Miya, A.; Kobayashi, K.; Yokozawa, T.; Matsuzuka, F.; Taniguchi, N.; Matsuura, N.; Kuma, K.; & Miyoshi, E. (2003). Expression of alpha1,6-fucosyltransferase (FUT8) in papillary carcinoma of the thyroid: its linkage to biological aggressiveness and anaplastic transformation. *Cancer Letters*, Vol.200, No.2, (October 2003), pp. 167-172, ISSN 0304-3835

Ito, Y.; Yoshida, H.; Tomoda, C.; Miya, A.; Kobayashi, K.; Matsuzuka, F.; Yasuoka, H.; Kakudo, K.; Inohara, H.; Kuma, K. & Miyauchi, A. (2005). Galectin-3 expression in follicular tumours: an immunohistochemical study of its use as a marker of follicular carcinoma. *Pathology*, Vol.37, No.4, (August 2005), pp. 296-298, ISSN 0031-3025

Iyer, S.P. & Hart, G.W. (2003). Roles of the tetratricopeptide repeat domain in O-GlcNAc transferase targeting and protein substrate specificity. *The Journal of Biological Chemistry*, Vol.278, No.27, (July 2003), pp. 24608-24616, ISSN 0021-9258

Jensen, M. & Berthold, F. (2007). Targeting the neural cell adhesion molecule in cancer. *Cancer Letters*, Vol.258, No.1, (December 2007), pp. 9-21, ISSN 0304-3835

Kamemura, K.; Hayes, B.K.; Comer, F.I. & Hart, G.W. (2002). Dynamic interplay between O-glycosylation and O-phosphorylation of nucleocytoplasmic proteins: alternative glycosylation/phosphorylation of Thr58, a known mutational hot spot of c-myc in lymphomas, is regulated by mitogens. *The Journal of Biological Chemistry*, Vol.277, No.21, (May 2002), pp. 19229-19235, ISSN 0021-9258

Kamoshida, S.; Ogane, N.; Yasuda, M.; Muramatsu, T.; Bessho, T.; Kajiwara, H. & Osamura, R.Y. (2000). Immunohistochemical study of type-1 blood antigen expressions in thyroid tumors: the significance for papillary carcinomas. *Modern Pathology*, Vol.13, No.7, (July 2000), pp. 736-741, ISSN 0893-3952

Kanai, T.; Amakawa, M.; Kato, R.; Shimizu, K.; Nakamura, K.; Ito, K.; Hama, Y.; Fujimori, M. & Amano, J. (2009). Evaluation of a new method for the diagnosis of alterations of Lens culinaris agglutinin binding of thyroglobulin molecules in thyroid carcinoma. *Clinical Chemistry and Laboratory Medicine*, Vol.47, No.10, (October 2009), pp. 1285-1290, ISSN 1434-6621

Kapran, Y.; Ozbey, N.; Molvalilar, S.; Sncer, E.; Dizdaroglu, F. & Ozarmagan, S. (2002). Immunohistochemical detection of E-cadherin, alpha- and beta-catenins in papillary thyroid carcinoma. *Journal of Endocrinological Investigation*, Vol.25, No.7, (July-August 2002), pp. 578–585, ISSN 0391-4097

Kato, N.; Tsuchiya, T.; Tamura, G. & Motoyama, T. (2002). E-cadherin expression in follicular carcinoma of the thyroid. *Pathology International*, Vol.52, No.1, (January 2002), pp. 13-18, ISSN 1320-5463

Kawachi, K.; Matsushita, Y.; Yonezawa, S.; Nakano, S.; Shirao, K.; Natsugoe, S.; Sueyoshi, K.; Aikou, T. & Sato, E. (2000). Galectin-3 expression in various thyroid neoplasms and its possible role in metastasis formation. *Human Pathology*, Vol.31, No.4, (April 2000), pp. 428-433, ISSN 0046-8177

Kebebew, E.; Peng, M.; Reiff, E. & McMillan, A. (2006). Diagnostic and extent of disease multigene assay for malignant thyroid neoplasms. *Cancer*, Vol.106, No.12, (June 2006), pp. 2592-2597, ISSN 0008-543X

Kholová, I.; Ludvíková, M.; Ryska, A.; Hanzelková, Z.; Cap, J.; Pecen, L. & Topolcan, O. (2003). Immunohistochemical detection of dipeptidyl peptidase IV (CD 26) in thyroid neoplasia using biotinylated tyramine amplification. *Neoplasma*, Vol.50, No.3, (2003), pp. 159-164, ISSN 0028-2685

Kiljański, J.; Ambroziak, M.; Pachucki, J.; Jazdzewski, K.; Wiechno, W.; Stachlewska, E.; Górnicka, B.; Bogdańska, M.; Nauman, J. & Bartoszewicz, Z. (2005). Thyroid sialyltransferase mRNA level and activity are increased in Graves' disease. *Thyroid*, Vol.15, No.7, (July 2005), pp. 645-652, ISSN 1050-7256

Kim, J.Y.; Cho, H.; Rhee, B.D. & Kim, H.Y. (2002). Expression of CD44 and cyclin D1 in fine needle aspiration cytology of papillary thyroid carcinoma. *Acta Cytologica*, Vol.46, No.4, (July-August 2002), pp. 679-683, ISSN 0001-5547

Komorowski, J.; Pasieka, Z.; Jankiewicz-Wika, J. & Stepien, H. (2002). Matrix metalloproteinases, tissue inhibitors of matrix metalloproteinases and angiogenic cytokines in peripheral blood of patients with thyroid cancer. *Thyroid*, Vol.12, No.8, (August 2002), pp. 655-662, ISSN 1050-7256

Kotacková, L.; Baláziová, E. & Sedo, A. (2009). Expression pattern of dipeptidyl peptidase IV activity and/or structure homologues in cancer. *Folia Biologica (Praha)*, Vol. 55, No.3, (2009), pp. 77-84, ISSN 0015-5500.

Kotani, T.; Asada, Y.; Aratake, Y.; Umeki, K.; Yamamoto, I.; Tokudome, R.; Hirai, K.; Kuma, K.; Konoe, K.; Araki, Y. & Ohtaki S. (1992). Diagnostic usefulness of dipeptidyl aminopeptidase IV monoclonal antibody in paraffin-embedded thyroid follicular tumours. *The Journal of Pathology*, Vol.168, No.1, (September 1992), pp. 41-45, ISSN 0022-3417

Krześlak, A.; Gaj, Z.; Pomorski, L. & Lipinska, A. (2007). Sialylation of intracellular proteins of thyroid lesions. *Oncology Reports*, Vol.17, No.5, (May 2007), pp. 1237-1242, ISSN 1021-335X

Krześlak, A.; Forma, E.; Bernaciak, M.; Romanowicz, H. & Bryś, M. (2011a). Gene expression of O-GlcNAc cycling enzymes in human breast cancers. *Clinical and Experimental Medicine*, (May 2011), DOI 10.1007/s10238-011-0138-5, ISSN 1591-8890

Krześlak, A.; Jóźwiak, P.; & Lipinska, A. (2011b). Down-regulation of β-N-acetyl-D-glucosaminidase increases Akt1 activity in thyroid anaplastic cancer cells. *Oncology Reports*, (May 2011), DOI: 10.3892/or.2011.1333, 1021-335X Vol.26, No.3,(September 2011), pp. 743-749

Krześlak, A. & Lipińska, A. (2004). Galectin-3 as a multifunctional protein. *Cellular & Molecular Biology Letters*, Vol.9, No.2, (2004), pp. 305-328, ISSN 1425-8153

Krześlak, A.; Pomorski, L.; Gaj, Z. & Lipińska, A. (2003). Differences in glycosylation of intracellular proteins between benign and malignant thyroid neoplasms. *Cancer Letters*, Vol.196, No.1, (June 2003), pp. 101-107, ISSN 0304-3835

Krześlak, A.; Pomorski, L. & Lipinska A. (2010). Elevation of nucleocytoplasmic beta-N-acetylglucosaminidase (O-GlcNAcase) activity in thyroid cancers. *International Journal of Molecular Medicine*, Vol.25, No.4, (April 2010), pp. 643-648, ISSN 1107-3756

Kufe, D.W. (2009). Mucins in cancer: function, prognosis and therapy. *Nature reviews. Cancer*, Vol.9, No.12, (December 2009), pp. 874-885, ISSN 1474-175X

Lambert, E.; Dassé, E.; Haye, B. & Petitfrère, E. (2004). TIMPs as multifacial proteins. *Critical Reviews in Oncology/Hematology*, Vol.49, No.3, (March 2004), pp. 187-198, ISSN 1040-8428

Lazarus, B.D.; Love, D.C. & Hanover, J.A. (2006). Recombinant O-GlcNAc transferase isoforms: identification of O-GlcNAcase, yes tyrosine kinase, and tau as isoform-specific substrates. *Glycobiology*, Vol.16, No.5, (May 2006), pp. 415-421, ISSN 0959-6658

Lin, J.D. (2008). Thyroglobulin and human thyroid cancer. *Clinica Chimica Acta*, Vol.388, No.1-2, (February 2008), pp. 15-21, ISSN 0009-8981

Liu, Y.Y.; Morreau, H.; Kievit, J.; Romijn, J.A.; Carrasco, N. & Smit, J.W. (2008). Combined immunostaining with galectin-3, fibronectin-1, CITED-1, Hector Battifora mesothelial-1, cytokeratin-19, peroxisome proliferator-activated receptor-{gamma}, and sodium/iodide symporter antibodies for the differential diagnosis of nonmedullary thyroid carcinoma. *European Journal of Endocrinology*, Vol.158, No.3, (March 2008), pp. 375-384, ISSN 0804-4643

Love, D.C.; Kochan, J.; Cathey, R.L.; Shin, S.H. & Hanover, J.A. (2003). Mitochondrial and nucleocytoplasmic targeting of O-linked GlcNAc transferase. *Journal of Cell Science*, Vol.116, No.4, (February 2003), pp. 647-654, ISSN 0021-9533

Lubas, W.A. & Hanover, J.A. (2000). Functional expression of O-linked GlcNAc transferase. Domain structure and substrate specificity. *The Journal of Biological Chemistry*. Vol.275, No.15, (April 2000), pp. 10983-10988, ISSN 0021-9258

Ma, B.; Simala-Grant, J.L. & Taylor, D.E. (2006). Fucosylation in prokaryotes and eukaryotes. *Glycobiology*, Vol.16, No.12, (December 2006), pp. 158R-184R, ISSN 0959-6658

Maeta, H.; Ohgi, S. & Terada, T. (2001). Protein expression of matrix metalloproteinases 2 and 9 and tissue inhibitors of metalloproteinase 1 and 2 in papillary thyroid carcinomas. *Virchows Archiv: An International Journal of Pathology*, Vol.438, No.2, (February 2001), pp. 121-128, ISSN 0945-6317

Magro, G.; Schiappacassi, M.; Perissinotto, D.; Corsaro, A.; Borghese, C.; Belfiore, A.; Colombatti, A.; Grasso, S.; Botti, C.; Bombardieri, E. & Perris, R. (2003). Differential expression of mucins 1-6 in papillary thyroid carcinoma: evidence for transformation-dependent post-translational modifications of MUC1 *in situ*. *The Journal of Pathology*, Vol.200, No.3, (July 2003), pp. 357-369, ISSN 0022-3417

Mariotti, S.; Barbesino, G.; Caturegli, P.; Marino, M.; Manetti, L.; Pacini, F.; Centoni, R. & Pinchera, A. (1995). Assay of thyroglobulin in serum with thyroglobulin autoantibodies: an unobtainable goal? *The Journal of Clinical Endocrinology and Metabolism*, Vol.80, No.2, (February 1995), pp. 468-472, ISSN 0021-972X

Maruta, J.; Hashimoto, H.; Yamashita, H.; Yamashita, H. & Noguchi, S. (2004). Immunostaining of galectin-3 and CD44v6 using fine-needle aspiration for distinguishing follicular carcinoma from adenoma. *Diagnostic Cytopathology*, Vol.31, No.6, (December 2004), pp. 392-396, ISSN 1097-0339

Maruyama, M.; Kato, R.; Kobayashi, S. & Kasuga, Y.A. (1998). Method to differentiate between thyroglobulin derived from normal thyroid tissue and from thyroid carcinoma based on analysis of reactivity to lectins. *Archives of Pathology & Laboratory Medicine*, Vol.122, No.8, (August 1998), pp. 715-720, ISSN 0003-9985

Matesa, N.; Samija, I. & Kusić, Z. (2007). Galectin-3 and CD44v6 positivity by RT-PCR method in fine needle aspirates of benign thyroid lesions. *Cytopathology*, Vol.18, No.2, (April 2007), pp. 112-116, ISSN 0956-5507

Matsuura, H.; Takio, K.; Titani, K.; Greene, T.; Levery, S.B.; Salyan, M.E. & Hakomori, S. (1988). The oncofetal structure of human fibronectin defined by monoclonal antibody FDC-6. Unique structural requirement for the antigenic specificity provided by a glycosylhexapeptide. *The Journal of Biological Chemistry*, Vol.263, No.7, (March 1988), pp. 3314-3322, ISSN 0021-9258

Mehrotra, P.; Okpokam, A.; Bouhaidar, R.; Johnson, S.J.; Wilson, J.A.; Davies, B.R. & Lennard, T.W. (2004). Galectin-3 does not reliably distinguish benign from malignant thyroid neoplasms. *Histopathology*, Vol.45, No.5, (November 2004), pp. 493-500, ISSN 0309-0167

Mi, W.; Gu, Y.; Han, C.; Liu, H.; Fan, Q.; Zhang, X.; Cong, Q. & Yu, W. (2011). O-GlcNacylation is a novel regulator of lung and colon cancer malignancy. *Biochimica et Biophysica Acta*, Vol.1812, No.4, (April 2011), pp. 514-519, ISSN 0006-3002

Miettinen, M. & Kärkkäinen, P. (1996). Differential reactivity of HBME-1 and CD15 antibodies in benign and malignant thyroid tumours. Preferential reactivity with malignant tumours. *Virchows Archiv: An International Journal of Pathology*, Vol.429, No.4-5, (November 1996), pp. 213-219, ISSN 0945-6317

Mills, L.J.; Poller, D.N. & Yiangou, C. (2005). Galectin-3 is not useful in thyroid FNA. *Cytopathology*, Vol.16, No.3, (June 2005), pp. 132-138, ISSN 0956-5507

Miyoshi, E.; Ito, Y. & Miyoshi, Y. (2010). Involvement of aberrant glycosylation in thyroid cancer. *Journal of Oncology*, Vol. 2010, (June 2010), DOI: 10.1155/2010/816595, ISSN 1687-8450

Miyoshi, E.; Moriwaki, K. & Nakagawa T. (2008). Biological function of fucosylation in cancer biology. *Journal of Biochemistry*, Vol.143, No.6, (June 2008), pp. 725-729, ISSN 0021-924X

Mlynek, M.L.; Richter, H.J. & Leder, L.D. (1985). Mucin in carcinomas of the thyroid. *Cancer*, Vol.56, No.1, (December 1985), pp. 2647-2650, ISSN 0008-543X

Morari, E.C.; Silva, J.R.; Guilhen, A.C.; Cunha, L.L.; Marcello, M.A.; Soares, F.A.; Vassallo, J. & Ward, L.S. (2010). Muc-1 expression may help characterize thyroid nodules but does not predict patients' outcome. *Endocrine Pathology*, Vol.21, No.4, (December 2010), pp. 242-249, ISSN 1046-3976

Naito, A.; Iwase, H.; Kuzushima, T.; Nakamura, T. & Kobayashi, S. (2001). Clinical significance of e-cadherin expression in thyroid neoplasms. *Journal of Surgical Oncology*, Vol.76, No.3, (March 2001), pp. 176-180, ISSN 0022-4790

Nam, K.H.; Noh, T.W.; Chung, S.H.; Lee, S.H.; Lee, M.K.; Won Hong, S.; Chung, W.Y.; Lee, E.J. & Park, C.S. (2011). Expression of the membrane mucins Muc4 and Muc15, potential markers of malignancy and prognosis, in papillary thyroid carcinoma. *Thyroid*, Vol.21, No.7, (May 2011), DOI: 10.1089/thy.2010.0339, ISSN 1050-7256

Nasir, A.; Catalano, E.; Calafati, S.; Cantor, A.; Kaiser, H.E. & Coppola, D. (2004). Role of p53, CD44V6 and CD57 in differentiating between benign and malignant follicular neoplasms of the thyroid. *In Vivo (Athens, Greece)*, Vol.18, No.2, (March-April 2004), pp. 189-195, ISSN 0258-851X

Nasr, M.R.; Mukhopadhyay, S.; Zhang, S. & Katzenstein, A.L. (2006). Immunohistochemical markers in diagnosis of papillary thyroid carcinoma: Utility of HBME1 combined with CK19 immunostaining. *Modern Pathology*. Vol.19, No.12, (December 2006), pp. 1631-1637, ISSN 0893-3952

Niedziela, M.; Maceluch, J. & Korman, E. (2002). Galectin-3 is not an universal marker of malignancy in thyroid nodular disease in children and adolescents. *The Journal of Clinical Endocrinology and Metabolism*, Vol.87, No.9, (September 2002) pp. 4411-4415, ISSN 0021-972X

Nikiel, B.; Chekan, M.; Jaworska, M.; Jarzab, M.; Maksymiuk, B. & Lange, D. (2006). Expression of the selected adhesive molecules (cadherin E, CD44, LGAL3 and CA50) in papillary thyroid carcinoma. *Polish Journal of Endocrinology*, Vol.57, No.4, (July-August 2006), pp.326-335, ISSN 0423-104X

Nozawa, Y.; Ami, H.; Suzuki, S.; Tuchiya, A.; Abe, R. & Abe, M. (1999). Distribution of sialic acid-dependent carbohydrate epitope in thyroid tumors: immunoreactivity of FB21 in paraffin-embedded tissue sections. *Pathology International*, Vol.49, No.5, (May 1999), pp. 403-407, ISSN 1320-5463

Ohashi, Y.; Dogru, M. & Tsubota, K. (2006). Laboratory findings in tear fluid analysis. *Clinica Chimica Acta*, Vol.369, No.1, (July 2006), pp. 17-28, ISSN 0009-8981

Oler, G.; Camacho, C.P.; Hojaij, F.C.; Michaluart, P. Jr; Riggins, G.J. & Cerutti, J.M. (2008). Gene expression profiling of papillary thyroid carcinoma identifies transcripts correlated with BRAF mutational status and lymph node metastasis. *Clinical Cancer Research*, Vol.14, No.15, (August 2008), pp. 4735-4742, ISSN 1557-3265

Orlandi, F.; Saggiorato, E.; Pivano, G.; Puligheddu, B.; Termine, A.; Cappia, S.; De Giuli, P. & Angeli, A. (1998). Galectin-3 is a presurgical marker of human thyroid carcinoma. *Cancer Research*. Vol.58, No.14, (July 1998), pp. 3015-3020, ISSN 0008-5472

Ozolins, A.; Narbuts, Z.; Strumfa, I.; Volanska, G. & Gardovskis, J. (2010). Diagnostic utility of immunohistochemical panel in various thyroid pathologies. *Langenbeck's Archives of Surgery*, Vol.395, No.7, (September 2010), pp.885-891, ISSN 1435-2443

Ożóg, J.; Jarząb, M.; Pawlaczek, A.; Oczko-Wojciechowska, M.; Włoch, J.; Roskosz, J. & Gubała, E. (2006). Expression of DPP4 gene in papillary thyroid carcinoma. *Polish Journal of Endocrinology*. Vol.57, Suppl. A, (2006), pp. 12-17, ISSN 0423-104X.

Pankov, R.; & Yamada, K.M. (2002). Fibronectin at a glance. *Journal of Cell Science*, Vol.115, No.Pt20, (October 2002) pp. 3861-3863, ISSN 0021-9533

Papotti, M.; Rodriguez, J.; De Pompa, R.; Bartolazzi, A. & Rosai, J. (2005). Galectin-3 and HBME-1 expression in well-differentiated thyroid tumors with follicular architecture of uncertain malignant potential. *Modern Pathology*, Vol.18, No.4, (April 2005), pp. 541-546, ISSN 0893-3952

Patel, K.N.; Maghami, E.; Wreesmann, V.B.; Shaha, A.R.; Shah, J.P.; Ghossein, R. & Singh B. (2005). Muc1 plays a role in tumor maintenance in aggressive thyroid carcinomas. *Surgery*, Vol.138, No.6, (December 2005), pp. 994-1001, ISSN 0039-6060

Pisani, T.; Vecchione, A. & Giovagnolii, M.R. (2004). Galectin-3 immunodetection may improve cytological diagnosis of occult papillary thyroid carcinoma. *Anticancer Research*, Vol.24, No.2C, (March-April 2004), pp. 1111-1112, ISSN 0250-7005

Ponta, H.; Sherman, L. & Herrlich, P.A. (2003). CD44: from adhesion molecules to signalling regulators. *Nature Reviews. Molecular Cell Biology*, Vol.4, No.1, (January 2003), pp.33-45, ISSN 1471-0072

Prasad, M.L.; Pellegata, N.S.; Huang, Y.; Nagaraja, H.N.; de la Chapelle, A. & Kloos, R.T. (2005). Galectin-3, fibronectin-1, CITED-1, HBME1 and cytokeratin-19 immunohistochemistry is useful for the differential diagnosis of thyroid tumors. *Modern Pathology*, Vol.18, No.1, (January 2005), pp. 48-57, ISSN 0893-3952

Pro, B. & Dang, N.H. (2004). CD26/dipeptidyl peptidase IV and its role in cancer. *Histology and Histopathology*, Vol.19, No.4, (October 2004), pp. 1345-1351, ISSN 0213-3911

Rangaswami, H.; Bulbule, A. & Kundu, G.C. (2006). Osteopontin: role in cell signaling and cancer progression. *Trends in Cell Biology*, Vol.16, No.2, (February 2006), pp. 79-87, ISSN 0962-8924

Ringel, M.D. & Ladenson, P.W. (2004). Controversies in the follow-up and management of well-differentiated thyroid cancer. *Endocrine Related Cancer*, Vol.11, No.1, (March 2004), pp. 97-116, ISSN 1351-0088

Ringel, M.D.; Balducci-Silano, P.L.; Anderson, J.S.; Spencer, C.A.; Silverman, J.; Sparling, Y.H.; Francis, G.L.; Burman, K.D.; Wartofsky, L.; Ladenson, P.W.; Levine, M.A, & Tuttle, R.M. (1999). Quantitative reverse transcription– polymerase chain reaction of circulating thyroglobulin messenger ribonucleic acid for monitoring patients with thyroid carcinoma. *The Journal of Clinical Endocrinology and Metabolism*, Vol.84, No.11, (November 1999), pp. 4037-4042, ISSN 0021-972X

Ringel, M.D.; Ladenson, P.W. & Levine, M.A. (1998). Molecular diagnosis of residual and recurrent thyroid cancer by amplification of thyroglobulin messenger ribonucleic acid in peripheral blood. *The Journal of Clinical Endocrinology and Metabolism*, Vol.83, No.12, (December 1998), pp. 4435-4442, ISSN 0021-972X

Rocha, A.S.; Soares, P.; Fonseca, E.; Cameselle-Teijeiro, J.; Oliveira, M.C. & Sobrinho-Simões, M. (2003). E-cadherin loss rather than beta-catenin alterations is a common feature of poorly differentiated thyroid carcinomas. *Histopathology*, Vol.42, No.6, (June 2003), pp. 580-587, ISSN 0309-0167

Rorive, S.; Eddafali, B.; Fernandez, S.; Decaestecker, C.; André, S.; Kaltner, H.; Kuwabara, I.; Liu, F.T.; Gabius, H.J.; Kiss, R. & Salmon, I. (2002). Changes in galectin-7 and cytokeratin-19 expression during the progression of malignancy in thyroid tumors: diagnostic and biological implications. *Modern Pathology*, Vol.15, No.12, (December 2002), pp. 1294-1301, ISSN 0893-3952

Saggiorato, E.; Aversa, S.; Deandreis, D.; Arecco, F.; Mussa, A.; Puligheddu, B.; Cappia, S.; Conticello, S.; Papotti, M. & Orlandi, F. (2004). Galectin-3: presurgical marker of thyroid follicular epithelial cell-derived carcinomas. *Journal of Endocrinological Investigation*, Vol.27, No.4, (April 2004), pp. 311-317, ISSN 0391-4097

Saggiorato, E.; Cappia, S.; De Giuli, P.; Mussa, A.; Pancani, G.; Caraci, P.; Angeli, A. & Orlandi, F. (2001). Galectin-3 as a presurgical immunocytodiagnostic marker of minimally invasive follicular thyroid carcinoma. *The Journal of Clinical Endocrinology and Metabolism*, Vol.86, No.11, (November 2001), pp. 5152-5158, ISSN 0021-972X

Sanabria, A.; Carvalho, A.L.; Piana de Andrade, V.; Pablo Rodrigo, J.; Vartanian, J.G.; Rinaldo, A.; Ikeda, M.K.; Devaney, K.O.; Magrin, J.; Augusto Soares, F.; Ferlito, A. & Kowalski, L.P. (2007). Is galectin-3 a good method for the detection of malignancy in patients with thyroid nodules and a cytologic diagnosis of "follicular neoplasm"? A critical appraisal of the evidence. *Head & Neck*, Vol.29, No.11, (November 2007), pp. 1046-1054, ISSN 1043-3074

Sato, H.; Ino, Y.; Miura, A.; Abe, Y.; Sakai, H.; Ito, K. & Hirohashi, S. (2003). Dysadherin: expression and clinical significance in thyroid carcinoma. *The Journal of Clinical Endocrinology and Metabolism*, Vol.88, No.9, (September 2003), pp. 4407-4412, ISSN 0021-972X

Satoh, F.; Umemura, S.; Yasuda, M. & Osamura, R.Y. (2001). Neuroendocrine marker expression in thyroid epithelial tumors. *Endocrine Pathology*, Vol.12, No.3, (Fall 2001), pp. 291-299, ISSN 1046-3976

Saussez, S.; Glinoer, D.; Chantrain, G.; Pattou, F.; Carnaille, B.; André, S.; Gabius, H.J. & Laurent, G. (2008). Serum galectin-1 and galectin-3 levels in benign and malignant nodular thyroid disease. *Thyroid*, Vol.18, No.7, (July 2008), pp. 705-712, ISSN 1050-7256

Savagner, F.; Rodien, P.; Reynier, P.; Rohmer, V.; Bigorgne, J.C. & Malthiery, Y. (2002). Analysis of Tg transcripts by real-time RT–PCR in the blood of thyroid cancer patients. *The Journal of Clinical Endocrinology and Metabolism*, Vol.87, No.2, (February 2002), pp. 635-639, ISSN 0021-972X

Scarpino, S.; Di Napoli, A.; Melotti, F.; Talerico, C.; Cancrini, A. & Ruco, L. (2007). Papillary carcinoma of the thyroid: low expression of NCAM (CD56) is associated with downregulation of VEGF-D production by tumour cells. *The Journal of Pathology*, Vol.212, No.4, (August 2007), pp. 411-419, ISSN 0022-3417

Scheumman, G.F.; Hoang-Vu, C.; Cetin, Y.; Gimm, O.; Behrends, J.; von Wasielewski, R.; Georgii, A.; Birchmeier, W.; von Zur Mühlen, A. & Dralle, H. (1995). Clinical significance of E-cadherin as a prognostic marker in thyroid carcinomas. *The Journal of Clinical Endocrinology and Metabolism*, Vol.80, No.7, (July 1995), pp. 2168-2172, ISSN 0021-972X

Seelentag, W.K.; Li, W.P.; Schmitz, S.F.; Metzger, U.; Aeberhard, P.; Heitz, P.U. & Roth, J. (1998). Prognostic value of beta1,6-branched oligosaccharides in human colorectal carcinoma. *Cancer Research*, Vol.58, No.23, (December 1998), pp. 5559-5564, ISSN 0008-5472

Serini, G.; Trusolino, L.; Saggiorato, E.; Cremona, O.; De Rossi, M.; Angeli, A.; Orlandi, F. & Marchisio, P.C. (1996). Changes in integrin and Ecadherin expression in neoplastic versus normal thyroid tissue. *Journal of the National Cancer Institute*, Vol.88, No.7, (April 1996), pp. 442-449, ISSN 0027-8874

Shafi, R.; Iyer, S.P.; Ellies, L.G.; O'Donnell, N.; Marek, K.W.; Chui, D.; Hart, G.W. & Marth, J.D. (2000). The O-GlcNAc transferase gene resides on the X chromosome and is essential for embryonic stem cell viability and mouse ontogeny. *Proceedings of the National Academy of Science of the United States of America*, Vol.97, No.11, (May 2000), pp. 5735-5739, ISSN 1091-6490

Shapiro, L. & Weis, W.I. (2009). Structure and biochemistry of cadherins and catenins. *Cold Spring Harbor Perspectives in Biology*, Vol.1, No.3, (September 2009), DOI: 10.1101/cshperspect.a003053, ISSN 1943-0264

Shi, Y.; Parhar, R.S.; Zou, M.; Hammami, M.M.; Akhtar, M.; Lum, Z.P.; Farid, N.R.; Al-Sedairy, S.T. & Paterson, M.C. (1999). Tissue inhibitor of metalloproteinases-1 (TIMP-1) mRNA is elevated in advanced stages of thyroid carcinoma. *British Journal of Cancer*, Vol.79, No.7-8, (March 1999), pp. 1234-1239, ISSN 0007-0920

Shi, Y.; Tomic, J.; Wen, F.; Shaha, S.; Bahlo, A.; Harrison, R.; Dennis, J.W.; Williams, R.; Gross, B.J.; Walker, S.; Zuccolo, J.; Deans, J.P.; Hart, G.W. & Spaner, D.E. (2010). Aberrant O-GlcNAcylation characterizes chronic lymphatic leukemia. *Leukemia*, Vol.24, No.9, (September 2010), pp. 1588-1598, ISSN 0887-6924

Shimizu, K.; Nakamura, K.; Kobatake, S.; Satomura, S.; Maruyama, M.; Kameko, F.; Tajiri, J. & Kato, R. (2007a). The clinical utility of Lens culinaris agglutinin-reactive thyroglobulin ratio in serum for distinguishing benign from malignant conditions of the thyroid. *Clinica Chimica Acta*, Vol.379, No.1-2, (April 2007), pp. 101-104, ISSN 0009-8981

Shimizu, K.; Nakamura, K.; Kobatake, S.; Satomura, S.; Maruyama, M.; Tajiri, J. & Kato, R. (2007b). Discrimination of thyroglobulin from thyroid carcinoma tissue and that from benign thyroid tissues with use of competitive assay between lectin and anti-thyroglobulin antibody. *Rinsho Byori*, Vol.55, No.5, (May 2007), pp. 428-433, ISSN 0047-1860

Slawson, C.; Zachara, N.E.; Vosseller, K.; Cheung, W.D.; Lane, M.D. & Hart, G.W. (2005). Perturbations in O-linked-beta-N-acetylglucosamine protein modification causes in severe defects in mitotic progression and cytokinesis. *The Journal of Biological Chemistry*, Vol.280, No.28, (September 2005), pp. 32944-32956, ISSN 0021-9258

Span, P.N.; Sleegers, M.J.; Van Den Broek, W.J.; Ross, H.A.; Nieuwlaat, W.A.; Hermus, A.R. & Sweep, C.G. (2003). Quantitative detection of peripheral thyroglobulin mRNA has limited clinical value in the follow-up of thyroid cancer patients. *Annals of Clinical Biochemistry*, Vol.40, No.Pt 1, (January 2003), pp. 94-99, ISSN 0004-5632

Spencer, C.A. (2004). Challenges of Serum Thyroglobulin (Tg) Measurement in the Presence of Tg Autoantibodies. *The Journal of Clinical Endocrinology and Metabolism*, Vol.89, No.8, (August 2004), pp. 3702–3704, ISSN 0021-972X

Stanley, P.; Schachter, H. & Taniguchi, N. N-Glycans. In: *Essentials of Glycobiology*, Varki, A.; Cummings, R.D.; Esko, J.D.; Freeze, H.H.; Stanley, P., Bertozzi, C.R.; Hart, G.W. &

Etzler, M.E.,: Cold Spring Harbor Laboratory Press; 2009, ISBN-13: 9780879697709, Cold Spring Harbor (NY)

Stetler-Stevenson, W.G. (2008). Tissue inhibitors of metalloproteinases in cell signaling: metalloproteinase-independent biological activities. *Science Signaling*, Vol.1, No.27, (July 2008), pp. re6, ISSN 1937-9145

Tajiri, M.; Yoshida, S. & Wada, Y. Differential analysis of site-specific glycans on plasma and cellular fibronectins: application of a hydrophilic affinity method for glycopeptide enrichment. *Glycobiology*, Vol.15, No.12, (December 2005), pp. 1332-1340, ISSN 0959-6658

Takano, T.; Ito, Y.; Matsuzuka, F.; Miya, A.; Kobayashi, K.; Yoshida, H. & Miyauchi, A. (2007). Expression of oncofetal fibronectin mRNA in thyroid anaplastic carcinoma. *Japanese Journal of Clinical Oncology*, Vol.37, No.9, (September 2007), pp. 647-651, ISSN 0368-2811

Takano, T.; Miyauchi, A.; Yokozawa, T.; Matsuzuka, F.; Liu, G.; Higashiyama, T.; Morita, S.; Kuma, K. & Amino, N. (1998). Accurate and objective preoperative diagnosis of thyroid papillary carcinomas by reverse transcription-PCR detection of oncofetal fibronectin messenger RNA in fine-needle aspiration biopsies. *Cancer Research*, Vol.58, No.21, (November 1998), pp. 4913-4917, ISSN 0008-5472

Takano, T.; Miyauchi, A.; Yokozawa, T.; Matsuzuka, F.; Maeda, I.; Kuma, K. & Amino, N. (1999). Preoperative diagnosis of thyroid papillary and anaplastic carcinomas by real-time quantitative reverse transcription-polymerase chain reaction of oncofetal fibronectin messenger RNA. *Cancer Research*, Vol.59, No.18, (September 1999), pp. 4542-4545, ISSN 0008-5472

Tanaka, T.; Umeki, K.; Yamamoto, I.; Sakamoto, F.; Noguchi, S. & Ohtaki, S. (1995). CD26 (dipeptidyl peptidase IV/DPP IV) as a novel molecular marker for differentiated thyroid carcinoma. *International Journal of Cancer*, Vol.64, No.5, (October 1995), pp. 326-331, ISSN 0020-7136

Tang, A.C.; Raphael, S.J.; Lampe, H.B.; Matthews, T.W. & Becks, G.P. (1996). Expression of dipeptidyl aminopeptidase IV activity in thyroid tumours: a possible marker of thyroid malignancy. *The Journal of Otolaryngology*, Vol.25, No.1, (February 1996), pp. 14-19, ISSN 0381-6605

Than, T.H.; Swethadri, G.K.; Wong, J.; Ahmad, T.; Jamil, D.; Maganlal, R.K.; Hamdi, M.M. & Abdullah, M.S. (2008). Expression of Galectin-3 and Galectin-7 in thyroid malignancy as potential diagnostic indicators. *Singapore Medical Journal*, Vol.49, No.4, (April 2008), pp. 333-338, ISSN 0037-5675

Toleman, C.; Paterson, A.J.; Whisenhunt, T.R. & Kudlow, J.E. (2004). Characterization of the histone acetyltransferase (HAT) domain of a bifunctional protein with activable O-GlcNAcase and HAT activities. *The Journal of Biological Chemistry*, Vol.279, No.51, (December 2004), pp. 53665-53673, ISSN 0021-9258

Türköz, H.K.; Oksüz, H.; Yurdakul, Z. & Ozcan, D. (2008). Galectin-3 expression in tumor progression and metastasis of papillary thyroid carcinoma. *Endocrine Pathology*, Vol.19, No.2, (Summer 2008), pp. 92-96, ISSN 1046-3976

Umeki, K.; Tanaka, T.; Yamamoto, I.; Aratake, Y.; Kotani, T.; Sakamoto, F.; Noguchi, S. & Ohtaki, S. (1996). Differential expression of dipeptidyl peptidase IV (CD26) and thyroid peroxidase in neoplastic thyroid tissues. *Endocrine Journal*, Vol.43, No.1, (February 1996), pp. 53-60, ISSN 0918-8959

Vali, M.; Rose, N.R. & Caturegli, P. (2000). Thyroglobulin as autoantigen: structure-function relationships. *Reviews in Endocrine & Metabolic Disorders*, Vol.1, No.1-2, (January 2000), pp. 69-77, ISSN 1389-9155

Varki, A.; Kannami, R.& Toole, B.P. (2009) Glycosylation Changes in Cancer. In: *Essentials of Glycobiology*, Varki, A.; Cummings, R.D.; Esko, J.D.; Freeze, H.H.; Stanley, P., Bertozzi, C.R.; Hart, G.W. & Etzler, M.E.,: Cold Spring Harbor Laboratory Press; 2009, ISBN-13: 9780879697709, Cold Spring Harbor (NY)

Verburg, F.A.; Lips, C.J.; Lentjes, E.G. & de Klerk, J.M. (2004). Detection of circulating Tg-mRNA in the follow-up of papillary and follicular thyroid cancer: how useful is it? *British Journal of Cancer*, Vol.91, No.2, (July 2004), pp. 200-204, ISSN 0007-0920

Vierbuchen, M.; Larena, A.; Schröder, S.; Hanisch, F.G.; Ortmann, M.; Larena, A.; Uhlenbruck, G. & Fischer, R. (1992). Blood group antigen expression in medullary carcinoma of the thyroid. An immunohistochemical study on the occurrence of type 1 chain-derived antigens. *Virchows Archiv. B, Cell pathology including molecular pathology*, Vol.62, No.2, (1992), pp. 79-88, ISSN 0340-6075

Volante, M.; Bozzalla-Cassione, F.; Orlandi, F. & Papotti, M. (2004). Diagnostic role of galectin-3 in follicular thyroid tumors. *Virchows Archiv: An International Journal of Pathology*, Vol.444, No.4, (April 2004), pp. 309-312, ISSN 0945-6317

von Wasielewski, R.; Rhein, A.; Werner, M.; Scheumann, G.F.; Dralle, H.; Pötter, E.; Brabant, G. & Georgii, A. (1997). Immunohistochemical detection of E-cadherin in differentiated thyroid carcinomas correlates with clinical outcome. *Cancer Research*, Vol.57, No.12, (June 1997), pp. 2501-2507, ISSN 0008-5472

Wai, P.Y. & Kuo, P.C. (2008). Osteopontin: regulation in tumor metastasis. *Cancer and Metastasis Reviews*, Vol.27, No.1, (March 2008), pp. 103-118, ISSN 0167-7659

Wang, X.; Chao, L.; Zhen, J.; Chen, L.; Ma, G.& Li, X. (2010). Phosphorylated c-Jun NH2-terminal kinase is overexpressed in human papillary thyroid carcinomas and associates with lymph node metastasis. *Cancer Letters*, Vol.293, No.2, (July 2010), pp. 175-180, ISSN 0304-3835

Wasenius, V.M.; Hemmer, S.; Kettunen, E.; Knuutila, S.; Franssila, K. & Joensuu, H. (2003). Hepatocyte growth factor receptor, matrix metalloproteinase-11, tissue inhibitor of metalloproteinase-1, and fibronectin are up-regulated in papillary thyroid carcinoma: a cDNA and tissue microarray study. Cl*inical Cancer Research*, Vol.9, No.1, (January 2003), pp.68-75, ISSN 1078-0432

Weber, K.B.; Shroyer, K.R.; Heinz, D.E.; Nawaz, S.; Said, M.S. & Haugen, B.R. (2004). The use of a combination of galectin-3 and thyroid peroxidase for the diagnosis and prognosis of thyroid cancer. *American Journal of Clinical Pathology*, Vol.122, No.4, (October 2004), pp. 524-531, ISSN 0002-9173

Wehmeier, M.; Petrich, T.; Brand, K.; Lichtinghagen, R. & Hesse, E. (2010). Oncofetal fibronectin mRNA is highly abundant in the blood of patients with papillary thyroid carcinoma and correlates with high-serum thyroid-stimulating hormone levels. *Thyroid*, Vol.20, No.6, (June 2010), pp. 607-613, ISSN 1050-7256

Wei, X, & Li, L. (2009). Comparative glycoproteomics: approaches and applications. *Briefings Functional Genomics & Proteomics*, Vol.8, No.2, (March 2009), pp. 104-113, ISSN 473-9550

Wierzbicka-Patynowski, I. & Schwarzbauer, J.E. (2003). The ins and outs of fibronectin matrix assembly. *Journal of Cell Science*, Vol.116, No.Pt16, (August 2003), pp. 3269-3276, ISSN 0021-9533

Wopereis, S.; Lefeber, D.J.; Morava, E. & Wevers, R.A. (2006). Mechanisms in protein O-glycan biosynthesis and clinical and molecular aspects of protein O-glycan biosynthesis defects: a review. *Clinical Chemistry*, Vol.52, No.4, (April 2006), pp. 574-600, ISSN 0009-9147

Wreesmann, V.B.; Sieczka, E.M.; Socci, N.D.; Hezel, M.; Belbin, T.J.; Childs, G.; Patel, S.G.; Patel, K.N.; Tallini, G.; Prystowsky, M.; Shaha, A.R.; Kraus, D.; Shah, J.P.; Rao, P.H.; Ghossein, R.; & Singh B. (2004). Genome-wide profiling of papillary thyroid cancer identifies Muc1 as an independent prognostic marker. *Cancer research*, Vol.64, No.11, (June 2004), pp. 3780-3789, ISSN 0008-5472

Xu, X.C.; el-Naggar, A.K. & Lotan, R. (1995). Differential expression of galectin-1 and galectin-3 in thyroid tumors. Potential diagnostic implications. *The American Journal of Pathology*, Vol.147, No.3, (September 1995), pp. 815-822, ISSN 0002-9440

Yang, S.X.; Pollock, H.G. & Rawitch, A.B. (1996). Glycosylation in human thyroglobulin: location of the N-linked oligosaccharide units and comparison with bovine thyroglobulin. *Archives of Biochemistry and Biophysics*, Vol.327, No.1, (March 1996), pp. 61-70, ISSN 0003-9861

Yang, W.H.; Kim, J.E.; Nam, H.W.; Ju, J.W.; Kim, H.S.; Kim, Y.S. & Cho, J.W. (2006). Modification of p53 with O-linked n-acetylglucosamine regulates p53 activity and stability. *Nature Cell Biology*, Vol.8, No.10, (October 2006), pp. 1074-1083, ISSN 1465-7392

Zachara, N.E. & Hart, G.W. (2006). Cell signaling, the essential role of O-GlcNAc! *Biochimica et Biophysica Acta*, Vol.1761, No.5-6, (May-June 2006), pp. 599-617, ISSN 0006-3002

Zeidan, Q. & Hart, G.W. (2010). The intersections between O-GlcNAcylation and phosphorylation: implications for multiple signaling pathways. *Journal of Cell Science*, Vol.123, No.Pt1, (January 2010), pp. 13-22; ISSN 0021-9533

Zeromski, J.; Dworacki, G.; Jenek, J.; Niemir, Z.; Jezewska, E.; Jenek, R. & Biczysko, M. (1999). Protein and mRNA expression of CD56/NCAM on follicular epithelial cells of the human thyroid. *International Journal of Immunopathology and Pharmacology*, Vol.12, No.1, (January-April 1999), pp. 23-30, ISSN 0394-6320

Zeromski, J.; Lawniczak, M.; Galbas, K.; Jenek, R. & Golusinnski, P. (1998). Expression of CD56/N-CAM antigen and some other adhesion molecules in various human endocrine glands. *Folia Histochemica et Cytobiologica*, Vol.36, No.3, (1998), pp. 119-125, ISSN 0239-8508

4

Insulin-Like Growth Factor Receptor Signaling in Thyroid Cancers: Clinical Implications and Therapeutic Potential

Geetika Chakravarty* and Debasis Mondal
Tulane University School of Medicine, Department of Pharmacology, New Orleans, LA, USA

1. Introduction

Human Thyroid Tumors represent a multistage model of epithelial tumorigenesis. Even though a majority of these tumors originate from follicular cells, they exhibit a broad spectrum with different phenotypic characteristics and variable clinical behavior. Our recent studies suggest that numerous growth factors and their receptors may be abnormally overexpressed or constitutively activated in thyroid tumors to influence their biological behavior. In this chapter we review our current understanding of the role of Insulin-like growth factors (IGFs) and their receptors in the pathogenesis of thyroid cancer and how expression of pIGF-IR may be an indicator of their clinical behavior [1]. Mechanistic evidence for direct involvement of IGF-I signaling in metastasis of anaplastic thyroid cancer & on tumor associated angiogenesis [2] is also discussed. Finally, as several small molecular inhibitors of IGF-IR signaling (peptide-based antagonists and monoclonal antibodies) are being tested, we will discuss the potential impact of utilizing IGF-I signaling pathway as a therapeutic target [2, 3] for aggressive thyroid cancers especially in cases where the current therapeutics have failed to show a favorable outcome.

Thyroid cancer (TC) is one of the most common endocrine malignancies worldwide. According to recent American Cancer Society (ACS) estimates, its incidence is rising in the US, with an average increase of 6% between 1975 & 2008[4]. Recent data further indicates that its incidence is three times higher in women than in men amongst all ethnic populations. Even though a majority of these tumors originate from follicular cells, they exhibit a broad spectrum with different phenotypic characteristics and variable clinical outcomes. Histopathological evaluation of TC specimens suggests that these tumors can be further sub-classified as differentiated thyroid carcinoma (DTC), undifferentiated (anaplastic) thyroid carcinoma (ATC) and medullary thyroid carcinoma (MTC). DTC and ATC are also referred to as nonmedullary thyroid cancer (NMTC) and may include subtypes like Hurthle cell carcinomas (HCC). Ninety to ninety three percent of all thyroid tumors are of differentiated phenotypes and have a papillary (PTC) or follicular (FTC)

* Corresponding Author

morphology. Usually these tumors follow a protracted clinical course with a 10-year survival rate of 92%. Another 5% are MTCs where the 5-year survival rate is approximately 50%. On the contrary, ATCs arise either de novo or may evolve from follicular or papillary carcinomas. These tumors are rare, occurring in only 1-2% of all TCs, and are invariably associated with fatal outcomes [5]. In the clinic, these patients present themselves with widely invasive local disease and are surgically incurable. The survival rate for ATCs which frequently metastasize to distant sites, is <10%. Severity of ATC is further underscored by the fact that even when these patients receive aggressive multimodal therapy such surgery, radiotherapy, and chemotherapy, more than 80% of patients die within months, especially those who are more than sixty years of age[6]. An in-depth understanding of thyroid cancer biology is therefore a necessary prerequisite to develop better management schemes for different types of thyroid cancers. Furthermore, the information gleaned could be utilized to make therapeutic advances that may improve the outcomes of thyroid cancer patients in the near future.

So far, study of genetic and epigenetic alterations in thyroid cancer cells has given us exciting new insights into the mechanisms that give rise to thyroid tumors [7]. Even though

Single TKIs	**Target**	**Ref**
gefitinib[67]	EGFR	Pennell et.al.
imatinib (STI571) [64]	c-kit	Ha et.al.
Multikinase inhibitors	**Target**	**Ref**
sorafenib[63, 66]	BRAF, VEGFR 1 and 2 and	Duntas et.al
	PDGFR, c-kit, Flt-3	Lam et.al.
sunitinib (SU11248) [60, 61]	Flt-3, c-kit, VEGFR,	Broutin, et.al.
	and PDGFR	Carr et.al.
Axitinib(AG-013736)[62]	All VEGFRs	Cohen et.al.
Motesanib (AMG 706)[69]	VEGFR 1–3, RET and c-KIT	Rosen et.al.
Vandetanib (ZD 6474)[68, 70]	VEGFR 2 and 3, RET and EGFR	Robinson et.al. Wells et.al.
Pazopanib (GW786034)[59]	VEGFR 1–3 and c-KIT	Bible et.al.
XL184 (Exelixis)[65]	RET, c-MET and VEGFR 1 and 2	Review by Kapiteijn et.al.
PLX 4032[65]	V600E mutant BRAF kinase, not wild type	Review by Kapiteijn et.al.
E7080[65]	VEGFRs, c-KIT and PDGFRß stem cell factor	Review by Kapiteijn et.al.

Table 1. Single and multi-kinase inhibitors under clinical development for treating thyroid cancer.

we may be far away from a clear understanding of the complete set of molecular events that transform benign thyroid cells into tumorigenic cells, a vast majority of literature indicates that signals originating from growth factors (GF) and their receptors play an important role in fueling the growth of aggressive cancer.

It is well established that GF signaling is required for maintaining the malignant phenotype through alteration of the cell cycle, induction of apoptosis, and modulation of the behaviour of tumor cell or its micro-environment [8]. It is no surprise then that GF and their receptors have become attractive candidates for targeted therapy of cancer[9]. Constitutive signaling through the receptor tyrosine kinases (RTKs), particularly the epidermal growth factor receptor (EGFR, erbB1), Her2/neu (c-erbB2), and vascular endothelial growth factor receptor (VEGFR) has been reported in multiple tumor types including TC. This has opened up the possibility of blocking them with small molecule tyrosine kinase inhibitors (TKIs) either as single agent or as a cocktail of multi-kinase complexes (see Table 1), or with human or humanized monoclonal antibodies (mAb) (see Table 2).

Trade name	Type of Ab	Target	Clinical Use
Trastuzumab	hmAb	against the juxtamembrane region of HER2	HER-2 over-expressing breast cancer
Cetuximab	mAb	competitive antagonist for EGFR	CRC, HNSCC
Bevacizumab	recom hmAb	specific for the VEGF A	CRC, NSCLC

Table 2. Monoclonal antibodies as inhibitors of receptor tyrosine kinases.

Insulin-like growth factor–I receptor (IGF-IR) is another candidate gene that has gained popularity as a viable RTK target in the last two decades for several different reasons [10, 11]. The most significant reason is that multiple oncogenes require the presence of IGF-IR to achieve cellular transformation[12]. In addition, IGF-I signaling confers resistance to many therapies that currently constitute the standard of care in oncology[13-15]. Furthermore, epidemiological studies have shown that elevated plasma levels of IGF-I are associated with higher risk of several cancers (breast, colon, prostate and lung) [16-19]. All of these data suggest that instead of using conventional cytotoxic chemotherapy, targeting the IGF-I axis may be an important, effective and well-tolerated therapeutic alternative for treating cancer[20]. Indeed, several anti-IGF-IR compounds are in Phase I and Phase II clinical trials[21] to measure their anti-tumor effects as single agents or when given in combination with chemotherapy or radiotherapy (Table 3). However, very few studies have looked at the role of IGF-IR signaling in TC or evaluated the potential of anti-IGF-IR therapy for in this cancer. We investigated whether enhanced IGF-IR signaling promotes

class	ID	Company	Phase of dev	Target organs
IGF-IR inhibition	IGF-IR specific Antisense oligonucleotides			
IGF-IR inhibition	IGF-IR specific Si or ShRNA			
IGF-IR specific Antibodies				
	CP-751,871 (figitumumab)	Pfizer	Phase III	NSCLC, and ovarian carcinoma, prostate, breast, colon
	IMC-A12	Imclone Systems	Phase II	neuroendocrine tumors, prostate, colorectal, breast, pancreatic, liver, and head and neck, HCC
	AMG 479 (ganitumab)	Amgen	Phase II	Ewing's/PNET, colorectal, breast, pancreatic, and small-cell lung cancer
	MK0646 (dalotuzumab)	Merck	Phase II	Colon, Pancreas, neuroendocrine tumors
	AVE1642	Sanofi_Aventis	Phase II	Breast, Liver, Multiple myeloma, Ewing's sarcoma
	R1507	Roche	Phase II	Lung, breast, sarcoma, advanced solid tumor
TKI	NVP-AEW541	Novartis	Phase I/II	Multiple myeloma, glioblastoma, Ewing's sarcoma and breast cancer
	NVP-ADW742	Novartis		
	NVP-TAE226	Novartis		
	BMS-536924	Bristel Myers Squibb		
	BMS-554417*	Bristel Myers Squibb		
	BMS-754807*	Bristel Myers Squibb		Breast, head and neck, advanced solid tumor
	OSI-906 (PQIP)	OSI Pharma	Phase III	Adrenocortical, ovarian, breast, advanced solid tumor, colon and liver
	A-928605	Abbott		
	XL-228**	Exelixis	Phase I	CML, lymphoma, cancer
	AXL1717	Axelar AB	Phase I/II	
Antibodies for the ligands	KM1468 KM3168 KM3002	Kyowa Hakko	preclinical	
IGFBPs	Recombinant human IGFBP3 protein SomatoKine/IPLEX	Imsmed Incorporated	Phase I/II	Myotonic dystrophy type 1
	cyclolignan picropodophyllin (PPP)	Biovitrum		
	nordihydroguaiaretic acid***	INSMED		

*Targets IR in addition to IGF-IR, **targets Abl, SFK,Src, Aurora kinase A, *** targets Her2

Table 3. Drugs targeting Type I insulin-like growth factor receptor.

thyroid cancer progression and if so, is it a viable candidate for RTK therapy in thyroid cancer. In this chapter, we review the basics of IGF-IR signaling, our experience with over-expression of IGF-IR signaling components in TC and how blockade of IGF-I signaling through its receptor has the potential to curb the growth of poorly differentiated FTC and ATC. Later sections of the chapter also describe important molecular changes resulting from IGF-IR blockade and their influence on tumor growth.

2. Brief overview of insulin-like growth factor receptor signaling

Major components of IGF signaling axis include the three ligands (IGF-I, IGF-II & Insulin), IGF binding proteins (IGFBPs) and the three tyrosine kinase receptors, namely, IGF-IR, IGF-IIR and Insulin receptor (IR). All of these ligands can act as circulating hormone or tissue growth factors. Similarly, the IGFBPs are also produced in the liver or other organs and

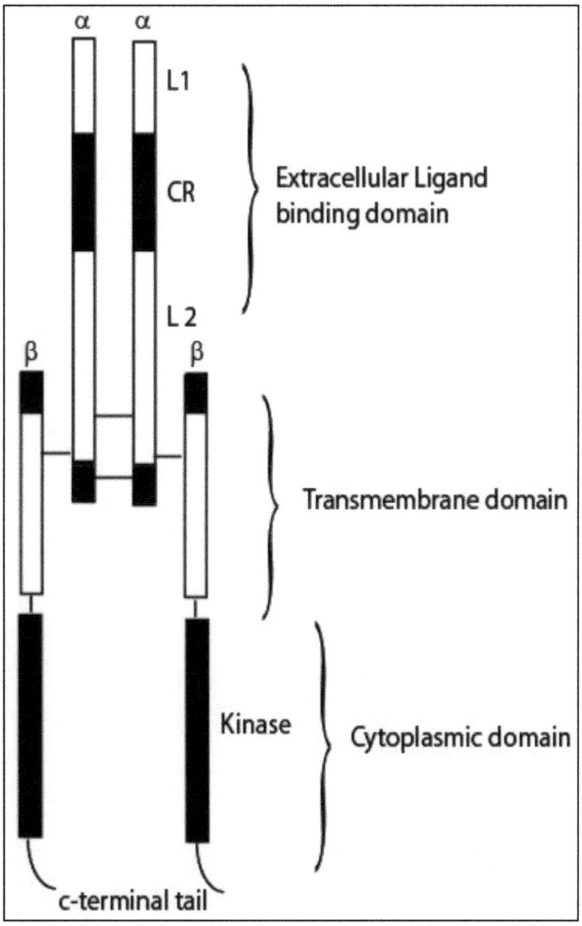

Fig. 1. Schematic of Insulin like growth factor receptor illustrating its different domains and the position of sulphide bonds. IGF-IR is a trans-membrane tyrosine kinase and consists of two αβ chains and has high affinity for its ligands IGF-I and IGF-II. Insulin can also bind and signal through this receptor although with much lower affinity.

delivered to the target tissue in an endocrine manner. The balance of IGF-I, either bound to IGFBP or its unbound form determine whether a cell will follow a survival pathway or follow an apoptotic course. Free IGF-I exerts its effects through the activation of IGF-IR, its preferred cell surface receptor. IGF-IR is synthesized as a precursor peptide of 1367 amino acid residues. It is then cleaved at residue 706, to dissociate the α chain containing the extracellular domain from the β-chain that encompasses the transmembrane and tyrosine kinase domains (Fig. 1).

It moves to the membrane fully assembled in the dimeric form with two α-chains and two β-subunits[22]. Signaling through IGF-IR is initiated when IGF-I and IGF-II produced by the liver and at many extra hepatic sites including tumor cells and stromal fibroblasts or insulin bind to IGF-IR. Upon ligand binding, IGF-IR is auto phosphorylated to stimulate its tyrosine kinase activity that subsequently phosphorylates additional intracellular substrates, including insulin receptor substrates-1 through 4 (IRS-1-4) and Shc (an SH2 domain containing adaptor protein). These early events activate multiple signaling pathways, including the mitogen-activated protein kinase [MAPK, extracellular signal-regulated kinase (ERK)] and phosphatidylinositide 3-kinase (PI3-K)/Akt-1 (protein kinase B) pathways (Fig. 2)[23, 24]. Signaling from IGF-IR is known to play a crucial role in organ development[25-27]during embryogenesis and regulation of mitogenesis through suppression of apoptosis and stimulation of proliferation[28].

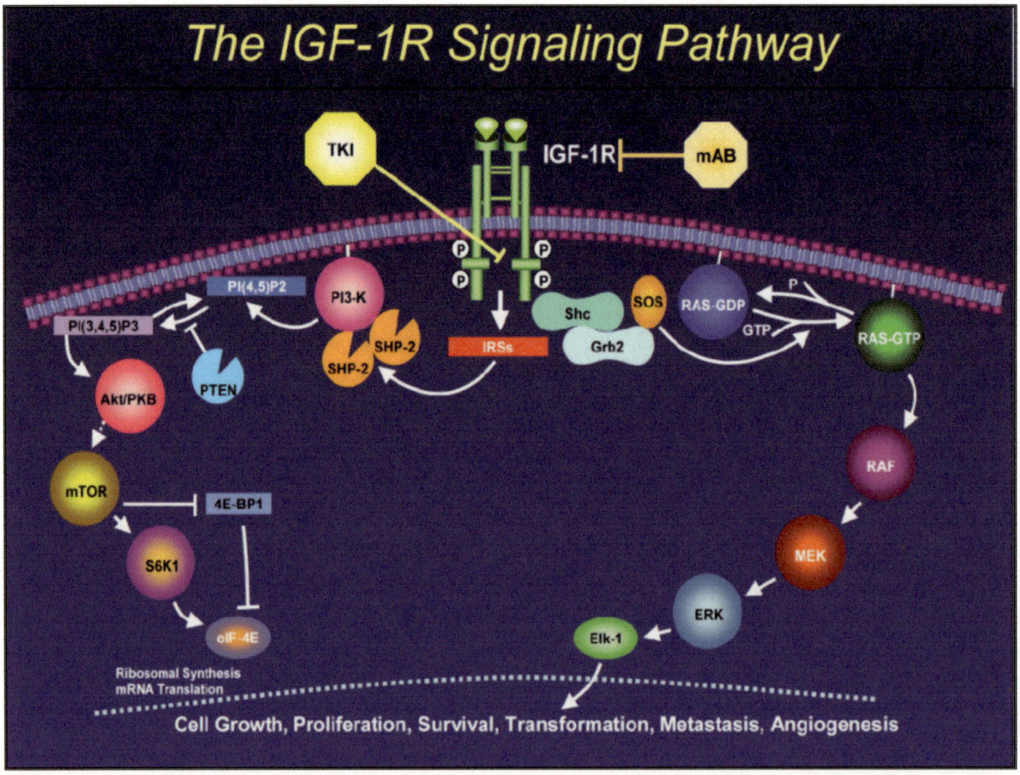

Fig. 2. IGF-IR signaling and two most frequently used IGF-IR inhibition strategies: In response to ligand binding, IGF-IRβ gets activated and phosphorylates adaptor proteins belonging to the IRS family or SHC. Activation of IRS and SHC leads to activation of extracellular signal-regulated kinase (ERK) 1/2 of the MAPK cascade via the growth factor

receptor binding protein 2 (Grb2)/Sos/Ras/Raf/MAPK extracellular signal–regulated kinase kinase (MEK) pathway. IRS proteins also bind to the p110 subunit of PI3K, leading to the generation of phosphatidylinositol 3,4.5-triphosphate (PIP3) and phosphorylation of Akt by phosphoinositide dependent kinase (PDK1). Phosphorylation of Akt leads to subsequent activation of mammalian target of rapamycin (mTOR), eukaryotic translation initiation factor 4E (eIF4E), and p70S6 kinase (S6K). Activation of these downstream signaling pathways leads to enhanced proliferation, survival, and metastasis in cancer cells. Similar signaling pathways are activated by IR and other IGF-IR/IR hybrid receptors.

In normal cells, the IGF/IGF-IR signaling is regulated at multiple levels (Fig. 3)[29]. Initially, Growth hormone-releasing hormone (GHRH) stimulates the expression of growth hormone (GH) produced in the pituitary gland. GH then stimulates the secretion of IGFs and IGFBPs from the hepatocytes [30]. As stated earlier, activation of IGF-IR is tightly regulated by amount of free forms of the ligands, which is controlled by the action of IGFBP and the type 2 IGF receptor (IGF-IIR) also known as mannose 6-phosphate receptor. This receptor can bind IGF-II but lacks tyrosine kinase activity. Accordingly, when IGF-II binds the receptor, it fails to transduce its signal and just serves as a sink for the IGF-II. This reduces the circulating levels of IGF-II thus enhancing the signalling of IGF-IR [31].

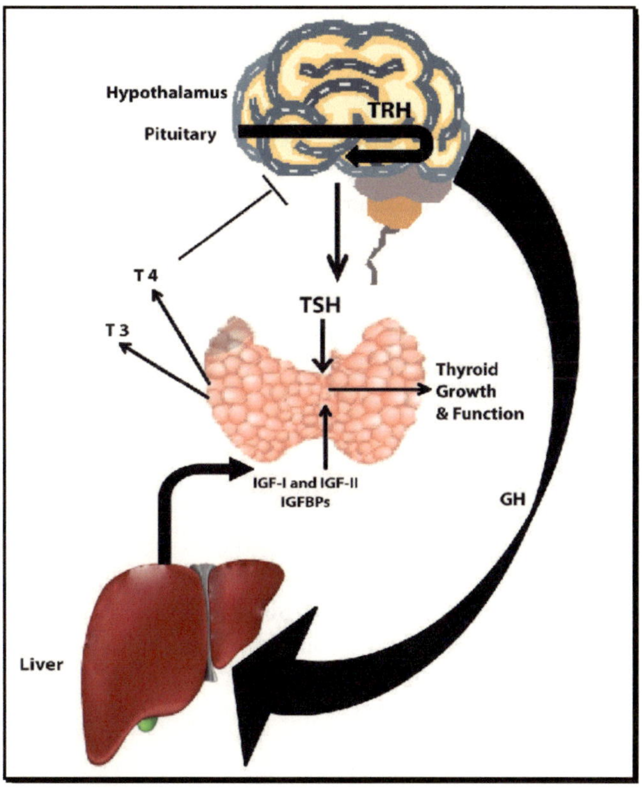

Fig. 3. Growth hormone (GH) and Thyroid stimulating hormone (TSH) are produced under the influence of hypothalamic factors. GH controls the secretion of IGF-I, IGF-II and IGFBPs from liver, whereas TSH controls the secretion of T3 & T4 that regulate thyroid growth. In normal thyroid cells TSH cooperates with IGF-I signaling to promote thyroid growth and

function. However, in some cases, excessive constitutive synthesis of IGF-I may be involved in abnormal growth of the thyroid.

In contrast, IGFBP 1-6 modulate IGF activity by reducing bioavailability of IGFs that may bind to the IGF-IR. The complex balance between the IGFs and the IGFBPs is modulated by specific IGFBP proteases, such as matrix metalloproteinase (MMP)[32]. Like IGF-I and IGF-II, Insulin can also signal through the IGF-IR, IR and the IGF-IR/IR hybrid receptor to induce a variety of biological effects in typical insulin target (adipocyte, hepatocyte, and myocyte) cells[33] and in cancer cells. Upon ligand binding, insulin/IGF-IR undergoes auto-phosphorylation on tyrosine residues, activating the same downstream signaling cascade as the ones initiated upon IGF-I binding. However, as insulin binds to the IGF-1R with 100- to 1000-fold lower affinity than IGF-I[34], most of the signaling from the IGF-IR may be assumed to be the result of IGF-I signaling. Nevertheless, the high degree of homology of IGF-IR to insulin receptor has been a considerable challenge for the development of anti-IGF-IR therapies that are specific to IGF-IR.

3. Role of IGF-IR signaling axis components in human thyroid cancers

Inappropriate IGF-IR signaling is implicated in the development and progression of several human malignancies [35] including those of the thyroid[36-38], and often correlates with poor prognosis[39, 40]. Activation of IGF-IR is essential for the mitogenic effects of TSH and for thyroid function [41-44]. Unlike other growth factor receptors, IGF-IR and insulin receptor (IR) are not inhibitory to thyroid function. Instead they cooperate with TSH to stimulate growth (Fig. 3). However, in some cases, excessive constitutive synthesis of IGF-I has been shown to be involved in abnormal growth of the thyroid[45]. Additional accumulated evidence from studies of other neoplasms suggests that in addition to the TSH-IGF-I nexus, there are several other mechanisms by which IGF-IR signaling may be dysregulated in human tumors. It can be constitutively activated through autocrine or paracrine signaling[39, 46]. Alternatively, ligand-independent mechanisms can result in the activation of the receptor[47]. By far, the most common occurrence is overexpression of IGF-IR. However, whether that is the case in thyroid cancer is unknown.

4. IGF-I and IGF-IRß expression is high in all histological subtypes of thyroid cancer and thyroid cancer cell lines

In recent studies, the authors measured the expression of IGF-I, IGF-IRß and phosphorylated IGF-IRβ (pIGF-IRβ) in normal and neoplastic human thyroid tissue to determine whether IGF-I axis plays a role in thyroid tumor progression. Evaluation of the distribution and abundance of IGF-l in human thyroid cancers with different histopathologic characteristics showed that immunoreactive IGF-l was present in all the thyroid tissues examined. Its expression was lowest in normal the thyroid tissues and highest in all thyroid carcinomas studied. Examination of expression level of IGF-IRβ in normal and neoplastic thyroid tissue on human tissue arrays showed that none of the normal thyroid tissue specimens stained positively for IGF-IRβ, whereas 60 out of 63 specimens of thyroid cancer were positive. The intensity of staining ranged from + to +++ (+ being low, ++ moderate and +++high). Compared to the normal thyroid tissue specimens, the positive staining rate of ATC (37/39, 94%) FTC (11/11, 100%) and PTC (12/13, 92%) specimens revealed statistically significant differences in IGF-IRß expression

($P < 0.001$). No statistical differences between ATC, FTC-and PTC-positive staining (Fig. 4A and Table 4) were noted.

Similar analysis of the thyroid cancer cell lines confirmed our findings from human tumor specimens. As per our expectation, most of the FTC and PTC cell lines showed little variability in IGF-IRβ expression. But its expression was comparatively lower in ATC cell lines. pIGF-IRβ expression on the other hand was variable. Overall, FTC and PTC cell lines had higher pIGF-IRβ levels compared to the normal thyroid cells or the anaplastic cell lines (Fig. 4B & C). It is important to mention here that the data presented is for representative cell lines only. More details can be accessed at Wang et.al. (2006)[2]. Nevertheless, despite the high IGF-IR content of several of the thyroid cancer cell lines tested, auto-phosphorylation of the receptor in response to IGF-I stimulation was observed only in cell lines that had an intact IGF-I axis. Evaluation of the phosphorylated form of the receptor (pIGF-IR) in surgical specimens of human FTC, PTC and ATC indicated that both FTC and PTC specimens had moderate to high levels of pIGF-IR. But neither the ATC specimens nor most of the ATC cell lines tested had detectable levels of pIGF-IR (Fig 4B). This data implied attenuated expression of growth-signaling components of the IGF system. In particular low pIGF-IR expression may be associated with malignant phenotype or more aggressive form of thyroid cancer. To test this hypothesis further, a quantitative immunohistochemical assay for pIGF-IR expression was developed[1] and archival human thyroid tumor microarrays containing specimens with 10 to 12 year follow up were analyzed as described.

Tissue type	No. of samples	IGF-IRß staining				
		Level of staining				Positive staining (%)
		0	+	++	+++	
Normal thyroid	8	8	0	0	0	0
Follicular thyroid cancer	11	0	0	4	7	100.0
Papillary thyroid cancer	13	1	7	4	1	92.3
Anaplastic thyroid cancer	39	2	12	15	10	94.9

Table 4. Level of immunohistochemical staining for IGF-IRβ in normal thyroid, follicular, papillary and anaplastic thyroid cancer tissue from 63 human surgical samples (including specimens on tissue array and permanent pathological slides) [2].

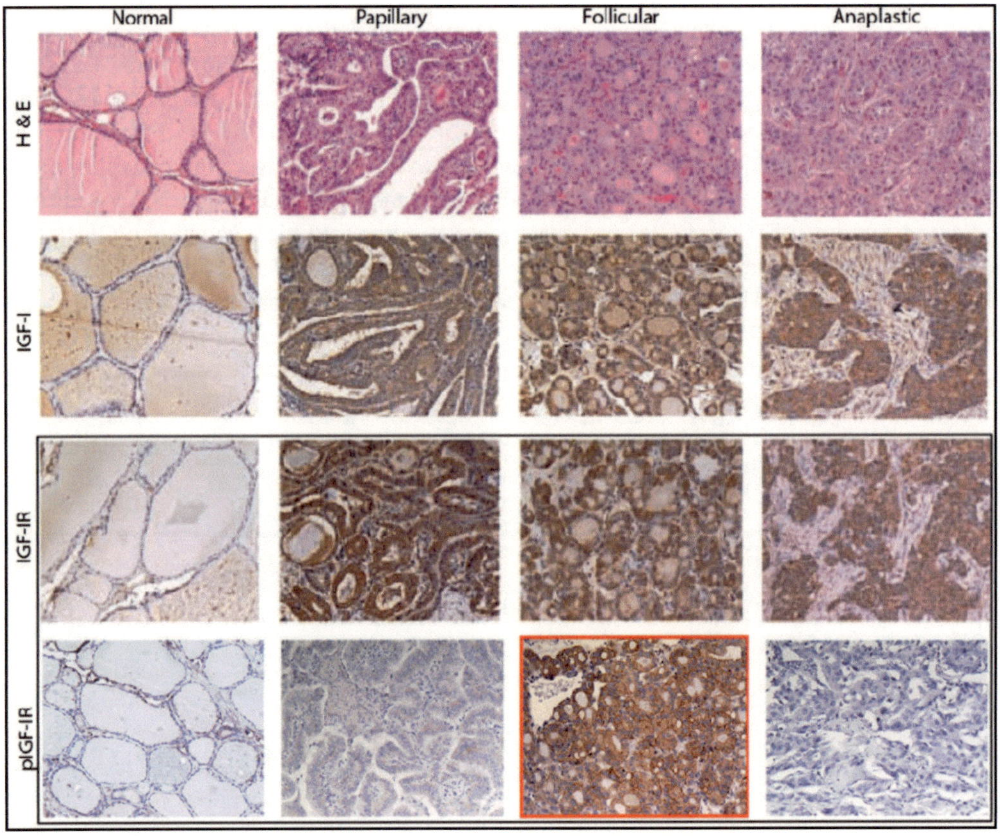

Fig. 4A. Expression of pIGF-IRβ is down regulated in majority of anaplastic and some papillary thyroid cancer specimens: Immunoperoxidase staining of thyroid tumor tissue sections to visualize expression of endogenous IGF-I, IGF-IRβ and pIGF-IRβ. The black boxed area indicates that as compared to normal thyroid tissue, PTC, FTC and ATC specimens show overexpression of IGF-IRβ, whereas expression of pIGF-IRβ is down regulated in majority of ATC and PTC specimens. In contrast pIGFIRβ expression (highlighted in red boxed specimen) is retained mostly in FTC specimens [1].

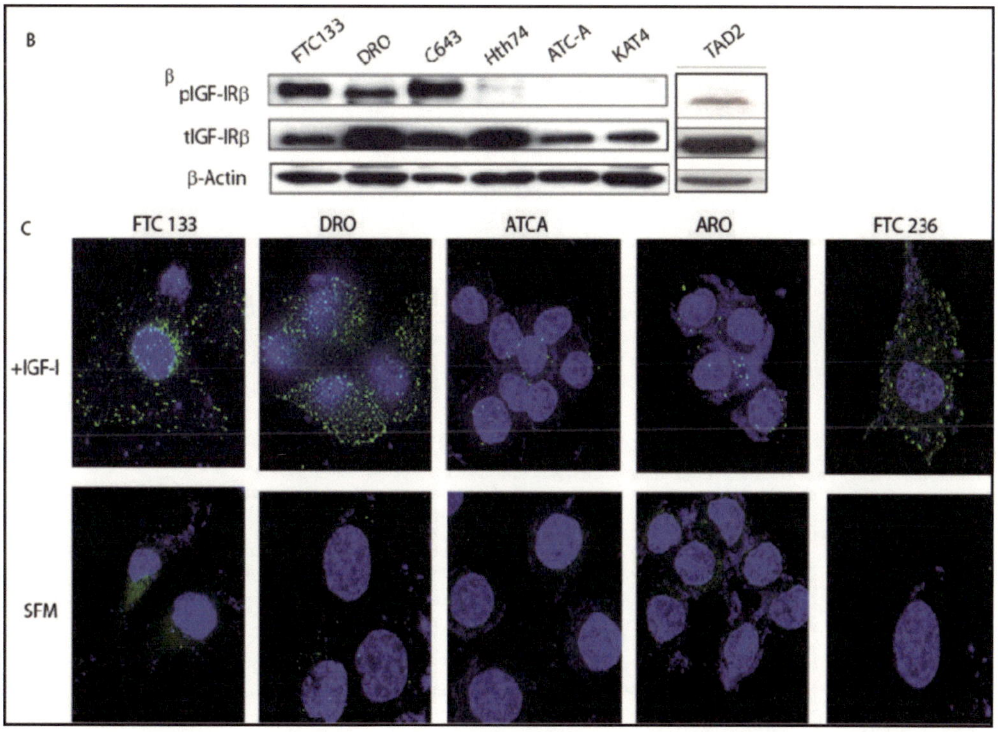

Fig. 4B. & C. IGF-IRβ/IRβ and pIGF-IRβ expression in representative thyroid cancer cell lines detected immunochemically using Western blotting (B) and Immunofluorescence (C). Total IGF-IRβ expression was detectable in all cell lines tested. pIGF-IRβ expression varied amongst cell lines and was almost undetectable in ATC cell lines. Its expression was lower in normal thyroid (TAD2) cells compared to the FTC cell lines. C) Immuno-fluorescent detection of pIGF-IRβ in FTC and ATC cell lines after stimulation with 10ng/ml IGF-I (top panels) or in serum free media (SFM). Green signal = pIGF-IR; Blue = DAPI.

4.1 pIGF-IR expression is high in differentiated thyroid cancers but its expression is attenuated in more aggressive thyroid cancers

Two thyroid tumor tissue arrays (TMA) containing 120 specimens on one and 84 specimens on the other, were analyzed in this study. One of the arrays also contained six pairs of normal thyroid tissue from the same patient. Detailed analysis of these tissue arrays (see Table 6 for demographics) confirmed that the pIGF-IR content of the differentiated component of the tumors was higher as compared to the matched pair of the normal tissue specimen. However, on the whole, all poorly differentiated tumor types, particularly the ATCs, showed negligible expression of pIGF-IR (Fig. 5).

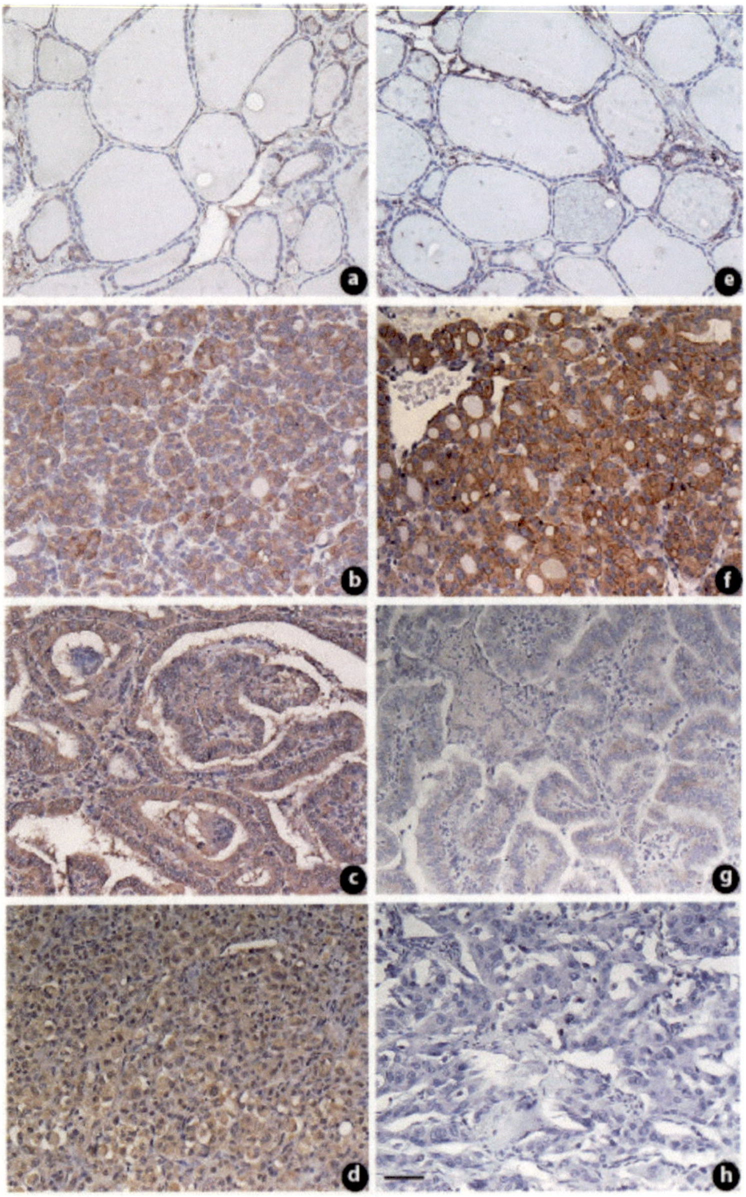

Fig. 5. Immunohistochemical analysis of IGF-IRβ and pIGF-IRβ/IRβ in histological subtypes of thyroid carcinoma: **A.** Representative paraffin-embedded sections of normal and histologcal subtypes of thyroid carcinoma treated with the anti-IGF-IRβ antibody (a – d) and anti-pIGF-IRβ/IRβ Ab (e-h). Panels a & e are sections from normal thyroid tissue treated with the two antibodies mentioned above. Note that the normal tissue has very low levels of IGF-IR or pIGF-IR/IR as compared to the adjacent panels showing intense staining in tumor tissues. Additionally, only follicular thyroid carcinoma samples and few papillary carcinoma were more often positive for anti-pIGF-IRβ/IRβ antibody staining even though all the tumor tissue types had detectable IGF-IRβ expression. Scale bar represents 50µm [1].

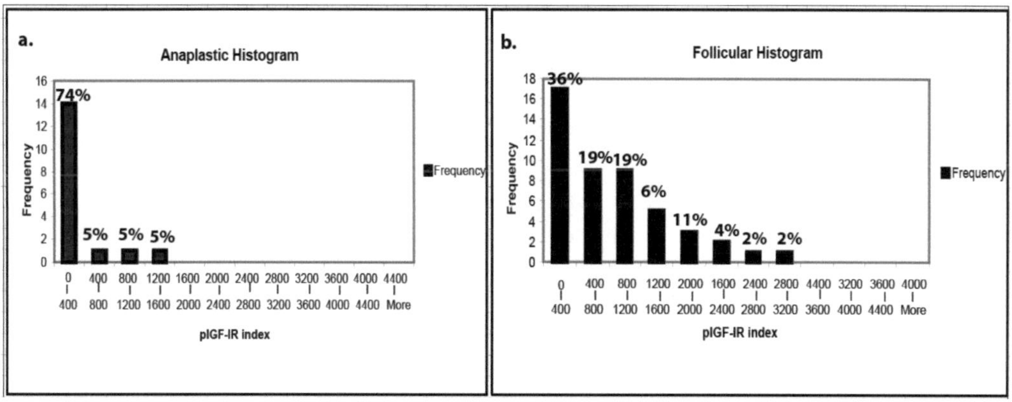

Fig. 6A. pIGF-IRβ/IRβ index of thyroid cancer specimens: Frequency distribution of pIGF-IR/IR index in a total of 17 Anaplastic (a) and 47 Follicular (b) thyroid carcinoma cases. Overall, more FTC specimens demonstrated a higher pIGF-IRβ index.

This was further substantiated by histogram analysis of all the morphological histotypes of thyroid cancer, where 74% of ATC specimens showed a pIGF-IR index below 400 as opposed to only 34% of the FTC (Fig. 6A). Furthermore, a significant difference was noted in the median pIGF-IR index of different histological subtypes of thyroid cancer ($P<0.001$) (Fig. 6A). When all thyroid cancers were stratified as differentiated [FTC, PTC and Hurthle cell carcinoma (HCC)] or other thyroid cancers (ATC and MTC), the median pIGF-IR index of differentiated thyroid cancer was significantly higher than the median index of other thyroid cancers (114 vs. 63, $P<0.001$, Fig. 6B).

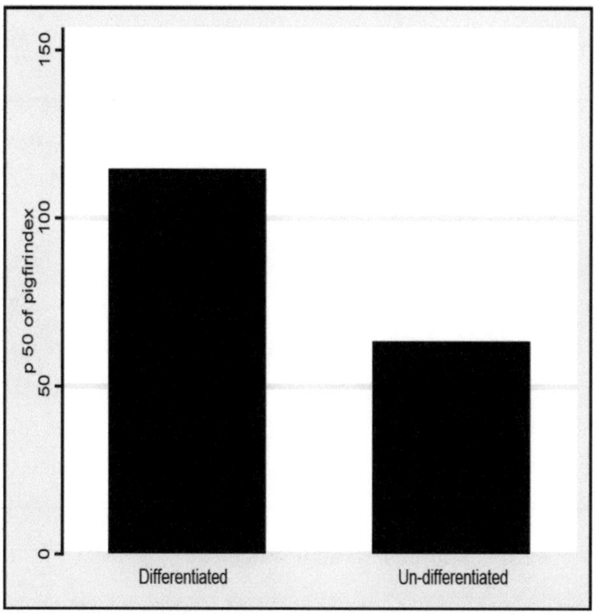

Fig. 6B. Median pIGF-IRβ/IRβ index of differentiated thyroid carcinoma was significantly higher than that of all other thyroid cancers $p<0.001$ (Mann-Whitney test).

To make the predictive power of our analysis more significant, additional parameters such as age, tumor size, tumor grade and lymph node metastasis were analyzed along with the pIGF-IR index of the specimen.

Our data showed that when patients with PTC or FTC were stratified according to their age, the mean pIGF-IR index of differentiated thyroid cancer patients above 45 years of age was significantly lower than the mean pIGF-IR index of patients below 45 years of age. However, due to the small sample size of our study, statistical significance couldn't be reached, although, a clear trend was noted (Table 5A). No significant difference was noted in the pIGF-IR index of tumors grouped by size or stage. Furthermore, although lymph node (LN) metastasis is not a good prognostic indicator in thyroid cancer, it does indicate recurrence and local control. Accordingly, when tumors were stratified based on their LN status, our analysis indicated that patients with differentiated thyroid cancer without lymph node metastases have a significantly higher pIGF-IR index (P = 0.03) as compared to patients with lymph node metastasis. Once again, no significant difference was noted among those patients with poorly differentiated thyroid cancer with or without lymph node metastasis (P = 0.12) (Table 5B)[1].

	Age	Median pIGF-IR	Mean pIGF-IR	P value
Follicular	<45 yrs (7)	948	1,273	0.84
	>45 yrs (10)	708	794	
Papillary	<45 yrs (7)	912	341	0.25
	>45 yrs (4)	64	59	
Differentiated	<45 (14)	991	807	0.71
	>45 (19)	125	451	

Table 5A. pIGF-IRβ/IRβ index variability by age in differentiated thyroid cancers.

Patient group	n	Median pIGF-IRß index	P value
Differentiated thyroid cancer with no lymph node metastasis	21	471.3	0.0329*
Differentiated thyroid cancer with lymph node metastasis	12	78.51	
Poorly differentiated thyroid cancer with no lymph node metastasis	7	37.5	0.1208
Poorly differentiated thyroid cancer with lymph node metastasis	15	69.07	

Table 5B. pIGF-IRβ/IRβ expression vs. patient outcome

Overall, low pIGF-IR expression was found to correlate with aggressive human thyroid carcinoma. It is thus likely that IGF-IR signaling may not be needed for progression of ATC as other cell signaling pathways may be activated in these cells thereby obviating the need for intact IGF-IR signaling. Nonetheless, as both IGF-IRβ & pIGF-IRβ were up-regulated in a majority of differentiated thyroid carcinomas, we hypothesized that IGF-IR may be a viable potential target for therapy in patients with more differentiated types of thyroid cancer.

	Specimens	Controls	statistically analyzed
Total number in study	126	6	58
Tumor histology	Specimens		Gender
Anaplastic	19		8 (4M, 4F)
Follicular	47		18 (7M, 11F)
Papillary	12		11 (1M, 10F)
Medullary	22		14 (4M, 10F)
Other (Hurthle & Sarcomatoid)	26		7 (5M, 2F)
			M: Male F: Female

Table 6. Demographics of thyroid cancer patient samples used in statistical analysis of pIGF-IR index of thyroid tumor microarray (TMA)

5. Targeting IGF-IR in thyroid cancer

Targeted therapies consisting of human monoclonal antibodies against IGFBPs and the IGF-IR, or, the small molecular tyrosine kinase inhibitors (SMTKI) that target the kinase domain of IGF-IR, are a new class of pharmacological agents that have been shown to be useful in the treatment of cancers with enhanced expression and activity of IGF-IR. Pharmacological inhibition of IGF-I signaling with these therapeutic agents has been shown to significantly decrease migration, invasion, metastatic spread, and angiogenesis with little toxicity in mouse tumor models. Similarly, inhibition of IGF-IR signaling has also been reported to sensitize cancer cells to radiation and chemotherapeutic agents[48-58]. Our objective therefore, was to build upon this knowledge and investigate whether targeted therapy directed at the IGF-IR, and given in combination with chemotherapy, can be an attractive new treatment strategy for thyroid cancer[20]. Given our findings on up-regulation of components of the IGF-I signaling pathway in thyroid cancer cell lines and in human thyroid carcinoma tissue microarrays, we proceeded to test this hypothesis both *in vitro* and *in vivo*.

5.1 Choice of anti-IGF-IR compounds in clinical development

Several therapeutic agents that specifically inhibit IGF-1R but do not affect IR signaling are in preclinical and clinical development. Some of the strategies being used to interfere with IGF-1R signaling (a) reduction of IGF-1R expression by antisense nucleotides (b) siRNA or antisense RNA against IGF-IR (c) monoclonal antibodies and (d) tyrosine kinase inhibitors. Altogether, 30 different IGF-1R targeting agents are in preclinical or clinical development [59-70] (Table 3) and at least 58 active clinical trials are evaluating anti-IGF-1R targeting agents alone or in various combinations (www.clinicaltrials.gov). However, the two main strategies employed to inhibit this pathway are antibodies directed against IGF-1R or small molecule TKIs. Both approaches have their inherent strengths and weaknesses, particularly their specificity for IGF-IR and issues related to side effects like hyperglycemia. Whether sparing IR is a good strategy or not is an important question to be considered as IR does play a role in IGF-I signaling and could compromise efficacy of anti-IGF-IR compounds. Nonetheless, we chose to evaluate the efficacy of A12 (a monoclonal Ab) and NVP-AEW541 (a SMTKI) in ATC and FTC respectively.

5.2 In vitro effects of anti - IGF-IR antibody A12 on signal transduction, cell proliferation and apoptosis of thyroid cancer cell lines

A12 is a high-affinity humanized monoclonal antibody that specifically binds to IGF-IR and blocks IGF-I and IGF-II signaling but does not block the binding of insulin to the insulin receptor. It has been shown to inhibit the growth of breast, colon, and pancreatic cancer cell lines, both *in vitro* and in subcutaneous tumors in nude mouse models by antibody-mediated blockade of ligand binding to IGF-IR. In a study of xenograft tumor model of breast, pancreas and colon cancer, A12 produced a marked increase in apoptosis with minimal toxicity [49].

In our studies, A12 was able to completely inhibit both IGF-I and IGF-II-induced phosphorylation of IGF-IR at high concentrations (100 nM) in TC cell lines (Fig 7). At lower concentrations (1 nM and 50 nM), it was able to inhibit the phosphorylation of IRS-I, Akt and MAPK. However, 10 fold more A12 was required to inhibit the IGF-2 mediated signaling (Fig. 7).

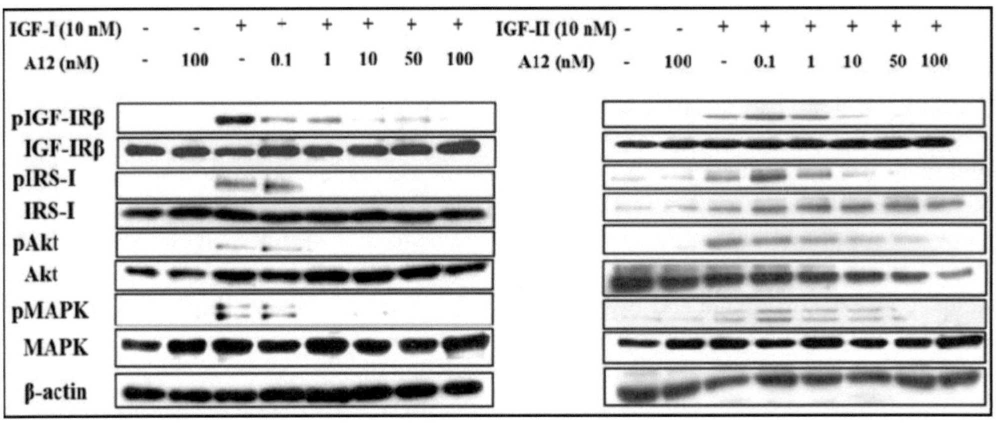

Fig. 7. Dose-dependent inhibition of IGF-1- and IGF-II-induced IGF-IRβ, IRS-I, Akt, and MAPK autophosphorylation in ARO cells after treatment with A12. Serum-starved ARO cells were treated with A12 (0-100 nM) for 2 hours and then incubated with or without IGF-I or IGF-II (10 nM) for 10 minutes. Total protein extracts were obtained to analyze IGF-IR signaling components by western blotting. Note that 10 times more A12 is required to inhibit IGF-II signaling in ARO cells [2].

Twenty-four hours after plating, the cells were treated with increasing concentrations of A12 (0-100 nM) without (A) or with (B) IGF-I stimulation for 72 hours. At the end of incubation, the inhibitory effect of A12 was measured using an MTT assay (Fig. 8).

With respect to its effect on cell proliferation, increasing the concentration of A12, with or without IGF-I, inhibited the proliferation of some TC cell lines (ARO, DRO & C643). Other TC cell lines (Hth74, KAT4 and ATC-A) were only minimally responsive to A12 treatment

(Fig. 8). To understand if this difference was due to differential induction of apoptosis, A12 treated cells were analyzed by Flowcytometry (FCM). Only minimal induction of apoptosis was observed in A12 treated cells, suggesting that growth inhibitory effects of A12 were driven through apoptosis independent pathways *in vitro*. Nonetheless, combining A12 with Irinotecan (chemotherapeutic drug of choice for head and neck cancers) was particularly useful in sensitizing ARO cells to the cytotoxic effects of Irinotecan (Fig. 9).

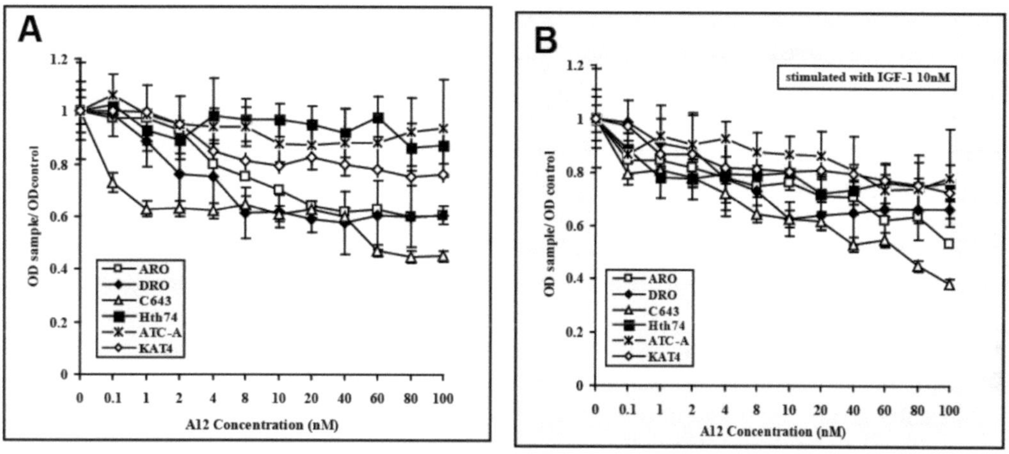

Fig. 8. Inhibition of survival and IGF-I induced proliferation by increasing concentration of A12 in ATC cell lines ARO, DRO, C643, Hth74, ATC-A, and KAT4. All ATC cell lines were plated in 96-well plates at a density of 2000 cells/well.

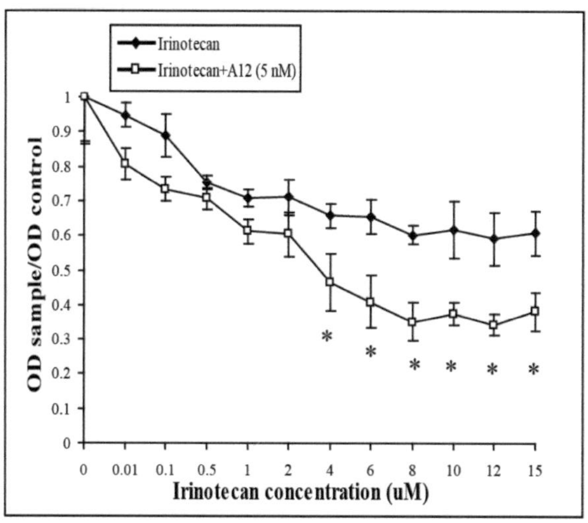

Fig. 9. Synergistic effect of A12 and Irinotecan on in vitro cell proliferation. ARO cells per well were grown in RPMI 1640 medium supplemented with 10% FBS for 24 hours. They were then treated with various concentrations of Irinotecan (0.01–15 mM) or with irinotecan with or without 5 nM A12. After a 3-day incubation period, number of metabolically active cells were determined with an MTT assay. Bars indicate mean values ± SE,. *P < .05 for cells treated with the combination versus vehicle-treated controls.

But, unlike Herceptin that down regulates ErbB2 receptor expression, IGF-IR expression remained unchanged in cells concomitantly treated with IGF-I and A12[2]. Similar findings have been reported for breast cancer cells[49].

5.3 In vivo A12 reduces tumor volume and prolongs survival in combination with irinotecan in an orthotopic nude mice model of ATC

Since it is the anaplastic thyroid carcinoma that is associated with poor clinical outcome and some ATC cell lines showed moderate IGF-IR and pIGF-IR expression [1], preclinical efficacy of A12 antibody as a single agent and in combination with chemotherapy was first evaluated in a nude mouse model of ATC[2]. Four groups [placebo (control), A12, irinotecan, and A12 plus irinotecan] of 10 mice each were analyzed. Treatment with A12 or irinotecan alone led to a 57% and 80% decrease respectively in the tumor volumes of ARO xenografts. The differences in the mean tumor volume compared with the control group were statistically significant ($P = 0.023$ [for A12] and 0.002 [irinotecan], respectively). However, the highest growth inhibition was achieved by the co-administration of A12 plus irinotecan. At the end of the 3-week treatment period, mice treated with A12 plus irinotecan showed a 93% decrease in the estimated mean tumor volumes compared with the control group ($P = 0.001$). The decrease in mean tumor volumes in mice receiving combination treatment was also significantly greater than that of the groups receiving A12 or irinotecan alone ($P < 0.01$) (Fig. 10A & B). A12 was well tolerated by the animals, without substantial adverse effects. The weights of the animals remained constant throughout the treatment period (data not shown) and none of the animals had to be killed before the end of the study. In the survival study, the survival rates of the mice treated with irinotecan alone and combination treatment was significantly greater than that of the mice in the control group with P values of 0.044 and 0.0003 respectively. The combination group also achieved a greater survival rate than mice treated with A12 alone ($P = 0.004$). However, there was no significant improvement in the survival rates between the group treated with A12 alone and the control group ($P = 0.356$) (Fig. 10C).

5.4 Therapeutic potential of IGF-IR specific small molecular tyrosine kinase inhibitor NVP-AEW541 in an orthotopic follicular thyroid carcinoma model

Small molecular tyrosine kinase inhibitors are another class of anti-tumor agents frequently used to inhibit IGF-IR signaling. They inhibit both ligand independent and ligand-dependent receptor phosphorylation and do not evoke immunogenic response on repeated exposure. Due to their small size, they also exhibit good tumor penetration. NVP-AEW541 (Caymen Chemical) is one such SMTKI that is a more potent inhibitor of IGF-IR (IC50 = 0.086 μM), eventhough, at high enough concentrations (IC50 = 2.3 μM) it can also inhibit the closely related insulin receptor. Structurally, NVP-AEW541 is a pyrrolo[2,3-d]pyrimidine derivative that can abrogate IGF-I-mediated survival and colony formation in soft agar at concentrations that are consistent with inhibition of IGF-IR auto-phosphorylation *in vitro*. *In vivo*, it has also been shown to inhibit IGF-IR signaling in tumor xenografts and significantly reduce the growth of IGF-IR-driven fibrosarcomas[54]. To evaluate its efficacy in thyroid cancer, human follicular thyroid cancer cell line stably expressing a constitutively activated form of IGF-IR with a downstream luciferase reporter were injected into the thyroid glands of 8-week-old athymic mice. We found that injection of 2.5×10^5 WRO cells was sufficient for

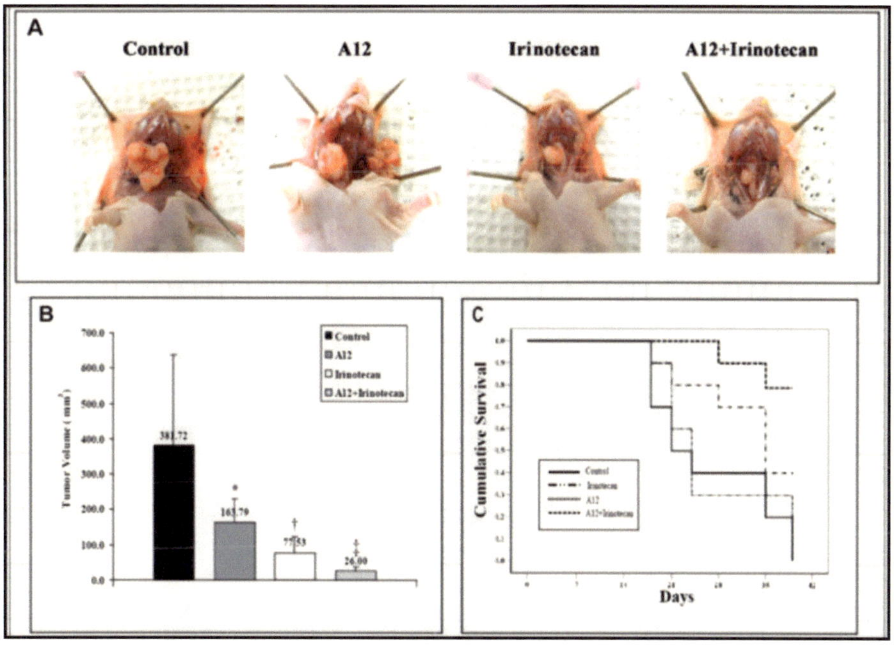

Fig. 10. In vivo antitumor effects of single drugs or simultaneous combination of irinotecan and A12 on tumor growth and survival in an orthotopic nu/nu model of ATC. ARO cells were injected into the right thyroid lobe of the mice. Four days after injection, the mice were randomized into 4 groups (10mice in each group) and the drugs were administered as follows: irinotecan (50 mg/kg i.p. every week) or A12 (1mg/250ul/mouse 2x weekly). A) After 3 weeks of treatment, all the mice were killed, and necropsy was performed. Representative images from each group of mice are shown to highlight the effect of drugs over control. B)At the end of the growth-inhibition study, the tumors were measured in three dimensions, and the mean tumor volumes were calculated in each group.* $P = 0.023$, compared with the control group; † $P = 0.002$, compared with the control group; ‡ $P = 0.001$, compared with the control group; and $P < 0.01$, compared with the A12-alone and irinotecan-alone groups (independent t-test). C, The combined treatment of A12 plus irinotecan prolonged the survival rate in the orthotopic nude mouse ATC model. Irinotecan alone or in combination with A12 significantly increased the survival rate compared with that of the control group ($P < 0.05$).

tumor development. Tumors were visualized via non-invasive real time imaging as early as 10 days post-implantation. After randomization into 3 separate groups with 10 mice in each group, they were either treated with placebo (25 mM tartaric acid solution), Irinotecan (50 mg/kg, I.P. once a week) or NVP-AEW541 (50 mg/kg PO twice daily). Real-time whole-body fluorescence imaging was carried out weekly to monitor tumor growth in response to the various treatments. After approximately three weeks, as the control group of mice became premorbid, mice from all the three groups were sacrificed and tumors harvested at necropsy. Time to premorbid condition varied between mice and was associated with primary tumor growth pattern (early local compression of the esophagus) rather than development of metastatic disease. Additionally, difficulty with oral gavage in mice with

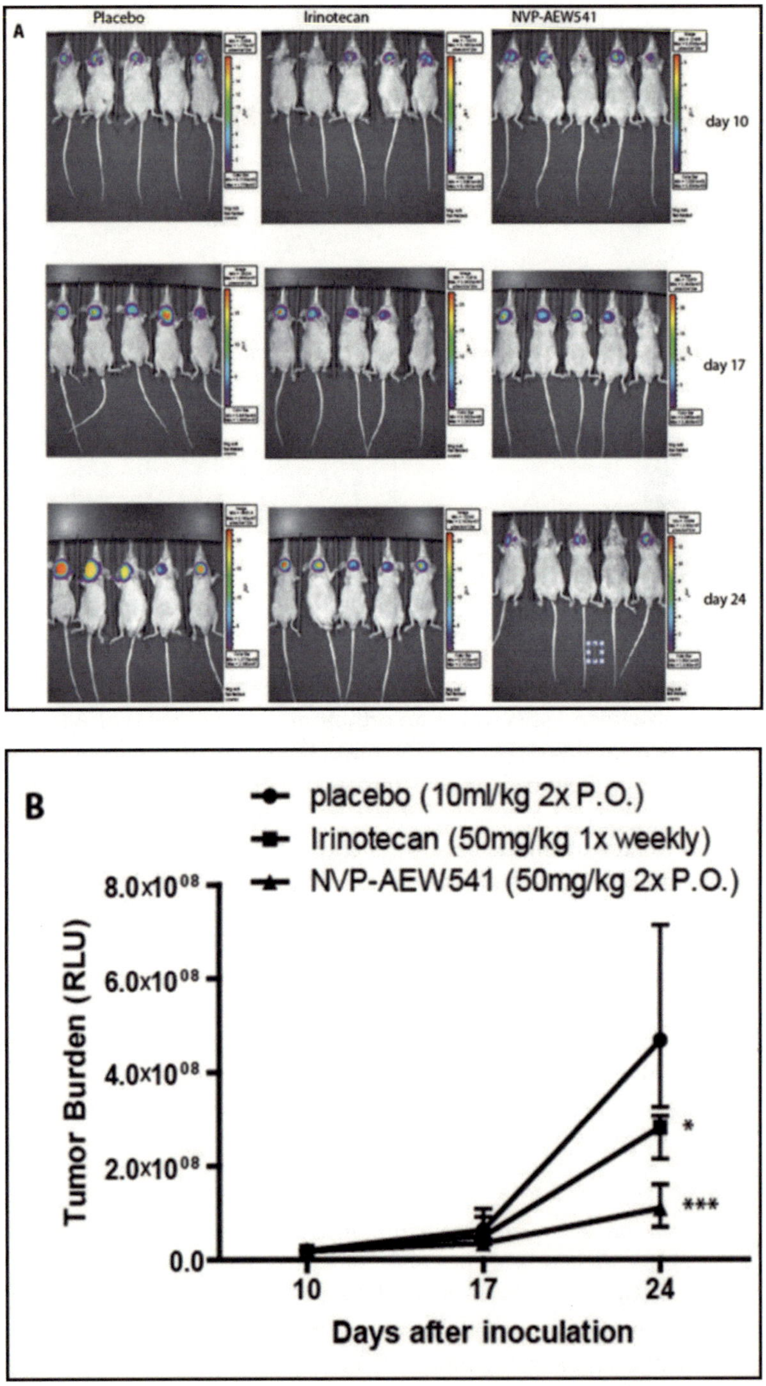

Fig. 11. Realtime bioluminescent imaging (BLI) to monitor the growth of orthotopically inoculated FTC cells treated with placebo, Irinotecan or NVP-AEW541. A) Representative images of mouse at days 10, 17, and 24 after inoculation. (B) Quantification of biochemically

measured luciferase activity (RLU), an indicator of tumor burden to assess the effect of drugs on the respective days shown in panel (A). Tumor growth was significantly inhibited in the NVP-AEW541 treated group as compared to the placebo treated group. Median and range is shown for each point on the graph. Statistics were performed by Student's t test, and significance ($P < 0.05$) relative to control is noted in the graph.

tumors obstructing the esophagus also partially affected the outcome of survival in these mice. Despite the difficulties, NVP-AEW541 significantly inhibited the growth of orthotopic Wro tumors in nude mice (Fig. 11A) as compared to control or Irinotecan-treated mice (Fig. 11B). Furthermore, microvessel density (MVD) was also significantly decreased after treatment with this compound (Fig. 12) and correlated with decreased VEGF secretion by vascular endothelial growth factors (VEGF) WRO cells treated with NVP-AEW541 in an in vitro ELISA assay (see below). These experiments were conducted only once. Pictorial data has been presented from a representative group of mice and quantitative analysis is based on data obtained from 6 – 8 mice/group.

5.5 Both IGF-IR antibody A12 and SMTKI inhibitor NVP-AEW541 inhibit IGF-I signaling and tumor angiogenesis in orthotopic ATC and FTC models

IGFs have been found to promote the growth, survival, and migration of tumor cells, as well as to induce the syntheses of vascular endothelial growth factors A and C and matrix metalloproteinase 2, which may favor the development of the blood supply essential for the progressive growth of primary malignancies and the development of metastases[71-73]. A recent study was conducted to determine whether anti IGF-IR therapy inhibits IGF-I signaling and tumor angiogenesis *in vivo*. Immunohistochemical analyses of ATC tumors treated with A12 or A12 and Irinotecan showed a decrease in pIGF-IRβ, pAkt, and PCNA staining and an increase in apoptosis in both the treatment groups *in vivo*[2]. These observations were in striking contrast to A12's effect *in vitro*, where treatment of ATC cell lines with A12 failed to induce an apoptotic response. A possible explanation for this discordance could be that A12's additional ability to induce antibody-dependent cell cytotoxicity (ADCC) and complement-mediated cell death (CDC) *in vivo* results in the activation of immune response and inhibition of tumor growth. Strangely enough, despite A12's ability to induce apoptosis in vivo, the survival rate of mice treated with A12 alone was not improved over that of the placebo-treated mice ($p=0.578$). Contrarily, mice in the combination treatment group showed significant survival advantage ($p=0.002$) over the mice in control group[2]. These observations suggest that anti-IGF-IR therapy when given in combination with other therapeutic strategies augments anti-tumor effects. To further determine if anti-IGF-IR therapies can be used to inhibit thyroid tumor angiogenesis, we sought to determine whether IGF-IR regulates any molecular targets of angiogenesis as has been reported for colorectal cancer cells[74]. In these studies, stimulation of IGF-IR in colorectal cells has been shown to induce the expression of VEGF to regulate development of new blood vessels[75]. Furthermore, blockade of IGF-IR led to significant down-regulation of VEGF and inhibition of tumor growth and lymph node metastasis of these tumors[76]. To test whether over-expression of IGF-IR in follicular carcinoma cells (WRO) increases VEGF secretion as reported for the colon carcinoma cells, 5×10^5 vector transfected (WRO-puro) or wild type IGF-IR over-expressing (WRO-wt) or constitutively active IGF-IR expressing (CA-IGF-IR) WRO cells were allowed to attach and grow for

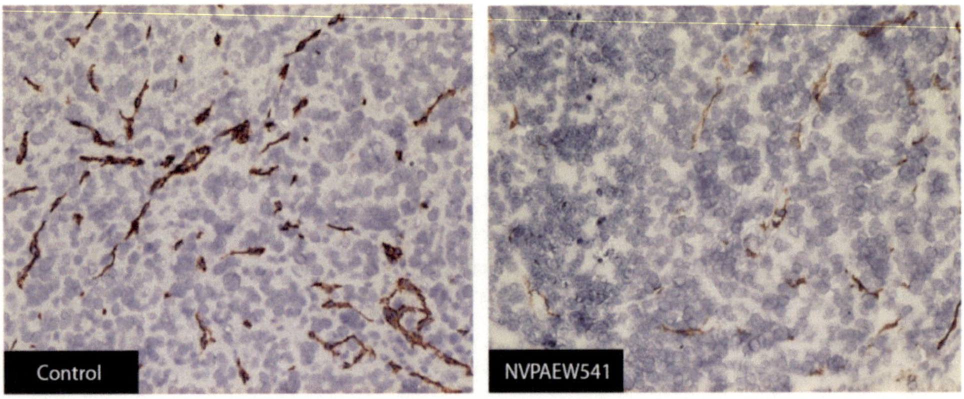

Fig. 12. Histological analysis of tumor sections from Wro-Cd8IGF-IR orthotopic tumors untreated or treated with NVP-AEW541. Tumor samples from representative animals were resected, fixed, and processed for immunohistochemistry with anti CD31 antibody. NVP-AEW541-treated samples showed noticeable reduction in angiogenesis compared to control. Magnification 200X.

24hrs. The supernatant was then replaced with 2 - 3 mL fresh 2% heat-inactivated fetal bovine serum containing culture medium and further cultured for 24 hours. The concentration of VEGF165 in each supernatant was determined using commercially available enzyme-linked immune-absorbent assay (ELISA) kit (R&D Systems, Minneapolis, MN). Culture supernatant from MDA1986 cells was used as positive control for VEGF-A secretion. Both the IGF-IR overexpressing WRO cells and the CA-IGF-IR cells secreted significantly higher levels of VEGF-A as compared to the vector control cells (WRO Puro). We further observed that the treatment of these cells with the SMTKI NVP-AEW541 partially suppressed IGF-IR induced up-regulation of VEGF secretion (Fig. 13; $P < 0.005$ in both cases), suggesting that VEGF secretion in part may be regulated through the IGF-IR signaling pathway.

However, even though NVP-AEW541 is highly sensitive to IGF-IR, it does demonstrate inhibitory activity towards IR, MAPK and PI3K. Thus involvement of other TKIs in the process cannot be overruled. Nonetheless these data does provide credence to our hypothesis that thyroid tumor angiogenesis may be the result of enhanced VEGF secretion in IGF-IR over-expressing tumors. Additional evidence for involvement of IGF-IR in thyroid tumor angiogenesis came from our observations in A12 treated orthotopic ATC specimens. Staining of these tumors for CD31 showed a significant decrease in microvessel density especially in tumors treated with A12 alone and in tumors treated in combination with Irinotecan. Additional staining for pIGF-IR in the tumor endothelium of these tumors confirmed that this response was due to the loss of phosphorylation of IGF-IR in tumor-associated endothelium of A12-treated tumors[2]. In summary, these studies suggest that thyroid tumor angiogenesis is partially regulated through IGF-IR signaling in both ATCs and FTC orthotopic xenografts. To further confirm if human thyroid specimens showed a correlation between IGF-IR signaling and local metastasis, we measured the pIGF-IR content of human thyroid cancer specimens with and without lymph node metastasis. We observed that pIGF-IR expression when computed as an index (pIGF-IR index) varied amongst thyroid tumors. Particularly, pIGF-IR index of thyroid tumors with lymph node metastasis was lower than for ones without lymph node metastasis, suggesting a direct role for IGF-I signaling in local thyroid tumor metastasis.

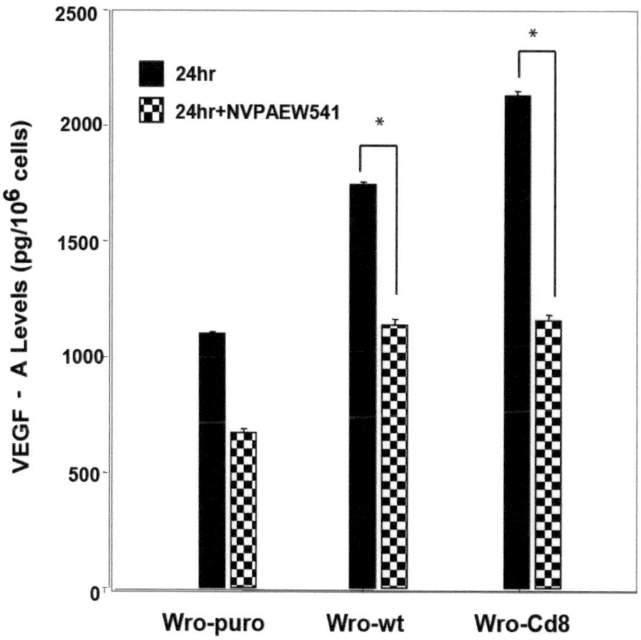

Fig. 13. Effect of NVP-AEW541 on VEGF - A secretion by follicular thyroid carcinoma cells that over express either the wt-IGF-IR or the constitutively activated IGF-IR or are vector transfected (Wro-puro). $5x10^5$ cells/ml were allowed to attach and grow for 24hrs in 6 well dishes. The supernatant was then replaced with 2 mL fresh culture medium containing 2% heat-inactivated fetal bovine serum and further cultured for 24 hours in the presence of IGF-IR inhibitor NVP-AEW541. The dose of NVP-AEW541 was predetermined using a standard MTT assay and was found to bring about 50% inhibition in cell growth at a concentration of 0.2uM. VEGF secretion was evaluated by ELISA in conditioned medium of the wro clones 24 hrs after exposing to the drug using commercially available enzyme-linked immuno-absorbent assay (ELISA) kits (R&D Systems, Minneapolis, MN). Results are presented in pg VEGF165 / 10^6 cells/24h for control and treated samples as mean ± STE from three separate experiments. MDA1986 cells were used as positive control for VEGF-A secretion. VEGF165 was undetectable in media without the cells (data for controls not shown)

6. Conclusions

IGF-I/IGF-IR axis plays a pivotal role in thyroid tumor progression, particularly by enhancing the angiogenic response of these tumors. Thus targeting IGF-1R signaling particularly in FTC, PTC and more differentiated ATCs could have significant therapeutic potential. Many compounds that directly target IGF-1R have now been developed and the two most investigated strategies to date have used IGF-1R tyrosine kinase inhibitors such as NVP-AEW541 and anti-IGF-1R monoclonal antibodies such as A12. We tested the specificity of both these compounds in orthotopic models of ATC and FTC and have presented data that shows their efficacy. Furthermore, blockade of IGF-IR suppressed IGF-I signaling, induced apoptosis in vitro and in vivo. Both compounds also suppressed angiogenesis although via different mechanisms. Combining A12 treatment with standard of care chemotherapeutic drug Irinotecan enhanced the cytotoxic effects of the chemotherapeutic drug. Our results are in agreement with previously reported data in other solid tumors and suggest that blocking IGF-IR with A12 or NVP-AEW541 seems to be a potential avenue for treating thyroid cancer through their direct antitumor effects and their effects on tumor vasculature. Additionally, we reviewed additional strategies that are under clinical development or in clinical trial for targeting this axis in cancer. Nevertheless, as clinical developmental programs progress careful attention must be paid to the potential side effects of this approach, especially since IGF-I signaling plays an equally important role in cell growth, energy metabolism and differentiation. A closer look on the effect of dose and schedule on toxicity are also warranted.

7. Acknowledgements

We thank Dr. M.N. Younes and S.A. Jasser for help with animal surgeries and VEGF ELISA assays respectively. These studies were carried out with funds from Louisiana Cancer Research Consortium and University of Texas M.D. Anderson Cancer Center Head and Neck Spore grant P50 CA097007 and CA016672. We also thank Dr. Sugoto Chakravarty and our colleagues at Tulane University for helpful discussions.

8. References

[1] Chakravarty, G., et al., Phosphorylated insulin like growth factor-I receptor expression and its clinico-pathological significance in histologic subtypes of human thyroid cancer. Exp Biol Med (Maywood), 2009. 234(4): p. 372-86.
[2] Wang, Z., et al., Growth-inhibitory effects of human anti-insulin-like growth factor-I receptor antibody (A12) in an orthotopic nude mouse model of anaplastic thyroid carcinoma. Clin Cancer Res, 2006. 12(15): p. 4755-65.
[3] Geetika Chakravarty, A.V.L., Jeffrey N. Myers, Essential role of Insulin like growth factor receptor signaling in transcriptional regulation of Id1 and Id2 in follicular thyroid carcinoma. Proceedings Annual Meeting of American Association of Cancer research, 2007.
[4] Howlader N, N.A., Krapcho M, Neyman N, Aminou R, Waldron W, Altekruse SF, Kosary CL, Ruhl J, Tatalovich Z, Cho H, Mariotto A, Eisner MP, Lewis DR, Chen HS, Feuer EJ, Cronin KA, Edwards BK (eds) (2011) SEER Cancer Statistics Review, 1975-2008. SEER Cancer Statistics Review.
[5] Sherman, S.I., Thyroid carcinoma. Lancet, 2003. 361(9356): p. 501-11.
[6] Kebebew, E., et al., Anaplastic thyroid carcinoma. Treatment outcome and prognostic factors. Cancer, 2005. 103(7): p. 1330-5.
[7] Kondo, T., S. Ezzat, and S.L. Asa, Pathogenetic mechanisms in thyroid follicular-cell neoplasia. Nat Rev Cancer, 2006. 6(4): p. 292-306.
[8] Weinberg, R.A., How cancer arises. Sci Am, 1996. 275(3): p. 62-70.
[9] Bianco, R., et al., Key cancer cell signal transduction pathways as therapeutic targets. Eur J Cancer, 2006. 42(3): p. 290-4.

[10] Baserga, R., The insulin-like growth factor I receptor: a key to tumor growth? Cancer Res, 1995. 55(2): p. 249-52.

[11] Sell, C., R. Baserga, and R. Rubin, Insulin-like growth factor I (IGF-I) and the IGF-I receptor prevent etoposide-induced apoptosis. Cancer Res, 1995. 55(2): p. 303-6.

[12] Sell, C., et al., Simian virus 40 large tumor antigen is unable to transform mouse embryonic fibroblasts lacking type 1 insulin-like growth factor receptor. Proc Natl Acad Sci U S A, 1993. 90(23): p. 11217-21.

[13] Abe, S., et al., Increased expression of insulin-like growth factor i is associated with Ara-C resistance in leukemia. Tohoku J Exp Med, 2006. 209(3): p. 217-28.

[14] Wan, X. and L.J. Helman, Effect of insulin-like growth factor II on protecting myoblast cells against cisplatin-induced apoptosis through p70 S6 kinase pathway. Neoplasia, 2002. 4(5): p. 400-8.

[15] Wiseman, L.R., et al., Type I IGF receptor and acquired tamoxifen resistance in oestrogen-responsive human breast cancer cells. Eur J Cancer, 1993. 29A(16): p. 2256-64.

[16] Chan, J.M., et al., Plasma insulin-like growth factor-I and prostate cancer risk: a prospective study. Science, 1998. 279(5350): p. 563-6.

[17] Hankinson, S.E., et al., Circulating concentrations of insulin-like growth factor-I and risk of breast cancer. Lancet, 1998. 351(9113): p. 1393-6.

[18] Ma, J., et al., Prospective study of colorectal cancer risk in men and plasma levels of insulin-like growth factor (IGF)-I and IGF-binding protein-3. J Natl Cancer Inst, 1999. 91(7): p. 620-5.

[19] Yu, H., et al., Plasma levels of insulin-like growth factor-I and lung cancer risk: a case-control analysis. J Natl Cancer Inst, 1999. 91(2): p. 151-6.

[20] Baserga, R., Targeting the IGF-1 receptor: from rags to riches. Eur J Cancer, 2004. 40(14): p. 2013-5.

[21] Scartozzi M, B.M., Maccaroni E, Giampieri R, Del Prete M, Berardi R, Cascinu S, State of the art and future perspectives for the use of insulin-like growth factor receptor 1 (IGF-1R) targeted treatment strategies in solid tumors. Discov Medicine, 2011. 57: p. 144-53.

[22] Ullrich, A., et al., Insulin-like growth factor I receptor primary structure: comparison with insulin receptor suggests structural determinants that define functional specificity. Embo J, 1986. 5(10): p. 2503-12.

[23] Butler, A.A., et al., Insulin-like growth factor-I receptor signal transduction: at the interface between physiology and cell biology. Comp Biochem Physiol B Biochem Mol Biol, 1998. 121(1): p. 19-26.

[24] Samani, A.A. and P. Brodt, The receptor for the type I insulin-like growth factor and its ligands regulate multiple cellular functions that impact on metastasis. Surg Oncol Clin N Am, 2001. 10(2): p. 289-312, viii.

[25] Laustsen, P.G., et al., Essential role of insulin and insulin-like growth factor 1 receptor signaling in cardiac development and function. Mol Cell Biol, 2007. 27(5): p. 1649-64.

[26] Liu, J.P., et al., Mice carrying null mutations of the genes encoding insulin-like growth factor I (Igf-1) and type 1 IGF receptor (Igf1r). Cell, 1993. 75(1): p. 59-72.

[27] Russo, V.C., et al., The insulin-like growth factor system and its pleiotropic functions in brain. Endocr Rev, 2005. 26(7): p. 916-43.

[28] LeRoith, D., et al., Molecular and cellular aspects of the insulin-like growth factor I receptor. Endocr Rev, 1995. 16(2): p. 143-63.

[29] Ferry, R.J., Jr., R.W. Cerri, and P. Cohen, Insulin-like growth factor binding proteins: new proteins, new functions. Horm Res, 1999. 51(2): p. 53-67.
[30] Kelijman, M., Age-related alterations of the growth hormone/insulin-like-growth-factor I axis. J Am Geriatr Soc, 1991. 39(3): p. 295-307.
[31] MacDonald, R.G., et al., A single receptor binds both insulin-like growth factor II and mannose-6-phosphate. Science, 1988. 239(4844): p. 1134-7.
[32] Clemmons, D.R., Role of insulin-like growth factor binding proteins in controlling IGF actions. Mol Cell Endocrinol, 1998. 140(1-2): p. 19-24.
[33] Rosen, O.M., After insulin binds. Science, 1987. 237(4821): p. 1452-8.
[34] Steele-Perkins, G., et al., Expression and characterization of a functional human insulin-like growth factor I receptor. J Biol Chem, 1988. 263(23): p. 11486-92.
[35] Baserga, R., F. Peruzzi, and K. Reiss, The IGF-1 receptor in cancer biology. Int J Cancer, 2003. 107(6): p. 873-7.
[36] Gydee, H., et al., Differentiated thyroid carcinomas from children and adolescents express IGF-I and the IGF-I receptor (IGF-I-R). Cancers with the most intense IGF-I-R expression may be more aggressive. Pediatr Res, 2004. 55(4): p. 709-15.
[37] Maiorano, E., et al., Insulin-like growth factor 1 expression in thyroid tumors. Appl Immunohistochem Mol Morphol, 2000. 8(2): p. 110-9.
[38] Yashiro, T., et al., Expression of insulin-like growth factor receptors in primary human thyroid neoplasms. Acta Endocrinol (Copenh), 1989. 121(1): p. 112-20.
[39] Kornprat, P., et al., Expression of IGF-I, IGF-II, and IGF-IR in gallbladder carcinoma. A systematic analysis including primary and corresponding metastatic tumours. J Clin Pathol, 2006. 59(2): p. 202-6.
[40] Parker, A.S., et al., High expression levels of insulin-like growth factor-I receptor predict poor survival among women with clear-cell renal cell carcinomas. Hum Pathol, 2002. 33(8): p. 801-5.
[41] Burikhanov, R., et al., Thyrotropin via cyclic AMP induces insulin receptor expression and insulin Co-stimulation of growth and amplifies insulin and insulin-like growth factor signaling pathways in dog thyroid epithelial cells. J Biol Chem, 1996. 271(46): p. 29400-6.
[42] Deleu, S., et al., IGF-1 or insulin, and the TSH cyclic AMP cascade separately control dog and human thyroid cell growth and DNA synthesis, and complement each other in inducing mitogenesis. Mol Cell Endocrinol, 1999. 149(1-2): p. 41-51.
[43] Van Keymeulen, A., J.E. Dumont, and P.P. Roger, TSH induces insulin receptors that mediate insulin costimulation of growth in normal human thyroid cells. Biochem Biophys Res Commun, 2000. 279(1): p. 202-7.
[44] Eggo, M.C., L.K. Bachrach, and G.N. Burrow, Interaction of TSH, insulin and insulin-like growth factors in regulating thyroid growth and function. Growth Factors, 1990. 2(2-3): p. 99-109.
[45] Williams, D.W., E.D. Williams, and D. Wynford-Thomas, Evidence for autocrine production of IGF-1 in human thyroid adenomas. Mol Cell Endocrinol, 1989. 61(1): p. 139-43.
[46] Schillaci, R., et al., Autocrine/paracrine involvement of insulin-like growth factor-I and its receptor in chronic lymphocytic leukaemia. Br J Haematol, 2005. 130(1): p. 58-66.
[47] Vella, V., et al., A novel autocrine loop involving IGF-II and the insulin receptor isoform-A stimulates growth of thyroid cancer. J Clin Endocrinol Metab, 2002. 87(1): p. 245-54.

[48] Zhang, H. and D. Yee, The therapeutic potential of agents targeting the type I insulin-like growth factor receptor. Expert Opin Investig Drugs, 2004. 13(12): p. 1569-77.
[49] Burtrum, D., et al., A fully human monoclonal antibody to the insulin-like growth factor I receptor blocks ligand-dependent signaling and inhibits human tumor growth in vivo. Cancer Res, 2003. 63(24): p. 8912-21.
[50] Mitsiades, C.S., et al., Inhibition of the insulin-like growth factor receptor-1 tyrosine kinase activity as a therapeutic strategy for multiple myeloma, other hematologic malignancies, and solid tumors. Cancer Cell, 2004. 5(3): p. 221-30.
[51] Warshamana-Greene, G.S., et al., The insulin-like growth factor-I receptor kinase inhibitor, NVP-ADW742, sensitizes small cell lung cancer cell lines to the effects of chemotherapy. Clin Cancer Res, 2005. 11(4): p. 1563-71.
[52] Maloney, E.K., et al., An anti-insulin-like growth factor I receptor antibody that is a potent inhibitor of cancer cell proliferation. Cancer Res, 2003. 63(16): p. 5073-83.
[53] Garcia-Echeverria, C., et al., In vivo antitumor activity of NVP-AEW541-A novel, potent, and selective inhibitor of the IGF-IR kinase. Cancer Cell, 2004. 5(3): p. 231-9.
[54] Scotlandi, K., et al., Antitumor activity of the insulin-like growth factor-I receptor kinase inhibitor NVP-AEW541 in musculoskeletal tumors. Cancer Res, 2005. 65(9): p. 3868-76.
[55] Benini, S., et al., Inhibition of insulin-like growth factor I receptor increases the antitumor activity of doxorubicin and vincristine against Ewing's sarcoma cells. Clin Cancer Res, 2001. 7(6): p. 1790-7.
[56] Cohen, B.D., et al., Combination therapy enhances the inhibition of tumor growth with the fully human anti-type 1 insulin-like growth factor receptor monoclonal antibody CP-751,871. Clin Cancer Res, 2005. 11(5): p. 2063-73.
[57] Girnita, A., et al., Cyclolignans as inhibitors of the insulin-like growth factor-1 receptor and malignant cell growth. Cancer Res, 2004. 64(1): p. 236-42.
[58] Goetsch, L., et al., A recombinant humanized anti-insulin-like growth factor receptor type I antibody (h7C10) enhances the antitumor activity of vinorelbine and anti-epidermal growth factor receptor therapy against human cancer xenografts. Int J Cancer, 2005. 113(2): p. 316-28.
[59] Bible KC, S.V., Molina JR, Smallridge RC, Maples WJ, Menefee ME, Rubin J, Sideras K, Morris JC 3rd, McIver B, Burton JK, Webster KP, Bieber C, Traynor AM, Flynn PJ, Goh BC, Tang H, Ivy SP, Erlichman C, Efficacy of pazopanib in progressive, radioiodine-refractory, metastatic differentiated thyroid cancers: results of a phase 2 consortium study. Lancet Oncol., 2010. 11(10): p. 962-72.
[60] Broutin, S., et al., Identification of soluble candidate biomarkers of therapeutic response to sunitinib in medullary thyroid carcinoma in preclinical models. Clin Cancer Res, 2011. 17(7): p. 2044-54.
[61] Carr, L.L., et al., Phase II study of daily sunitinib in FDG-PET-positive, iodine-refractory differentiated thyroid cancer and metastatic medullary carcinoma of the thyroid with functional imaging correlation. Clin Cancer Res, 2010. 16(21): p. 5260-8.
[62] Cohen, E.E., et al., Axitinib is an active treatment for all histologic subtypes of advanced thyroid cancer: results from a phase II study. J Clin Oncol, 2008. 26(29): p. 4708-13.
[63] Duntas, L.H. and R. Bernardini, Sorafenib: rays of hope in thyroid cancer. Thyroid, 2010. 20(12): p. 1351-8.
[64] Ha, H.T., et al., A phase II study of imatinib in patients with advanced anaplastic thyroid cancer. Thyroid, 2010. 20(9): p. 975-80.

[65] Kapiteijn, E., et al., New treatment modalities in advanced thyroid cancer. Ann Oncol, 2011.

[66] Lam, E.T., et al., Phase II clinical trial of sorafenib in metastatic medullary thyroid cancer. J Clin Oncol, 2010. 28(14): p. 2323-30.

[67] Pennell, N.A., et al., A phase II study of gefitinib in patients with advanced thyroid cancer. Thyroid, 2008. 18(3): p. 317-23.

[68] Robinson BG, P.-A.L., Krebs A, Vasselli J, Haddad R., Vandetanib (100 mg) in patients with locally advanced or metastatic hereditary medullary thyroid cancer. J Clin Endocrinol Metab., 2010. 95(6): p. 2664-71.

[69] Rosen, L.S., et al., Safety, pharmacokinetics, and efficacy of AMG 706, an oral multikinase inhibitor, in patients with advanced solid tumors. J Clin Oncol, 2007. 25(17): p. 2369-76.

[70] Wells SA, J., Gosnell JE, Gagel RF, Moley J, Pfister D, Sosa JA, Skinner M, Krebs A, Vasselli J, and Schlumberger, M., Vandetanib for the treatment of patients with locally advanced or metastatic hereditary medullary thyroid cancer. J Clin Oncol, 2010. 28 p. 767-772.

[71] Han, R.N., et al., Insulin-like growth factor-I receptor-mediated vasculogenesis/angiogenesis in human lung development. Am J Respir Cell Mol Biol, 2003. 28(2): p. 159-69.

[72] Delafontaine, P., Y.H. Song, and Y. Li, Expression, regulation, and function of IGF-1, IGF-1R, and IGF-1 binding proteins in blood vessels. Arterioscler Thromb Vasc Biol, 2004. 24(3): p. 435-44.

[73] Zhang, D., A.A. Samani, and P. Brodt, The role of the IGF-I receptor in the regulation of matrix metalloproteinases, tumor invasion and metastasis. Horm Metab Res, 2003. 35(11-12): p. 802-8.

[74] Hakam, A., et al., Expression of insulin-like growth factor-1 receptor in human colorectal cancer. Hum Pathol, 1999. 30(10): p. 1128-33.

[75] Akagi, Y., et al., Regulation of vascular endothelial growth factor expression in human colon cancer by insulin-like growth factor-I. Cancer Res, 1998. 58(17): p. 4008-14.

[76] Reinmuth, N., et al., Blockade of insulin-like growth factor I receptor function inhibits growth and angiogenesis of colon cancer. Clin Cancer Res, 2002. 8(10): p. 3259-69.

5

Principles and Application of Microarray Technology in Thyroid Cancer Research

Walter Pulverer, Christa Noehammer,
Klemens Vierlinger and Andreas Weinhaeusel
Austrian Institute of Technology GmbH
Health &Environment Department, Molecular Medicine
Vienna,
Austria

1. Introduction

In recent decades, ongoing development of microarrays and microarray platforms has revolutionized biological research. Especially in cancer research, microarray technology has brought forth many new insights and has been widely applied for the elucidation of biological interrelations, effects, pathways and aetiology of cancers such as thyroid cancer (Kundel et al., 2010; Williams et al., 2011; Rousset et al., 2011; Cheng et al., 2011; Vierlinger et al., 2011). Microarrays have initiated a new era of research for scientists, with new challenges. Moreover, these assays have contributed to the elucidation of potential therapeutic targets for drug development, and elucidate biomarker candidates for improving diagnostics. Therefore microarrays will help to improve therapy and to enable personalized medicine.

We start this chapter by summarizing the flow of information from DNA to protein, and discussing points of interest for cancer research and cancer diagnostics.

The biological information of all eukaryotic organisms is stored in the DNA, which is arranged in chromosomes to achieve a compact structure. The DNA offers multiple points of interest for cancer research. These comprise on the one hand sequence based variations including structural and copy number variations, and on the other hand epigenetic variations, which have a regulatory effect on gene expression, without causing any changes to the DNA sequence (Bird, 2007). In this chapter, we focus mainly on points of interest which can be experimentally examined and analyzed by microarray technology. Therefore, microarrays detecting sequence variations (SNP arrays) as well as copy number alterations (array CGH) and DNA methylation will be discussed. There are also microarrays for histone acetylation studies based on chromatin immunoprecipitation (ChIP), where the fragmented (by sonication or enzyme digestion) chromatin is precipitated by specific antibodies and the DNA-precipitate is hybridized then onto microarrays (chips). Thus this technique is called "ChIP on chip" and used to identify DNA sequences within chromatin regions having bound modified histones. ChIP on chip technology is the method of choice for the investigation of histone modifications - which are major players of epigenetic regulatory mechanisms of gene expression, together with DNA methylation (Collas, 2010; Russo et al., 2011). This method is also useful for studying (non-epigenetic) gene regulation, but we are not going to discuss that technology in detail in this chapter and would refer the reader to a review on "The current state of chromatin immunoprecipitation" written by Philippe Collas (Collas, 2010). Also, Russo et al., in a recently published paper, reviewed the important role of epigenetic changes in thyroid tumorigenesis (Russo et al., 2011). They summarized epigenetic effects on many genes involved in thyroid carcinogenesis, including those involved in the reduced ability of the tumour to concentrate radioiodine.

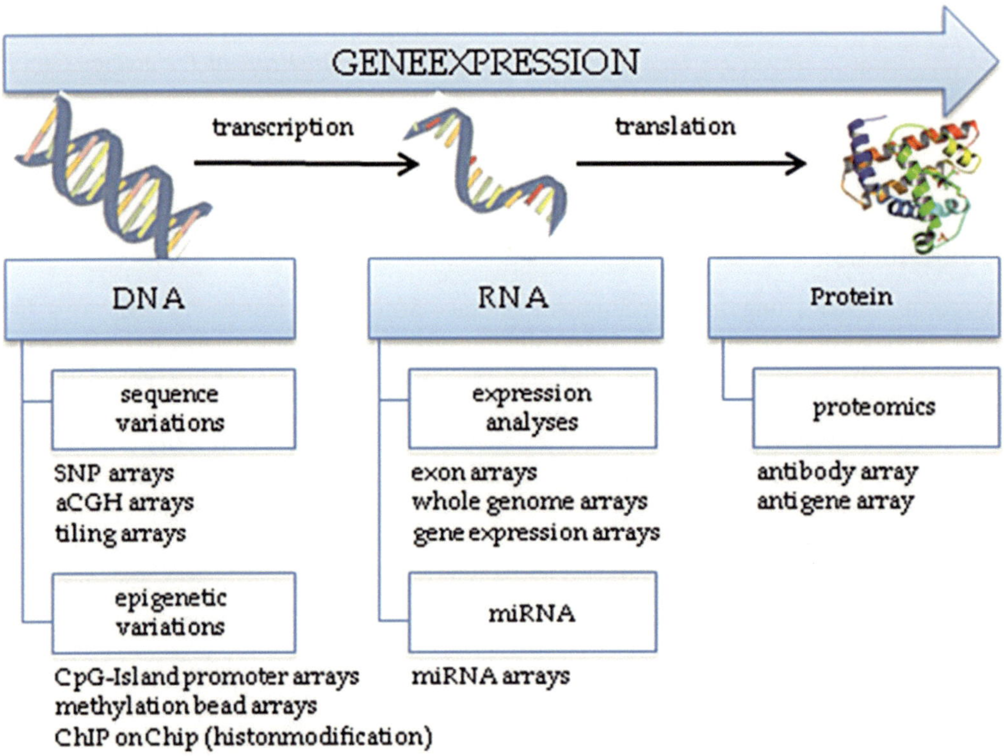

Fig. 1. Microarray applications used in cancer research enabling genomics (DNA), epigenetics (DNA methylation and epigenetic modification), transcriptomics (RNA) and antibody based proteomics (a special application in proteomics).

The most prominent example of microarrays being used in cancer research is gene expression profiling of mRNA, whereby the expression levels of the entire transcriptome can be measured simultaneously. This, however, does not account for post-transcriptional gene silencing which occurs when a small piece of RNA (miRNA) interacts with mature mRNA. The result is a double stranded RNA, which cannot be read by the ribosome, and hence the production of protein is disabled (Fire et al., 1998; Bagasra and Prilliman, 2004; MacRae et al., 2006; MacRae et al., 2007). Dysregulation of miRNAs has been associated with cancer (L. He et al., 2005; Mraz et al., 2009). Mazeh et al., for example elucidated the feasibility of the mir-221 miRNA for the detection of papillary thyroid carcinoma in fine needle aspiration biopsy (FNAB) samples (Mazeh et al., 2011). Another study, performed by

Kitano et al. aimed to evaluate the power of miRNAs for distinguishing papillary from follicular thyroid carcinoma. They elucidated two miRNAs (miR-126 and miR-7) with high diagnostic accuracy (0.81 and 0.77) (Kitano et al., 2011).

Although until now most protein-based studies are done by mass spectrometry, protein-microarrays offer highly multiplexed analyses of protein abundance, as well as identification of tumour autoantibodies. Tumour antibodies are produced as a result of a humoral immune response to antigens of the tumour itself (Tan et al., 2009). On microarrays we can either immobilize the antigens, to detect tumour specific antibodies in the sample, or we can immobilize antibodies on the microarray, to identify the antigens or proteins and their modification within a sample.

In the following sections of this chapter, we will discuss the general principles of microarray technology as wells as commercially available platforms used in connection with thyroid cancer research.

2. The development of the microarray technology

The most prominent and most commonly used molecules in microarray technology are nucleic acids (DNA and RNA). In 1953, Watson and Crick laid the cornerstone for microarray technology by their description of the DNA double helix (Watson and Crick, 1953). Further knowledge of DNA in biological as well as technical contexts was obtained soon after, as it was found out that the DNA could be separated by heat or alkali treatment (cavalieri et al., 1962; Uhlenhopp and Krasna, 1969). The overall main principle of DNA hybridization is based on denaturation and the corresponding reverse process, renaturation. Renaturation processes were first described by Marmur and Doty and are highly specific under proper conditions (Marmur and Doty, 1961). Analysis of nucleic acids by hybridization has been a key method since the early 1960s. Another cornerstone for improving DNA-hybridization was established in the 70's by Ed Southern (Southern, 1975), who introduced the pioneering technology of Southern blotting. This method combines the separation of DNA based on fragment length by electrophoresis with subsequent hybridization of a probe for the specific detection of DNA fragments. A few years later, scientists developed a technology in which they immobilized known molecules on a nitrocellulose membrane or glass plate (Bains and Smith, 1988; Drmanac et al., 1989; Khrapko et al., 1989). One of the first scientists, using such membranes with high feature density was Jörg Hoheisel (Hoheisel et al., 1994). It was also Hoheisel who increased the feature density on the surfaces by the simple replacement of manual procedures by robotics for the production of the so-called macroarrays. That invention took the technology a substantial step further, as it not only increased the feature density, but also removed human errors and made the microarray technology reproducible and accurate (Wheelan et al., 2008).

The term microarray was first introduced by Schena et al. (Schena et al., 1995) in 1995 and the first genome of an eukaryotic species completely investigated (Saccharomyces cerevisiae) by a microarray was published in 1997 (Lashkari et al., 1997). In the last few years, further improvements were made especially when substituting the immobilized DNA-probes derived from clone-libraries by chemically synthesized oligonucleotides. These improvements were possible after elucidation of entire genomes by large consortia projects, like the Human

Genome project. The sequence information from these projects laid the groundwork for generations of arrays covering entire genomes and transcriptomes which are available today. Some of the commercially available arrays cover genomes at a density of several hundred thousands and even millions of features which can be analysed in parallel in a single experiment. With the growing number of microarray applications and cost reductions, publications using microarray technologies in thyroid cancer research as well as in life sciences increased enormously in recent years (Figure 3). Yet, the applications and answerable questions of microarrays are still growing and have become a standard in all areas of life sciences.

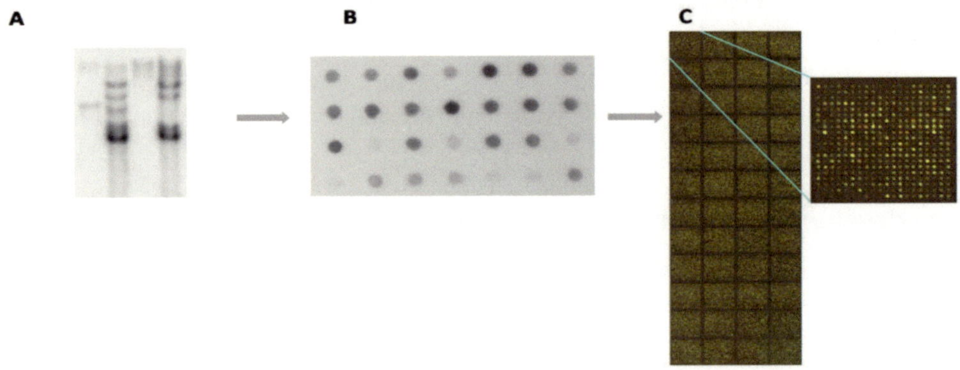

Fig. 2. Development (upscaling and simultaneous miniaturization) of molecular hybridization techniques: (A) Southern Blot, (B) dot blot, (C) microarray.

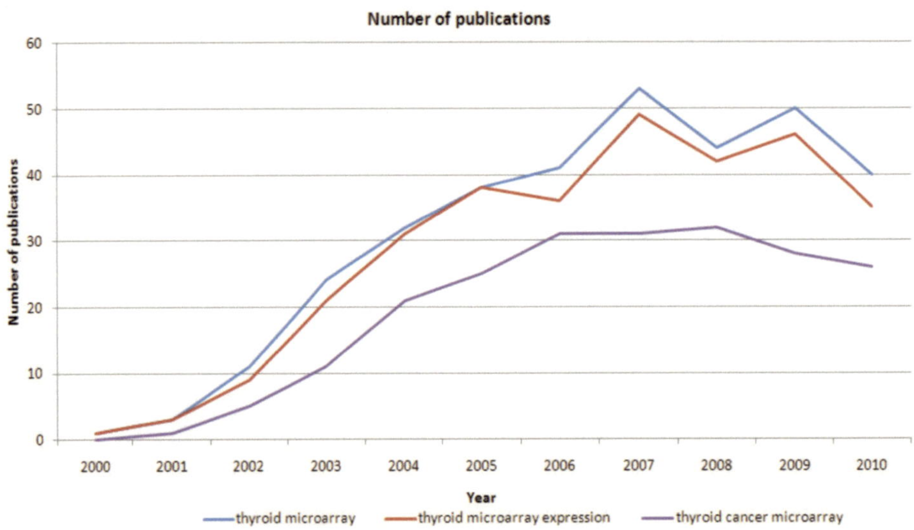

Fig. 3. Number of published papers in the National Center for Biotechnology Information (NCBI) database (www.ncbi.nlm.nih.gov).

3. Principles of microarray analyses

The collective term "microarray" describes a state-of-the-art technology in molecular biology which allows high-throughput and highly parallel analyses of up to several thousand points of interest (e.g. genes, mRNA, proteins). With some platforms, up to several hundred thousands of parallel measures (Sandoval et al., 2011) using nanogram amounts of sample material can be produced in one experiment. Parallel to the increase in throughput, quality also increased due to technical improvements of the array production process and molecular methods for labelling (Leung and Cavalieri, 2003; Priness et al., 2007; Thirlwell et al., 2010; Karakach et al., 2010; McCall et al., 2011).

The microarray itself consists of a carrier material. A very common, easy to handle surface is glass. The surfaces of the glass slides are usually modified with different reactive molecules (e.g. aldehyde or epoxy groups) onto which the biomolecules (probes) can be immobilized. These probes are either printed on the surfaces using microarray-spotters or directly synthesized using automated synthesizers (the reactive area between spots has to be blocked before starting hybridization of the targets). The latter process is used by several commercial microarray providers and enables production of high density array. Most microarray formats are of the size of a standard microscopic slide and can be easily handled. This allows the processing of many samples per assay and results in the generation of a high amount of data (Howbrook et al., 2003; Karakach et al., 2010).

An overview of the necessary experimental steps is given in Figure 4. Although different types of biomolecules and different strategies are used to generate microarray-data, the technical workflows are almost identical. The key event in the microarray-processing is the interaction between a probe (e.g. oligonucleotide) immobilized on the surface of the array and the target (e.g. fluorescent-labelled DNA). The immobilized molecules on the surfaces are referred to as probes, whereas the molecules which are being detected upon hybridization and binding towards the probes are called targets (Wheelan et al., 2008).

Every microarray study starts with the isolation of the respective targets (e.g. DNA or RNA). In principle nucleic acids are isolated upon cell disruption by mechanical or enzymatic methods and precipitated at increased salt concentrations or ethanol. State of the art methods use selective binding onto silicamembranes or silica coated magnetic beads at high salt or ethanol concentrations, proteins are washed off and nucleic acids are eluted from the silica-resins using water or low salt buffers (e.g. 10mM Tris.Cl, pH 8). The next step is labelling of the molecules with fluorescent dyes; for that step various methods exist. Often the labelling step is done during the enzymatic amplification reaction at which fluorescently labelled nucleotides or primers are incorporated into the newly synthesized amplicons (Schaferling and Nagl, 2006). Nowadays a broad range of fluorescent dyes with different absorption and excitation wavelengths are available. The different absorption and excitation maxima allow the combination of fluorescent dyes. In microarray analyses the fluorescent dyes Cy3 and Cy5 are widely used (Liang et al., 2003). After purification of the labelled amplicons, these molecules are mixed with a hybridization buffer and are subsequently applied to the microarrays and incubated over night. After the hybridization procedure, unbound molecules have to be washed off before the detection can be done by laser-scanning with dye specific wavelengths. The detection step generates an image of the microarray, which is employed for raw data extraction. Thus fluorescent intensities of each single spot of the microarrays are measured and written in a results file along with the spot coordinates and the specific "gene" identifier. The intensity of the generated signal depends on the amount of molecules (targets), which have bound to the probe-molecules within one spot (also called feature). The last step in a microarray experiment is the bioinformatic analysis of the data of a single slide (as in aCGH; see following chapters) or data from many samples of distinct classes (e.g. n x tumour samples vs. n x normal tissues) processed in parallel within one experiment. Dealing with that high amount of data is very challenging and requires high computer power as well as well established bioinformatics tools for – just to mention a few examples - image acquisition/analysis, normalization, statistical analyses like class prediction and pathway analysis (Leung and Cavalieri, 2003).

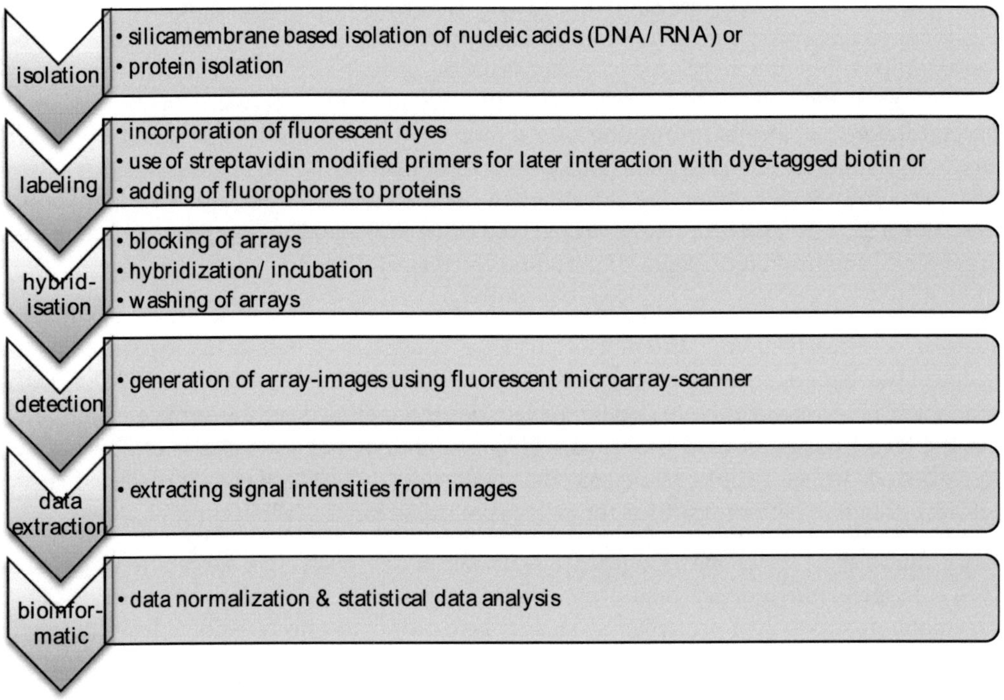

Fig. 4. Overview of the typical steps in a microarray experiment

Experimental strategies of microarray analyses have to be planned carefully to permit the generation of conclusive results. In principle, experiments can be conducted as either single colour or dual colour experiments. As already mentioned the commonly used Cy3 (green - excitation 535nm) and Cy5 (red – excitation 635nm) dyes enable distinct colour separation, thus 2 targets can be hybridized in parallel on a single array. Therefore the combination of both colours can be used for paralleled hybridization of e.g. a tumour-sample (red) and a reference sample (green). These so called two-colour experiments are less error prone. The result is a ratio of the 2 colours, depending on the contribution of sample 1 and sample 2 to the total amount of bound molecules, labelled with different fluorescent dyes (Patterson et al., 2006). Single colour experiments are conducted by using different arrays for every sample and also every reference sample. Both single and dual colour experiments are dependent on the array platform used and the specific experimental aims. These prerequisites have to be taken into account for experimental planning and therefore the interested reader should refer to specialist literature (Simon et al., 2003).

3.1.1 RNA expression microarrays

Analysis of mRNA expression profiles is still one of the most prominent examples in microarray technology. In expression profiling experiments, the mRNA is typically isolated from two samples (e.g. the normal tissue and tumour tissue of one individual) and, subsequently, reverse transcribed in an enzymatic reaction by reverse transcriptase polymerase chain reaction (RT-PCR) to generate complementary DNA (cDNA). The two cDNA samples are fluorescently labelled with different dyes (usually with Cy3, and Cy5). Subsequently the labelled cDNAs are pooled and cohybridized onto the arrays. Finally, dual colour images are generated upon scanning the microarrays (Figure 5) (Schena et al., 1995; Duggan et al., 1999).

Prominent commercially available platforms are Affymetrix, Nimblegen, Agilent and Illumina, with the technology being pioneered by Affymetrix. At the time of writing this article (June 2011), Affymetrix offers five different arrays for expression analyses on human samples and nine for mouse and rat. Affymetrix arrays have been successfully applied in a number of studies on thyroid cancer.

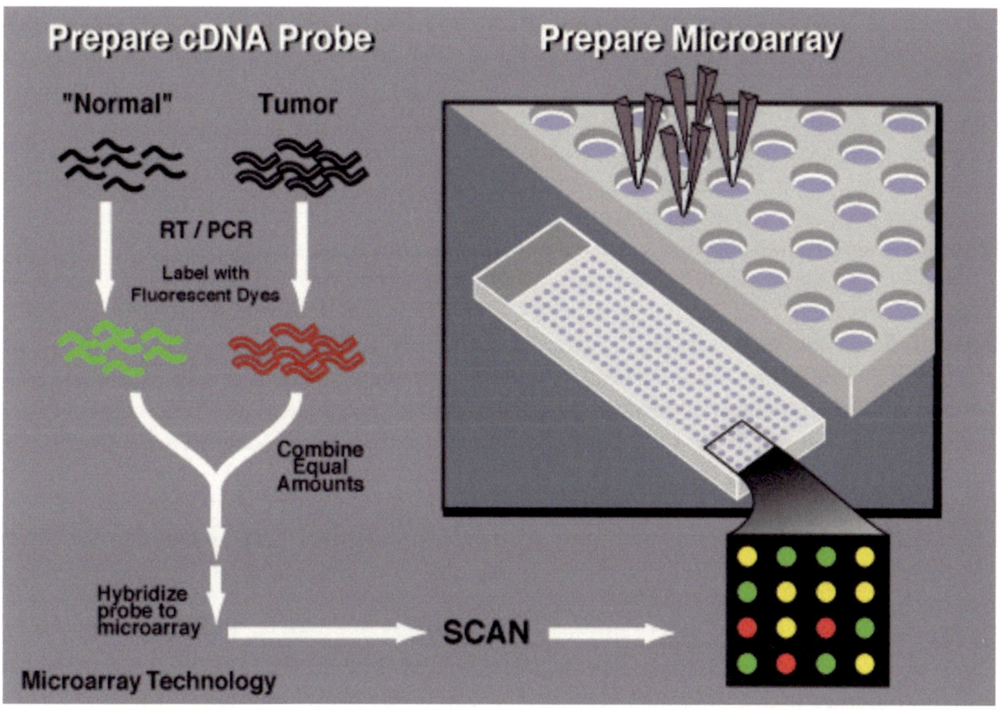

Fig. 5. Overview of a two-colour gene expression experiment. Picture from "National Human Genome Research Institute", Division of Intramural Research http://bioinfoworld.files.wordpress.com/2008/10/microarray_technology.gif?w=480&h=319

3.1.2 RNA expression microarrays in thyroid cancer research

Most research on thyroid cancer utilizing microarrays has been conducted using gene expression microarrays. For thyroid cancer in general, but also for the different subtypes of thyroid cancer, a number of gene expression studies have been performed. In Table 1 we mention some interesting gene expression studies with a high impact on thyroid cancer research. The different studies followed different objectives, such as the elucidation of biological processes involved in cancerogenesis, pathway analysis and defining new diagnostic, prognostic and predictive markers. Barden et al. (Barden et al., 2003) for example, aimed to elucidate differences in the gene expression profile of follicular thyroid adenomas (FTAs) and follicular thyroid carcinomas (FTCs) using Affymetrix chips (GeneChip Hu95 array). Their main result described a gene list containing 105 genes with different expression profiles between the two thyroid nodules. With those genes they were able to classify five follicular tumours correctly, which had an undisclosed final diagnosis. In 2004, Finley et al. (Finley et al., 2004) subjected different thyroid nodules to gene expression profiling with Affymetrix's U95 GeneChip with the objective of creating gene lists capable of distinguishing between malignant and benign cases. Their analysis was able to classify the 62 utilized samples into the malignant and benign groups with high sensitivity and high specificity. Gene expression profiling has not only confirmed known thyroid cancer associated genes, but also revealed genes which until now have not been known to be associatied with thyroid cancer. Mazzanti et al. (Mazzanti et al., 2004) tried to discriminate between benign and malignant thyroid tumours by using fine needle aspirations (FNA). They were able to set up a gene list with high discrimination power (87.1% accuracy; 12.9% error rate) between benign and malignant thyroid nodules. Translating these findings into routine clinical practice could improve the accuracy of diagnosis and hence patient care. With the increasing use of FNAs, Kundel et al. in 2010 (Kundel et al., 2010) investigated the usability of FNAs compared to tissue specimens in microarray experiments, utilizing the U133 GeneChip from Affymetrix. They concluded that FNAs are a good alternative to tissue specimens, as clustering analysis could pair together the concordant pairs with perfect sensitivity and specificity. In 2005, Eszlinger et al. (Eszlinger et al., 2005) used Affymetrix Gene Chips to demonstrate that RAS-MAPK signalling does not contribute to cold thyroid nodules (CTN), which was in question for that subtype of thyroid cancer. In addition, this study described 31 differentially regulated genes between CTN and the surrounding tissue. Lacroix et al. (Lacroix et al., 2005) and Giordano et al. (Giordano et al., 2006) investigated whether a subset of FTCs with a PAX8/PPARG translocation possess a unique gene expression profile compared to other thyroid tumours. While Lacroix et al. used a custom array system from Agilent; Giordano et al. used the Affymetrix U133A GeneChip. Both studies revealed a distinct gene expression profile of FTCs with the PAX8/PPARG translocation. Lacroix et al. defined a list of 93 genes which also included non-thyroid-specific genes and Giordano et al. described four genes (ANGPTL4, AQP7, ENO3, PGF) with high translocation association. Finn et al. (Finn et al., 2007b) used a genome wide gene expression microarray system from Applied Biosystems to search for marker to discriminate between PTC and the "follicular variant" of PTC (FVPTC), a subtype of PTC which is difficult to diagnose. They were able to identify 15 new genes (CD14, CD74, CTSC, CTSH, CTSS, DPP6, ETHE1, HLA-A, HLA-DMA, HLADPB1, HLA-DQB1, HLA-DRA, OSTF1, TDO2 and 1 uncharacterized/unnamed gene) which were associated with FVPTC and a narrow repertoire of functions of the identified genes.

Since the Chernobyl disaster in 1986, an increased incidence of thyroid carcinomas, especially in the juvenile population has been observed. For this reason, Stein et al. and Kim et al. (among others) performed studies to assess the radiation-induced DNA damage. Stein et al. (Stein et al., 2010) revealed a set of differentially regulated genes in radiation-induced papillary thyroid carcinoma in Chernobyl paediatric patients, and Kim et al. (Kim et al., 2010) tried to define a gene list which could distinguish between papillary thyroid carcinomas and papillary thyroid microcarcinomas (PTM). For that purpose, Kim et al. used Affymetrix's Human Genome U133A Chip, comparing PTCs and PTMs with the corresponding normal tissue counterparts. They elucidated over 200 statistically significant upregulated genes and over 150 downregulated genes in both groups, but they did not find any statistically significant differentially expressed genes when comparing the expression profiles of PTC and PTM. Kim's study demonstrated that a great deal of information from the different groups could be obtained in a simple but well-planned experiment. In a very recent study, Williams et al. (Williams et al., 2011) subjected thyroid nodules to the U133 Affymetrix GeneChip with the aim of setting up gene lists with discriminatory power between aggressive and nonaggressive follicular carcinomas. They revealed three gene lists which discriminated between histologically normal thyroid tissue and follicular neoplasms (421 genes), between FTCs and FTAs (94 genes) and between aggressive FTC and nonaggressive FTC (4 genes; NID2, TM7SF2, TRIM2, and GLTSCR2). Recently Rousset et al. (Rousset et al., 2011) elucidated 19 genes to distinguish between malignant and benign thyroid tumours which can be applied for improved diagnostic testing using molecular methods.

Due to the bulk of publically available data dealing with thyroid cancer, we have used meta-analysis using publically available gene expression data from microarray experiments. A meta-analysis combines the data from different studies and applies statistical methods to remove the bias from the data, which is caused by the different origins (laboratories, array-types, etc.) of the data sets.

Study Author	**Pub date**	**Purpose**	**Result**
Barden et al.	2003	Identification of differentially expressed genes in follicular thyroid carcinomas and adenomas.	105 genes were differentially expressed between FTA and FTC.
Finley et al.	2004	Discrimination between malignant and benign thyroid nodules (PTC, follicular variant of PTC, FTC, FTA and hyperplastic nodules) by gene expression profiling.	627 differentially expressed genes which distinguish between "malignant" and benign with 92% sensitivity and 96% specificity.
Mazzanti et al.	2004	Differentiation between benign and malignant thyroid tumours by fine needle aspiration.	Gene set which discriminates between benign and malignant thyroid carcinomas.
LaCroix et al.	2005	Comparison of the gene expression profile of normal tissue, thyroid adenomas and FTCs with and without the PAX8 and PPARG translocation (PPFP).	A genelist with 93 genes which discriminates between morphologically indistinguishable FTCs with and without the translocation. The list included no thyroid-specific genes.

Study Author	Pub date	Purpose	Result
Eszlinger et al.	2005	Genome wide expression analyses of cold thyroid nodules (CTN) with respect to the RAS-MAPK signalling pathway.	Cell cycle-associated genes show an increased gene-expression in CTN, but no RAS-MAPK signalling in CTNs was found. In addition a list of 31 differentially expressed genes was defined.
Giordano et al.	2006	Elucidation of genes associated with the gene product of the PAX8 and PPARG translocation (PPFP) in a subset of follicular thyroid carcinomas.	The expression of four genes (ANGPTL4, AQP7, ENO3, PGF) was highly associated with the PPFP product.
Finn et al.	2007	Discrimination between PTC and its subtype FVPTC.	Validation of well-known marker and identification of fifteen genes associated with FVPTC.
Kundel et al.	2010	Evaluation of the interchangeable use of thyroid fine needle aspirates and tissue specimen in microarray experiments.	Fine needle aspirates can be used as alternative to tissue samples.
Stein et al.	2010	Investigation of radiation-induced papillary thyroid carcinomas (PTC) induced by the Chernobyl fallout	Elucidation of 141 genes with different expression profiles in radiation-induced PTC.
Kim et al.	2010	Differentiation of PTC from papillary thyroid microcarcinomas (PTM) by gene expression.	No significantly regulated genes between PTC and PTM were found, but they found 200 upregulated and 180 downregulated genes in PTM compared to the normal counterpart tissue, similar changes were also found in PTC compared to the normal counterpart.
Williams et al.	2011	Discrimination between aggressive and nonaggressive follicular carcinomas	Genelists with discriminating power between normal thyroid tissue vs. follicular neoplasms; follicular carcinomas vs. follicular adenomas; aggressive vs. nonaggressive follicular carcinomas.
Rousset et al.	2011	Development of a molecular test based on 19 genes for the identification of malignant and benign thyroid tumours for diagnostics.	-

Table 1. Examples of some thyroid cancer microarray expression studies.

Conventionally, discrimination between benign and malignant thyroid nodules is done by fine needle aspiration biopsy (FNAB) followed by cytological assessment. Thyroid nodules are typically classified by their histology into benign types such as Nodular Goiter (NG) and Follicular Thyroid Adenoma (FTA) and the malignant entities are defined as Follicular Thyroid Carcinoma (FTC), Papillary Thyroid Carcinoma (PTC), Medullary Thyroid Carcinoma (MTC) and Anaplastic Thyroid Carcinoma (ATC). Only approximately 5% - 10% of thyroid nodules are malignant (Mazzaferri, 1992), the majority of which are papillary carcinomas. Despite many advances in the diagnosis and treatment of thyroid nodules and thyroid cancer, conventionally used diagnostic methods have a well-known low specificity (Cooper et al., 2006), resulting in an "indeterminate" or "suspicious" diagnosis in 10%-20% of cases. These patients usually undergo surgery, although the nodules are actually malignant in only 20% of these cases (Chang et al., 1997; Ravetto et al., 2000). This leads to a number of patients treated unnecessarily for malignant disease. Accordingly, we therefore followed the approach of using microarray gene expression profiles to obtain a diagnostic gene signature, with the potential of allowing a precise and reliable diagnosis from fine needle aspirates in the future. Before starting our own gene expression experiments in the lab by applying 44k whole genome arrays we used publically available microarray data sets from four studies (Huang et al., 2001; Jarzab et al., 2005; H. He et al., 2005) on PTC and applied an adopted meta-analysis approach. The methodology included bias removal between the four different studies using distance weighted discrimination (DWD) (Benito et al., 2004) (Figure 6).

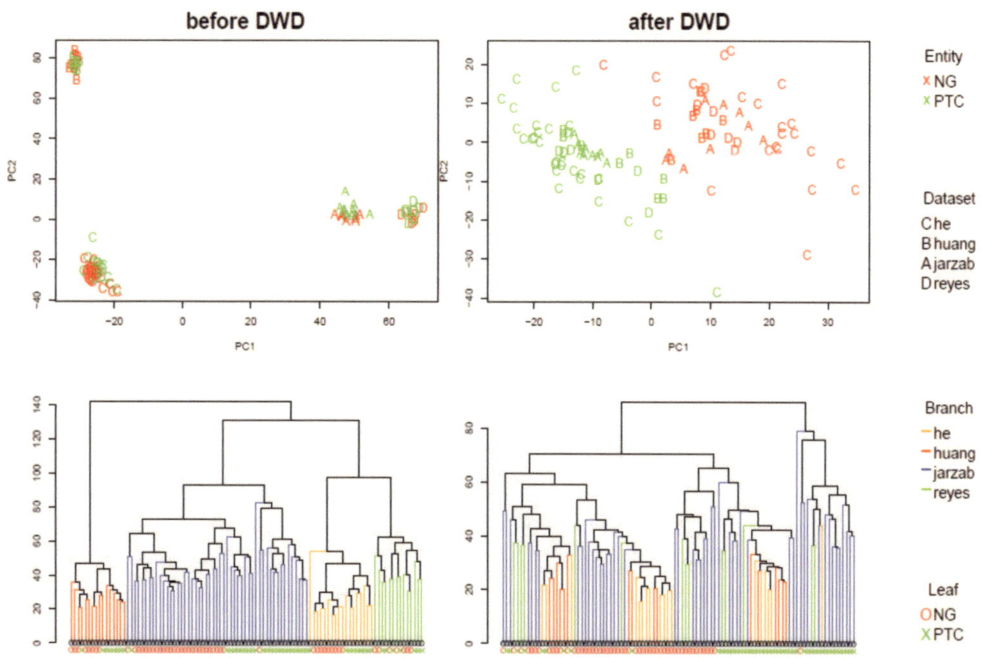

Fig. 6. DWD integration. The effect of DWD on the first two principal components (PC) and hierarchical clustering of the data. DWD was able to remove the separation between the datasets as indicated by the PC-plots and by the mixing of the branches in the dendrogram. The PC plots show that biological information is preserved after DWD integration (Samples cluster by dataset before integration and by tumour entity thereafter). Leaves in the dendrogram are coloured by tumour entity and branches are coloured according to dataset.

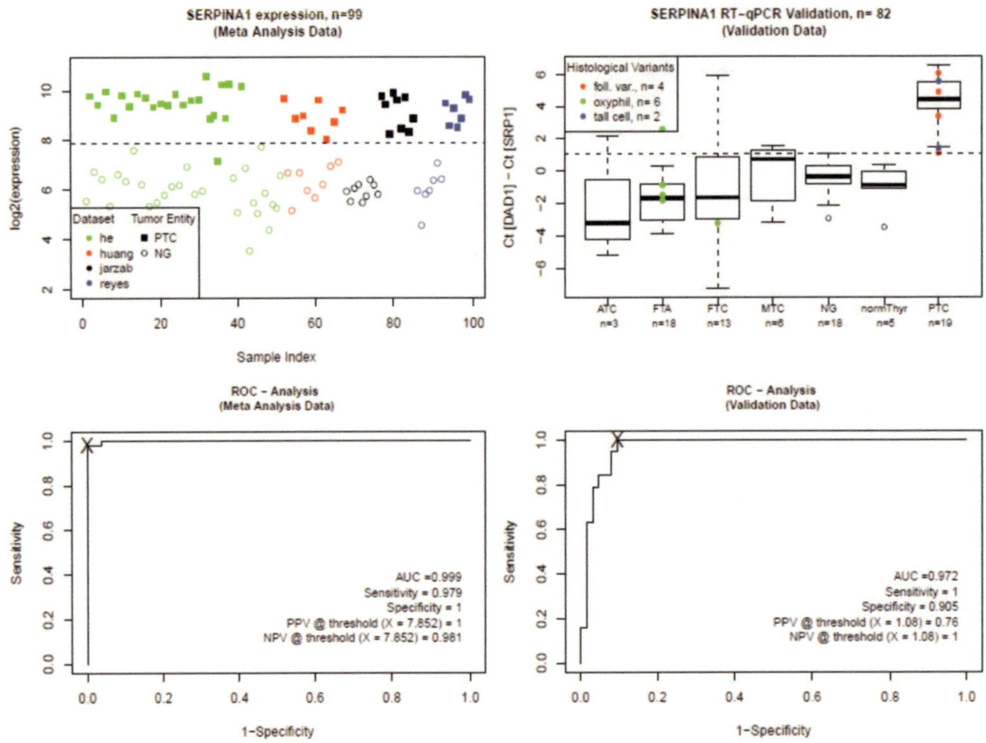

Fig. 7. SERPINA1 expression. Expression values and receiver-operating-characteristics (ROC) analysis of the SERPINA1 gene in the meta-analysis data (left) and the real-time (RT)-qPCR independent validation data (right). Classification thresholds were chosen from ROC analysis (shown as 'X' in the ROC plots). Positive Predictive Values (PPV) were calculated as number of true positives/number of all positives, Negative Predictive Values (NPV) as number of true negatives/ number of all negatives, both at the chosen threshold.

From this meta-analysis, we could identify a one-gene classifier (SERPINA1) for PTC (Vierlinger et al., 2011). Identification of papillary thyroid disease was further validated by rigorous study-crossvalidation, where the classification of papillary thyroid disease with SERPINA 1 as a single marker was achieved with 99% accuracy in leave-one-out crossvalidation and 93% accuracy by external real-time PCR validation using a data set generated in our own laboratory. In the latter dataset we analysed 82 thyroid samples from different entities: PTC (n=19), NG (n=18), FTC (n=13), FTA (n=18), ATC (n=3), MTC (n=6) and normal thyroid tissue (n=5) and tested for the discriminative power of SERPINA1. Figure 7 shows the signal intensities and ROC plots of the SERPINA1 probe across the different entities in the meta-analysis data and our real-time PCR validation.

Encouraged by the results from our meta-analysis on papillary carcinoma, which indicated a huge potential for future diagnostic applications, we performed microarray analysis on 49 N_2-frozen thyroid tumours in our laboratory from all major histological entities using Agilent 44k whole genome microarrays. From these data, we successfully selected features which had, in combination, a high discriminative power between (1) benign and malignant nodules and (2) follicular adenoma and follicular carcinoma. These two sets of features (20 genes for malignancy and 23 genes for the follicular classification task) were then tested on independent published datasets using leave-one-out crossvalidation (nearest shrunken centroid classification). We successfully tested the genes for classification task 1 (malignancy) on a total of 246 samples from eight different studies with an accuracy of 92% (19 misclassified) and the genes for classification task 2 (FTC vs. FTA) on 60 samples from three studies with an accuracy of 98% (one sample misclassified).

3.2.1 aCGH

Array comparative genomic hybridization (aCGH) is a method to detect copy number alterations in a genome (Shinawi and Cheung, 2008). The aCGH technology is an alternative of comparative/chromosomal genomic hybridization, which is a cytogenetic method to detect copy number variations in DNA (Cheung et al., 2005).

The process employs a test (e.g. cancerous tissue) DNA and a normal reference DNA. Those DNA samples are labelled with two different fluorescent dyes and are subsequently hybridized to the microarray. The result is a colour ratio of the two samples, of which copy number changes (gain or loss) can be detected along all the chromosomes (Figure 8). Early CGH based methods used entire chromosomes which were painted (using in principle fluorescent in situ hybridization - FISH techniques) - and colour ratios measured along the chromosomes. These methods had several limitations, like a low optical resolution, compared to the modern microarray based approaches. To detect single copy losses within a genome, the losses had to be at least 5-10 Mb in length. On array platforms, copy number variations of 5-10 Kb can be detected. Today, there are high-resolution arrays available which allow for the detection of copy number variations as small as 200 bp (Urban et al., 2006). Therefore, even the detection of microdeletions and duplications in different diseases (e.g. cancer) is possible.

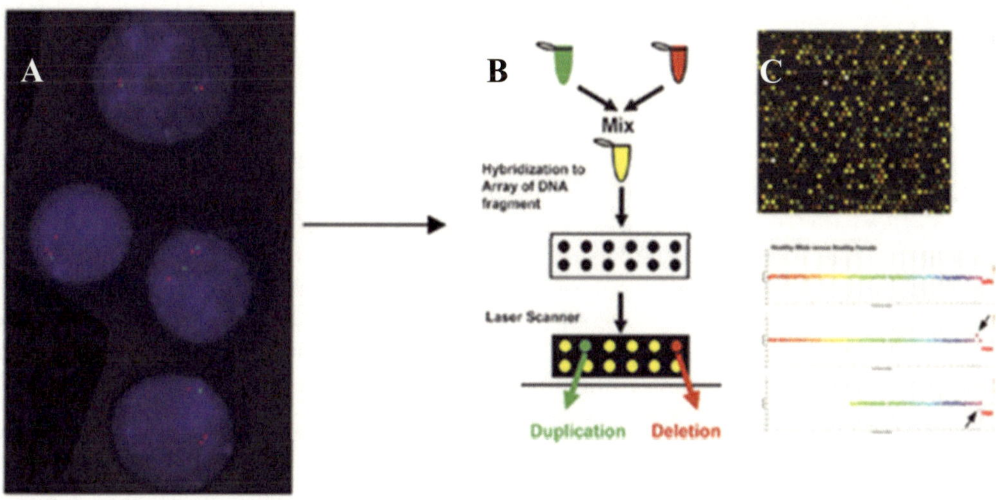

Fig. 8. (A) Cytogenetic method: Interphase FISH, (B) the principle of array CGH, (C) hybridized and scanned array. Adopted after Shinawi et al. „The aCGH and its clinical applications".

3.2.2 aCGH applications in thyroid cancer

In 2007, Rodriguez et al. (Rodrigues et al., 2007) screened for copy number variations within aneuploid PTC. They found copy number gains as well as losses in all analyzed samples. Nine gains in DNA copy number occurred in at least 50% of the analyzed cases, and the most frequent gain in the 5q region was determined in over 70% of cases followed by gains of 7p, 7q and 12q in 65% of the carcinomas. The degree of copy number losses was much lower than the gains, and fewer samples were affected by those losses. Only one loss (9q) occurred in more than 50% of the cases and five losses (1p, 9q, 22q, 11q, 13q) were found in 35–50% of the samples. Finn et al. (Finn et al., 2007a) investigated copy number gains and losses in PTC, where they found that chromosomal imbalances are more frequent than previously assumed, and that a gain in PDGFB alone was seen in tumours free of the BRAF mutation (the BRAF mutation had been identified as contributing to sporadic PTC). Finn et al. correlated the over expression of FGF4 and PDGF with a gain in copy numbers. But also in ATCs copy number changes were identified. Lee et al. (Lee et al., 2008) investigated ATCs in aCGH studies and also found copy number changes in all his analysed ATCs, especially in the genes CCND1 and UBCH10; a characteristic of ATC is the overexpression the CCND1 gene product, which is due to a gain in copy number. The previously mentioned study by Stein et al. (Stein et al., 2010) in addition to expression analyses, also employed aCGH analyses to examine the genomic effects of radiation from Chernobyl disaster. They were able to detect a number of regions with copy number alterations, including regions which had never before been associated with PTCs and are therefore unique to radiation-induced PTCs. They also came to the conclusion that gains are more frequent than deletions.

3.3.1 SNP arrays

A single nucleotide polymorphism (SNP) is a variation in a single base pair in DNA. The human genome contains approximately 10 million SNPs, which are conserved during evolution and within populations. SNP arrays, such as those from Affymetrix (Genome-Wide Human SNP Array 6.0, www.affymetrix.com), cannot only be applied to detect polymorphisms throughout the entire human genome, but also as an aCGH platform using the allele-ratios as an indicator for copy number variations. SNP arrays use the “single base extension” (SBE) principle. In single base extension dideoxy- instead of deoxy-NTPs (ddNTP vs. dNTP) are used. Due to its chemical structure just one fluorescently labelled ddNTP can be attached to the SBE-primer by the polymerase, further elongation is not possible. For each SNP-variant (e.g. C or T at a singular genomic location) a specific probe is present (e.g. thus 2 probes would be necessary for detection of that amplified C/T variant). The elongated ddNTP is complementary to the investigated SNP. Thus a signal on a specific spot is generated only when the complementary ddNTP can be bound to that microarray spot. SNP arrays are offered also by Illumina using a similar principle of detection. Nowadays these two companies offer the most comprehensive types of SNP arrays at different resolution and for different organisms.

3.3.2 SNP array application in thyroid cancer

SNPs are not well investigated in thyroid cancer, although SNPs could contribute to cancer development. Hence, not many papers investigating SNPs in thyroid cancer have been published so far - only one genome wide association study has been done. The study investigated 192 cases and 37196 controls (both Icelandic) and elucidated two SNPs (9q22.3 (nearest gene FOXE1), 14q13.3 (nearest gene TTF1)) which are highly associated with thyroid cancer. The risk of developing PTC and FTC is 5.7 times higher in carriers of the mutation than in non-carriers. The study also discovered that both alleles contributes to low concentrations of thyroid stimulating hormone (TSH) and the 9q22.3 gene is also associated with low T4 and high T3 concentrations (Gudmundsson et al., 2009).

3.4.1 DNA methylation arrays

Major players of epigenetic regulation are CpG methylation of DNA and histone modifications like methylation, acetylation and phosphorylation (Huang et al., 2010). These changes do not affect the DNA-sequence itself, but affect gene transcription due to structural changes of the chromatin conformation, enabling/disabling access of transcription factors. Both DNA methylation and histone modification interact with each other and clarifying these mechanisms is a relatively young area of research. Histone-modifications can be analysed by "ChIP on chip", using promoter- and CpG islands,- as well as tiling- arrays (those have immobilized probes presenting the specified genomic DNA regions). These methods are comparable to those used in aCGH but require initially performing a chromatin immunopreciptiation with a specific antibody.

In this part we want to focus at DNA methylation, which occurs at the 5'-carbon position of cytosine. Epigenetic events play a major role in gene expression (Sandoval et al., 2011) and aberrant DNA methylation changes are an early event as well a key event in human cancer development affecting transcriptional regulation (Berdasco and Esteller, 2010).

Many research groups have investigated DNA methylation, which was first discovered in the late 40s of the last century (Hotchkiss, 1948). Further important knowledge about DNA methylation with respect to cancer research was generated 40 years later by Adrian Bird, who elucidated the genomic regions with a high density of CG nucleotides, called CpG-islands (Bird, 1986). In the vertebrate genome only cytosine residues within CpG dinucleotides can be methylated, creating a 5-methyl cytosine (mC). Methylation of CpG-dinucleotides within CpG-islands is associated with transcriptional silencing of genes. In mammalian development, DNA methylation regions have a major impact in X-Inactivation and imprinting of genes (Senner, 2011). The great advantage of analyzing DNA methylation compared to other epigenetic modifications is its stability (Senner, 2011) in the various types of biological and clinical material available to the researcher. A number of studies have elucidated a linkage between hypermethylation of CpG-islands of promoter regions and tumorigenesis (Kass et al., 1997; Baylin and Herman, 2000). Since then, research activity dealing with DNA methylation with respect to cancer research has increased dramatically. This development goes along with the need for improved high throughput techniques, and companies responded with the manufacture of DNA methylation arrays. Methods to analyse the DNA methylation patterns throughout the genome are the methylated-DNA immunoprecipitation (MeDIP, similar to ChIP using an antibody specific to mC), or based on sodium-bisulfite based DNA deamination (cytosine is converted to uracil by deamination, methylated cytosines are not converted), as well as by methyl sensitive restriction enzymes (MSREs, which are enzymes blocked by methylated DNA). DNA processed by these methods can either be subjected to promoter arrays (which investigate DNA methylation within the CpG-island or promoter regions of genes, e.g. Agilent or

Affymetrix promoter arrays) or to microarrays using bead-based technology (e.g. Illumina). Upon bisulfite deamination single CpG methlylation events (C vs. U has to be differentiated) are detected by methods similar to SNP arrays. At the moment Illumina offers the Illumina Infinium 450k BeadChip; which is currently the most comprehensive microarray for genome wide DNA methylation studies. This chip allows the simultaneous investigation of 450000 CpGs throughout the entire human genome and is not restricted to the promoter regions of the genes (www.illumina.com).

3.4.2 DNA methylation in thyroid cancer

A number of studies have revealed the potency of DNA methylation profiles in tumour diagnostics. In the last decade several studies dealing with epigenetic modifications leading to, or affecting thyroid cancer, were performed, however large microarray based studies are missing. The first PCR based (not microarray) studies were performed in 1998 and 2004 from Elisei et al. (Elisei et al., 1998) and Xing et al. (Xing et al., 2004). p16INK4A was investigated by Elisei et al. and RASSF1A by Xing et al. Elisei et al. found 30% of the thyroid carcinomas with hypermethylated regions of p16INK4A. Xing et al. found over 25% of the RASSF1A alleles methylated in 20% of the PTCs, in 44% of the benign thyroid tumours and in 75% of the FTCs, hypothesizing that RASSF1A methylation contributes to the development of tumours. In the following years more studies were performed, focusing on the different subtypes of thyroid cancer. Those studies elucidated the impact of hypermethylated genes with varying occurrence in thyroid cancer subtypes. Zuo et al. (Zuo et al., 2010) published a study in which they reported a hypermethylated Rap1GAP gene in 71% of all PTCs. Alvarez-Nunez et al. (Alvarez-Nunez et al., 2006) published a study showing that a modulator of the PI3K/akt pathway (the PTEN gene) was hypermethylated in 100% of the FTCs and in 50% of the PTC cases. The studies by Guan et al. (Guan et al., 2008) and Hu et al. (Hu et al., 2006) identified five genes (hMLH1, SLC5A8, TIMP-3, DAPK, RARβ2) that were hypermethylated in PTCs and associated with BRAF mutations. Although the hypermethylation of these five genes was found to a varying degree in PTC (starting from 22% of RARβ2 to 53% of TIMP-3 genes), all of them were associated with BRAF mutations. All of the mentioned studies focused on a few genes since large genome wide DNA methylation studies are still missing, or not yet published.

Recently we performed a microarray based methylation study with the aim of elucidating methylation markers for different thyroid nodules. We used a self-manufactured targeted microarray called the "AIT CpG 360 cancer array" which targets CpG-islands of 323 genes (patent number: WO2010086389A1). Six histological classes (normal thyroid tissue [SD]; struma nodosa [SN, benign]; FTA; FTC; PTC; MTC) were subjected to microarray analyses. The elucidation of methylation markers which could distinguish in general between benign (struma nodosa, FTA) and malignant (FTC, PTC) thyroid tissue were brought into focus, but we also aimed for the elucidation of methylation markers which are capable of distinguishing between the FTC and FTA (diagnostically difficult to specify), PTC and FTA as well as between struma nodosa and FTC and PTC, respectively. We generated 10 classifiers (Table 2) which have high discrimination powers between the different groups of thyroid nodules (patent number: WO2010086389A1). The classifiers were created by applying a statistical method for class prediction classifications and contained between 5 and 37 genes, with which a correct classification of samples is possible with high specificity and sensitivity.

In this context we wish to point out to cluster 7, where we defined an 18-gene classifier for the discrimination between FTA and FTC, which can be difficult to differentially diagnose by cytology. With the defined classifiers, a correct classification of 100% of the FTA and FTC samples (n=37) was observed. The classifiers of cluster 2 and 3 also offer a high correct discriminatory power of 93% between the predefined groups.

cluster	discriminates between	genes/ genelist	classifiers
1*	SD, SN and FTA vs. FTC and PTC	7	PITX2, TJP2, CD24, ESR1, TNFRSF10D, RPA3, RASSF1
2*	SD vs. SN, FTA, FTC and PTC.	5	GATA5, RASSF1, HIST1H2AG, NPTX1, UNC13B
3*	SD, SN, FTA, FTC, and PTC vs. MTC	9	SMAD3, NANOS1, TERT, BCL2, SPARC, SFRP2, MGMT, MYOD1, LAMA1
4*	FTC, PTC and FTA vs. SN	5	TJP2, CALCA, PITX2, TFPI2, CDKN2B
5*	FTA vs. FTC and PTC	8	PITX2, TNFRSF10D, PAX8, RAD23A, GJB2, F2R, NTHL1, TP53,
6*	FTC vs. PTC	8	ARRDC4, DUSP1, SMAD9, HOXA10, C3, ADRB2, BRCA2, SYK
7**	FTA vs. FTC	18	PITX2, MT3, RPA3, TNFRSF10D, PTEN, TP53, PAX8, TGFBR2, HIC1, CALCA, PSAT1, MBD2, NTF3, PLAGL1, F2R, GJB2, ARRDC4, NTHL1
8**	FTA vs. PTC	11	PITX2, PAX8, CD24, TP53, ESR1, TNFRSF10D RAD23A, SCGB3A1, RARB, TP53, LZTS1
9**	SN vs. FTC	37	DUSP1, TFPI2, TJP2, S100A9, BAZ1A, CPEB4, AIM1l, CDKN2A, PITX2, ARPC1B, RPA3, SPARC, SFRP4, LZTS1, MSH4, PLAGL1, ABCB1, C13orf15, XIST, TDRD6, CCDC62, HOXA1, IRF4, HSD12B4, S100A9, MT3, KCNJ15, BCL2A1, S100A8, THBD, NANOS1, SYK, SMAD2, GNAS, HRAS, RARRES1, APEX1
10**	SN vs. PTC	14	TJP2, CALCA, PITX2, ESR1, EFS, SSMAD3, ARRDC4, CD24, FHL2, RDHE2, KIF5B, C3, KRT17, RASSF1

* $p<0.01$ **$p<0.05$

Table 2. Genelists derived from the "AIT CpG 360 cancer array" studies.

3.5 High density protein microarrays for tumour autoantibody detection

In recent years, a great deal of effort has gone into developing a screen for biomarkers at the proteomic level. Great improvement in proteomics using separation techniques based on high resolution 2D-gel-electrophoresis, HPLC and others, as well as improved detection limits in the femtogram range of target molecules by developments in mass spectrometry and combined bioinformatics data-analysis have been achieved. These technical improvements will help generate new insights in cancer biology and enable future diagnostic applications. With respect to microarray applications there is a growing interest in using serum tumour-associated antigen (TAA) antibodies as serological cancer biomarkers. The persistence and stability of autoantibodies in the serum of cancer patients is an advantage over other potential markers, including the TAAs themselves, some of which are released by tumours but rapidly degrade or are cleared after circulating in the serum for a limited time. Antibody-profiles of patient's serum can be easily detected using protein-microarrays with spotted antigens. Immunglobulins in serum bind to the immobilized antigens and can be detected using a fluorescent-labelled detection-antibody. Because of the simple test principle minimal invasive testing using serum autoantibody profiles has a great potential for improving early diagnosis, which is an unequivocal prerequisite for successful and efficient cancer therapy.

It had been shown for several cancers that panels of auto-antigens rather than individual antigens enhance the likelihood of detecting cancer antigens with diagnostic potential (Fernandez, 2005). Therefore our research group went on to establish high-density protein microarrays which can be used for autoantibody screening. For method optimization and proof of principle we started off with a microarray which included candidate marker proteins which were identified by previous SEREX (serological identification of antigens by recombinant expression cloning, screening of brain and lung cancer and screening macroarrays of a fetal brain cDNA expression library (Sahin et al., 1995). First "antigens" for microarray printing had to be generated. Thus recombinant candidate protein expression from E.coli expression clones was set up and optimized in a 96 well plate format. His-(histidine)-tagged recombinant proteins were purified using Ni-NTA (nickel immobilized onto agarose resin via nitrilo triacetic acid) sepharose and then printed onto epoxy-coated glass slides for the production of protein microarrays. Those were incubated with minute amounts (10µl of serum diluted 1:10) of serum from brain and lung tumour patients. Within this experiment we could show that using SEREX derived expression clones are suitable for microarray-based classification of patients. Repetitive serum-testing on different microarray slides confirmed the high reproducibility of the antibody signal patterns obtained and resulted in correlation coefficients ranging from 0.92 to 0.96 thereby clearly demonstrating the potential of protein microarrays (Stempfer et al., 2010).

Recently, protein microarray technologies have improved and arrays with either spotted antibodies or antigens are available for research. Especially, developments in microarrays for the elucidation of tumour-specific autoantibody profiles have been found to be very useful in enabling diagnostics, and many studies have been published regarding their utility in different (non-cancerous) diseases, as well as in cancer. Table 3 illustrates the potential of this testing principle highlighting "colon cancer" studies (Table 3) (Carpelan-Holmstrom et al., 1995; Ran et al., 2008; Liu et al., 2009; Babel et al., 2009; Chan et al., 2010). To the best of our knowledge, systematic studies using this approach are lacking for thyroid cancer diagnostics, although this approach may enable minimally invasive early diagnostic and even pres-symptomatic screening of patients.

Study	Antibody specificity	samples	Study Size (patients)	Sensitivity (%)	Specificity (%)
Carpelan-Holmstrom et al.	CEA	CRC vs.healthy	259	34	90
Ran et al.	6 SEREX clones	Colon cancer vs. healthy	48	91.7	91.7
	6 SEREX clones + CEA			91.7	95.2
Liu et al.	5 anti-TAAs: Imp1, p62, Koc, p53 and c-myc	Colon cancer vs. healthy	46	60.9	89.7
	5 anti-TAAs + CEA			82.6	89.7
Babel et al.	MAPKAPK3 and ACVR2B	CRC vs.healthy	64	83.3	73.9
Chan et al.	CCCAP, HDAC5, p53, NMDAR, NY-CO-16	Colon cancer vs. healthy	94	77.6	58.5

Table 3. Examples of the diagnostic potential using immunological and tumour-autoantibody based studies for serum based testing of colorectal cancer (CRC).

4. Bioinformatics

Microarray experiments require very careful planning and the use of proper statistical methods to analyze the highly multiplexed data (Simon, 2009). The fundamental idea behind microarray based studies in (thyroid) cancer research is the elucidation of genes which behave differently between distinct classes (e.g. tumour versus reference). Because of the high numbers of different features measured on a single sample and the great number of data points generated in parallel experiments of multiple samples, there is a serious consequence of performing statistical tests on many genes in parallel. This is known as multiplicity of p-values. Thus when analyzing 10000 genes one would detect 100 significant genes by chance with a p-value less than 0.01. Although there is a trade-off between controlling false positive and false negative results, the only way to improve both rates is to increase the number of individuals analysed in a (microarray) study. Thus for microarray experimental planning, the sample size for microarray experiments has to be defined prior to analysis for elucidation of statistically significant differences between groups at an acceptable statistical power. This corresponds to the percentage of the differentially expressed genes that are likely to be detected by the experiment. In addition the sample size depends on how large a difference someone wants to be able to detect. The classical way to estimate the number of replicates (sample size) in a microarray experiment is with power analyses. Therefore solutions are implemented in statistical software, which enables estimation of individuals needed per group in a microarray experiments. The number of replicates per group also affects data analysis, because the number of replicates can be used to determine the fold change to be detected in a gene or feature. For data analyses of the various microarray applications, different bioinformatic concepts and solutions exist and have filled many specialists books over recent years.

Most microarray experiments aim to 1) elucidate differentially "expressed" genes in one class of samples versus another class, 2) elucidate the relationship between "genes" or "samples", and 3) to classify new samples based on a classifier generated in an array experiment (Stekel, 2004). To address aim (1) various parametric and non-parametric t-tests are frequently used to analyse the differences between the 2 groups. For analyses of more complex experiments in which there might be more than 2 groups, ANOVA and linear models are the methods of choice. These are also suitable for analysis of experiments in which the response to more than one variable is measured. To study aim (2) - the relationship between genes or samples that behave in a similar manner, - correlation of parameters are identified by different distant measures. For visualization of the high-dimensional data, principal component analyses and multidimensional scaling are best suited for illustration of the distance matrix between multiple genes and/or samples. In addition, clustering is a widely used analysis tool for arranging gene and sample profiles into a tree so that concordant genes or samples are located close together. Thus clusters of genes and/or samples are built with minimal differences between the genes/samples within the respective clusters than between the different clusters. Clustering and cluster-trees, or dendrograms, enable unsupervised elucidation of similarities and associations as well as "visualization" and simplification of complex data. Especially for improving diagnostics (3) classification of patients and samples is a very exciting area of microarray analyses. Using supervised learning, a training set with well known classes (e.g. benign vs. malignant) is applied to the statistical analyses and examines the differences between the groups aiming to find a classifier consisting of a small number of "genes" (biomarkers) in the training set, that can predict to which group each individual belongs. Based on those data a prediction rule is established which enables the classification of new samples. The "classifier" genes or biomarkers can then be used in future molecular tests - like targeted microarrays or qPCR and other simpler methods for diagnostic testing. Classification algorithms applied in microarray analyses include compound covariate predictor, diagonal linear discriminant analysis, k-nearest neighbor-, nearest centroid -predictor, and support vector machines. These methods are powerful for classifying samples, each with advantages and disadvantages. After building a classifier by either of these methods the classifiers have to be validated by using training and test-set samples or by cross-validation. In bioinformatic tools options defining training and test-set samples as well as several cross-validation strategies are implemented. Although these analyses are computationally intensive, today's standard personal computers usually have sufficient performance for analyses of an experiment of 100 whole genome expression arrays with more than 40000 features. Data analyses principles established along with microarray developments (especially gene expression analyses) will also be useful for most other applications like miRNA, DNA-methylation, copy number variation, protein-arrays as well as for analyses of genome-sequencing derived highly paralleled data. For aCGH, SNP, ChIPChip several other aspects of data analysis have to be considered that are not discussed here.

For further information the interested reader should consult specific publications dealing with these type of microarrays (and companies selling the specific tools) as well as books about statistical bioinformatics and microarray analyses (e.g.(Lee, 2010); (Simon et al., 2003)).

5. Genome sequencing technologies

Since the invention of Sanger's chain-terminating DNA sequencing approach as the standard method in 1975 (Sanger and Coulson, 1975; Sanger et al., 1977), many technological improvements have been made in the field of DNA sequencing. Those improvements have made DNA sequencing more effective and affordable to a broad range of scientists. While the sequencing of the whole human genome by Sanger-Sequencing required billions of dollars, currently even a $1000 genome has come into reach (Rusk, 2009). The so-called next generation sequencing (NGS) technologies offer great applications for research, and many microarray-based analyses of interest in cancer research are detectable by genome sequencing approaches. Thus gene-mutations and sequence variations, RNA expression, DNA methylation, and also ChIPChip (then called ChIP-Seq) can be elucidated in a genome-wide manner by NGS. The NGS technology became commercially available in 2004, and the platforms of Roche, Illumina and Applied Biosystems are currently the three big players in the field using different biochemical principles for sequencing (Mardis, 2008). These and other companies are working on improving technologies that might enable increased sequencing throughput at decreased costs. All of the upcoming third-generation sequencing technologies have in common that the results can be monitored in real time. One of those three platforms is already commercially available (Helico Genetic Analysis) and one is ready to launch (Pacific Biosciences). Both platforms utilize a single-molecule sequencing approach, by incorporating fluorescently labelled nucleotides (Rusk, 2009;McCarthy, 2010). The third technology developed by Oxford Nanopore uses nanopores where nucleotides of a DNA strand are pulled base by base through a nanopore. The sequence is read via signal changes when nucleotides migrate through the nanopore and block an electrical current in the nanopore. No labeling of the nucleotides is required, and even methylcytosine can be detected without any prior DNA modification, such as bisulfite conversion (Clarke et al., 2009; Schadt et al., 2010)

6. Conclusion

In this chapter we have described various molecular-genetic high throughput analyses based on microarray technology, which have been widely applied over the past decade in clinical research. These techniques have provided considerable insights into biological processes and pathways for elucidation of disease mechanisms. Although many gene-expression studies have been conducted in thyroid cancer patients, studies for elucidation of epigenetic changes are lacking. In addition integration and combination of genomic and transcription data already available as well as integration of other -omics data (like epigenomics, proteomics, metabolomics, etc.) would enable a "systems biology approach in thyroid cancer", and might help to increase knowledge of thyroid cancer biology and uncover novel biological clues in cancer development and progression.

Although genome-sequencing technologies have developed rapidly over the last 10 years and have become more affordable over time, application of microarrays is still a state-of-the art technology. Genome sequencing approaches will improve life science research and replace microarrays in several applications. For future research, the aims, experimental design as well as costs will have to be considered when making the decision to use array- or sequencing approaches. Microarray technologies will likely maintain a role in thyroid cancer research in the future, since microarray technologies are already "mature technologies".

7. References

Affymetrix Inc. Date of access: June 2011, Available from: http://www.affymetrix.com

Alvarez-Nunez, F., Bussaglia, E., Mauricio, D., Ybarra, J., Vilar, M., Lerma, E., de, L. A. & Matias-Guiu, X. (2006). PTEN promoter methylation in sporadic thyroid carcinomas. *Thyroid,* 16, 17-23.

Babel, I., Barderas, R., az-Uriarte, R., Martinez-Torrecuadrada, J. L., Sanchez-Carbayo, M. & Casal, J. I. (2009). Identification of tumor-associated autoantigens for the diagnosis of colorectal cancer in serum using high density protein microarrays. *Mol.Cell Proteomics.,* 8, 2382-2395.

Bagasra, O. & Prilliman, K. R. (2004). RNA interference: the molecular immune system. *J.Mol.Histol.,* 35, 545-553.

Bains, W. & Smith, G. C. (1988). A novel method for nucleic acid sequence determination. *J.Theor.Biol.,* 135, 303-307.

Barden, C. B., Shister, K. W., Zhu, B., Guiter, G., Greenblatt, D. Y., Zeiger, M. A. & Fahey, T. J., III (2003). Classification of follicular thyroid tumors by molecular signature: results of gene profiling. *Clin.Cancer Res.,* 9, 1792-1800.

Baylin, S. B. & Herman, J. G. (2000). DNA hypermethylation in tumorigenesis: epigenetics joins genetics. *Trends Genet.,* 16, 168-174.

Benito, M., Parker, J., Du, Q., Wu, J., Xiang, D., Perou, C. M. & Marron, J. S. (2004). Adjustment of systematic microarray data biases. *Bioinformatics.,* 20, 105-114.

Berdasco, M. & Esteller, M. (2010). Aberrant epigenetic landscape in cancer: how cellular identity goes awry. *Dev.Cell,* 19, 698-711.

Bird, A. (2007). Perceptions of epigenetics. *Nature,* 447, 396-398.

Bird, A. P. (1986). CpG-rich islands and the function of DNA methylation. *Nature,* 321, 209-213.

Carpelan-Holmstrom, M., Haglund, C., Kuusela, P., Jarvinen, H. & Roberts, P. J. (1995). Preoperative serum levels of CEA and CA 242 in colorectal cancer. *Br.J.Cancer,* 71, 868-872.

Cavalieri, L. F., Small, T. & Sarkar, N. (1962). The renaturation of denatured DNA. *Biophys.J.,* 2, 339-350.

Chan, C. C., Fan, C. W., Kuo, Y. B., Chen, Y. H., Chang, P. Y., Chen, K. T., Hung, R. P. & Chan, E. C. (2010). Multiple serological biomarkers for colorectal cancer detection. *Int.J.Cancer,* 126, 1683-1690.

Chang, H. Y., Lin, J. D., Chen, J. F., Huang, B. Y., Hsueh, C., Jeng, L. B. & Tsai, J. S. (1997). Correlation of fine needle aspiration cytology and frozen section biopsies in the diagnosis of thyroid nodules. *J.Clin.Pathol.,* 50, 1005-1009.

Cheng, S., Serra, S., Mercado, M., Ezzat, S. & Asa, S. L. (2011). A high-throughput proteomic approach provides distinct signatures for thyroid cancer behavior. *Clin.Cancer Res.,* 17, 2385-2394.

Cheung, S. W., Shaw, C. A., Yu, W., Li, J., Ou, Z., Patel, A., Yatsenko, S. A., Cooper, M. L., Furman, P., Stankiewicz, P., Lupski, J. R., Chinault, A. C. & Beaudet, A. L. (2005). Development and validation of a CGH microarray for clinical cytogenetic diagnosis. *Genet.Med.,* 7, 422-432.

Clarke, J., Wu, H. C., Jayasinghe, L., Patel, A., Reid, S. & Bayley, H. (2009). Continuous base identification for single-molecule nanopore DNA sequencing. *Nat Nanotechnol.,* 4, 265-270.

Collas, P. (2010). The current state of chromatin immunoprecipitation. *Mol.Biotechnol.,* 45, 87-100.

Cooper, D. S., Doherty, G. M., Haugen, B. R., Kloos, R. T., Lee, S. L., Mandel, S. J., Mazzaferri, E. L., McIver, B., Sherman, S. I. & Tuttle, R. M. (2006). Management guidelines for patients with thyroid nodules and differentiated thyroid cancer. *Thyroid,* 16, 109-142.

Drmanac, R., Labat, I., Brukner, I. & Crkvenjakov, R. (1989). Sequencing of megabase plus DNA by hybridization: theory of the method. *Genomics,* 4, 114-128.

Duggan, D. J., Bittner, M., Chen, Y., Meltzer, P. & Trent, J. M. (1999). Expression profiling using cDNA microarrays. *Nat Genet.,* 21, 10-14.

Elisei, R., Shiohara, M., Koeffler, H. P. & Fagin, J. A. (1998). Genetic and epigenetic alterations of the cyclin-dependent kinase inhibitors p15INK4b and p16INK4a in human thyroid carcinoma cell lines and primary thyroid carcinomas. *Cancer,* 83, 2185-2193.

Eszlinger, M., Krohn, K., Berger, K., Lauter, J., Kropf, S., Beck, M., Fuhrer, D. & Paschke, R. (2005). Gene expression analysis reveals evidence for increased expression of cell cycle-associated genes and Gq-protein-protein kinase C signaling in cold thyroid nodules. *J.Clin.Endocrinol.Metab.,* 90, 1163-1170.

Fernandez, M. F. (2005). Autoantibodies in breast cancer sera: candidate biomarkers and reporters of tumorigenesis. *Cancer Lett.,* 230, 187-198.

Finley, D. J., Zhu, B., Barden, C. B. & Fahey, T. J., III (2004). Discrimination of benign and malignant thyroid nodules by molecular profiling. *Ann.Surg.,* 240, 425-436.

Finn, S., Smyth, P., O'Regan, E., Cahill, S., Toner, M., Timon, C., Flavin, R., O'Leary, J. & Sheils, O. (2007a). Low-level genomic instability is a feature of papillary thyroid carcinoma: an array comparative genomic hybridization study of laser capture microdissected papillary thyroid carcinoma tumors and clonal cell lines. *Arch.Pathol.Lab Med.,* 131, 65-73.

Finn, S. P., Smyth, P., Cahill, S., Streck, C., O'Regan, E. M., Flavin, R., Sherlock, J., Howells, D., Henfrey, R., Cullen, M., Toner, M., Timon, C., O'Leary, J. J. & Sheils, O. M. (2007b). Expression microarray analysis of papillary thyroid carcinoma and benign thyroid tissue: emphasis on the follicular variant and potential markers of malignancy. *Virchows Arch.,* 450, 249-260.

Fire, A., Xu, S., Montgomery, M. K., Kostas, S. A., Driver, S. E. & Mello, C. C. (1998). Potent and specific genetic interference by double-stranded RNA in Caenorhabditis elegans. *Nature,* 391, 806-811.

Giordano, T. J., Au, A. Y., Kuick, R., Thomas, D. G., Rhodes, D. R., Wilhelm, K. G., Jr., Vinco, M., Misek, D. E., Sanders, D., Zhu, Z., Ciampi, R., Hanash, S., Chinnaiyan, A., Clifton-Bligh, R. J., Robinson, B. G., Nikiforov, Y. E. & Koenig, R. J. (2006). Delineation, functional validation, and bioinformatic evaluation of gene expression in thyroid follicular carcinomas with the PAX8-PPARG translocation. *Clin.Cancer Res.,* 12, 1983-1993.

Guan, H., Ji, M., Hou, P., Liu, Z., Wang, C., Shan, Z., Teng, W. & Xing, M. (2008). Hypermethylation of the DNA mismatch repair gene hMLH1 and its association with lymph node metastasis and T1799A BRAF mutation in patients with papillary thyroid cancer. *Cancer,* 113, 247-255.

Gudmundsson, J., Sulem, P., Gudbjartsson, D. F., Jonasson, J. G., Sigurdsson, A., Bergthorsson, J. T., He, H., Blondal, T., Geller, F., Jakobsdottir, M., Magnusdottir, D. N., Matthiasdottir, S., Stacey, S. N., Skarphedinsson, O. B., Helgadottir, H., Li, W., Nagy, R., Aguillo, E., Faure, E., Prats, E., Saez, B., Martinez, M., Eyjolfsson, G. I., Bjornsdottir, U. S., Holm, H., Kristjansson, K., Frigge, M. L., Kristvinsson, H., Gulcher, J. R., Jonsson, T., Rafnar, T., Hjartarsson, H., Mayordomo, J. I., de la, C. A., Hrafnkelsson, J., Thorsteinsdottir, U., Kong, A. & Stefansson, K. (2009). Common variants on 9q22.33 and 14q13.3 predispose to thyroid cancer in European populations. *Nat Genet.,* 41, 460-464.

He, H., Jazdzewski, K., Li, W., Liyanarachchi, S., Nagy, R., Volinia, S., Calin, G. A., Liu, C. G., Franssila, K., Suster, S., Kloos, R. T., Croce, C. M. & de la, C. A. (2005a). The role of microRNA genes in papillary thyroid carcinoma. *Proc.Natl.Acad.Sci.U.S.A,* 102, 19075-19080.

He, L., Thomson, J. M., Hemann, M. T., Hernando-Monge, E., Mu, D., Goodson, S., Powers, S., Cordon-Cardo, C., Lowe, S. W., Hannon, G. J. & Hammond, S. M. (2005b). A microRNA polycistron as a potential human oncogene. *Nature,* 435, 828-833.

Hoheisel, J. D., Ross, M. T., Zehetner, G. & Lehrach, H. (1994). Relational genome analysis using reference libraries and hybridisation fingerprinting. *J.Biotechnol.,* 35, 121-134.

Hotchkiss, R. D. (1948). The quantitative separation of purines, pyrimidines, and nucleosides by paper chromatography. *J.Biol.Chem.,* 175, 315-332.

Howbrook, D. N., van der Valk, A. M., O'Shaughnessy, M. C., Sarker, D. K., Baker, S. C. & Lloyd, A. W. (2003). Developments in microarray technologies. *Drug Discovery Today,* 8, 642-651.

Hu, S., Liu, D., Tufano, R. P., Carson, K. A., Rosenbaum, E., Cohen, Y., Holt, E. H., Kiseljak-Vassiliades, K., Rhoden, K. J., Tolaney, S., Condouris, S., Tallini, G., Westra, W. H., Umbricht, C. B., Zeiger, M. A., Califano, J. A., Vasko, V. & Xing, M. (2006). Association of aberrant methylation of tumor suppressor genes with tumor aggressiveness and BRAF mutation in papillary thyroid cancer. *Int.J.Cancer,* 119, 2322-2329.

Huang, Y., Prasad, M., Lemon, W. J., Hampel, H., Wright, F. A., Kornacker, K., LiVolsi, V., Frankel, W., Kloos, R. T., Eng, C., Pellegata, N. S. & de la, C. A. (2001). Gene expression in papillary thyroid carcinoma reveals highly consistent profiles. *Proc.Natl.Acad.Sci.U.S.A,* 98, 15044-15049.

Huang, Y. W., Huang, T. H. & Wang, L. S. (2010). Profiling DNA methylomes from microarray to genome-scale sequencing. *Technol.Cancer Res.Treat.*, 9, 139-147.

Illumina Inc. Date of access: June 2011, Available from: https://www.illumina.com

Jarzab, B., Wiench, M., Fujarewicz, K., Simek, K., Jarzab, M., Oczko-Wojciechowska, M., Wloch, J., Czarniecka, A., Chmielik, E., Lange, D., Pawlaczek, A., Szpak, S., Gubala, E. & Swierniak, A. (2005). Gene expression profile of papillary thyroid cancer: sources of variability and diagnostic implications. *Cancer Res.*, 65, 1587-1597.

Karakach, T. K., Flight, R. M., Douglas, S. E. & Wentzell, P. D. (2010). An introduction to DNA microarrays for gene expression analysis. *Chemometrics and Intelligent Laboratory Systems*, 104, 28-52.

Kass, S. U., Pruss, D. & Wolffe, A. P. (1997). How does DNA methylation repress transcription? *Trends Genet.*, 13, 444-449.

Khrapko, K. R., Lysov, Y., Khorlyn, A. A., Shick, V. V., Florentiev, V. L. & Mirzabekov, A. D. (1989). An oligonucleotide hybridization approach to DNA sequencing. *FEBS Lett.*, 256, 118-122.

Kim, H. Y., Park, W. Y., Lee, K. E., Park, W. S., Chung, Y. S., Cho, S. J. & Youn, Y. K. (2010). Comparative analysis of gene expression profiles of papillary thyroid microcarcinoma and papillary thyroid carcinoma. *J.Cancer Res.Ther.*, 6, 452-457.

Kitano, M., Rahbari, R., Patterson, E. E., Xiong, Y., Prasad, N. B., Wang, Y., Zeiger, M. A. & Kebebew, E. (2011). Expression Profiling of Difficult-to-diagnose Thyroid Histologic Subtypes Shows Distinct Expression Profiles and Identify Candidate Diagnostic microRNAs. *Ann.Surg.Oncol.*.

Kundel, A., Zarnegar, R., Kato, M., Moo, T. A., Zhu, B., Scognamiglio, T. & Fahey, T. J., III (2010). Comparison of microarray analysis of fine needle aspirates and tissue specimen in thyroid nodule diagnosis. *Diagn.Mol.Pathol.*, 19, 9-14.

Lacroix, L., Lazar, V., Michiels, S., Ripoche, H., Dessen, P., Talbot, M., Caillou, B., Levillain, J. P., Schlumberger, M. & Bidart, J. M. (2005). Follicular thyroid tumors with the PAX8-PPARgamma1 rearrangement display characteristic genetic alterations. *Am.J.Pathol.*, 167, 223-231.

Lashkari, D. A., DeRisi, J. L., McCusker, J. H., Namath, A. F., Gentile, C., Hwang, S. Y., Brown, P. O. & Davis, R. W. (1997). Yeast microarrays for genome wide parallel genetic and gene expression analysis. *Proc.Natl.Acad.Sci.U.S.A*, 94, 13057-13062.

Lee, J. J., Au, A. Y., Foukakis, T., Barbaro, M., Kiss, N., Clifton-Bligh, R., Staaf, J., Borg, A., Delbridge, L., Robinson, B. G., Wallin, G., Hoog, A. & Larsson, C. (2008). Array-CGH identifies cyclin D1 and UBCH10 amplicons in anaplastic thyroid carcinoma. *Endocr.Relat Cancer.*, 15, 801-815.

Lee, J. K. (2010). *Statistical Bioinformatics - For biomedical and life science researchers.* (1st edition) Wiley-Blackwell, ISBN 978-0-471-69272-0, New Jersey

Leung, Y. F. & Cavalieri, D. (2003). Fundamentals of cDNA microarray data analysis. *Trends in Genetics*, 19, 649-659.

Liang, M., Briggs, A. G., Rute, E., Greene, A. S. & Cowley, A. W., Jr. (2003). Quantitative assessment of the importance of dye switching and biological replication in cDNA microarray studies. *Physiol Genomics*, 14, 199-207.

Liu, W., Wang, P., Li, Z., Xu, W., Dai, L., Wang, K. & Zhang, J. (2009). Evaluation of tumour-associated antigen (TAA) miniarray in immunodiagnosis of colon cancer. *Scand.J.Immunol.*, 69, 57-63.

MacRae, I. J., Zhou, K. & Doudna, J. A. (2007). Structural determinants of RNA recognition and cleavage by Dicer. *Nat Struct.Mol.Biol.*, 14, 934-940.

MacRae, I. J., Zhou, K., Li, F., Repic, A., Brooks, A. N., Cande, W. Z., Adams, P. D. & Doudna, J. A. (2006). Structural basis for double-stranded RNA processing by Dicer. *Science*, 311, 195-198.

Mardis, E. R. (2008). Next-generation DNA sequencing methods. *Annu.Rev Genomics Hum.Genet.*, 9, 387-402.

Marmur, J. & Doty, P. (1961). Thermal renaturation of deoxyribonucleic acids. *J.Mol.Biol.*, 3, 585-594.

Mazeh, H., Mizrahi, I., Halle, D., Ilyayev, N., Stojadinovic, A., Trink, B., Mitrani-Rosenbaum, S., Roistacher, M., Ariel, I., Eid, A., Freund, H. R. & Nissan, A. (2011). Development of a microRNA-based molecular assay for the detection of papillary thyroid carcinoma in aspiration biopsy samples. *Thyroid*, 21, 111-118.

Mazzaferri, E. L. (1992). Thyroid cancer in thyroid nodules: finding a needle in the haystack. *Am.J.Med.*, 93, 359-362.

Mazzanti, C., Zeiger, M. A., Costouros, N. G., Umbricht, C., Westra, W. H., Smith, D., Somervell, H., Bevilacqua, G., Alexander, H. R. & Libutti, S. K. (2004). Using gene expression profiling to differentiate benign versus malignant thyroid tumors. *Cancer Res.*, 64, 2898-2903.

McCall, M. N., Murakami, P. N., Lukk, M., Huber, W. & Irizarry, R. A. (2011). Assessing affymetrix GeneChip microarray quality. *BMC.Bioinformatics.*, 12, 137.

McCarthy, A. (2010). Third generation DNA sequencing: pacific biosciences' single molecule real time technology. *Chem.Biol.*, 17, 675-676.

Mraz, M., Pospisilova, S., Malinova, K., Slapak, I. & Mayer, J. (2009). MicroRNAs in chronic lymphocytic leukemia pathogenesis and disease subtypes. *Leuk.Lymphoma*, 50, 506-509.

National Center for Biotechnology. Date of access: June 2011, Available from: http://www.ncbi.nlm.nih.gov

Patterson, T. A., Lobenhofer, E. K., Fulmer-Smentek, S. B., Collins, P. J., Chu, T. M., Bao, W., Fang, H., Kawasaki, E. S., Hager, J., Tikhonova, I. R., Walker, S. J., Zhang, L., Hurban, P., de, L. F., Fuscoe, J. C., Tong, W., Shi, L. & Wolfinger, R. D. (2006). Performance comparison of one-color and two-color platforms within the MicroArray Quality Control (MAQC) project. *Nat.Biotechnol.*, 24, 1140-1150.

Priness, I., Maimon, O. & Ben-Gal, I. (2007). Evaluation of gene-expression clustering via mutual information distance measure. *BMC.Bioinformatics.*, 8, 111.

Ran, Y., Hu, H., Zhou, Z., Yu, L., Sun, L., Pan, J., Liu, J. & Yang, Z. (2008). Profiling tumor-associated autoantibodies for the detection of colon cancer. *Clin.Cancer Res.*, 14, 2696-2700.

Ravetto, C., Colombo, L. & Dottorini, M. E. (2000). Usefulness of fine-needle aspiration in the diagnosis of thyroid carcinoma: a retrospective study in 37,895 patients. *Cancer*, 90, 357-363.

Rodrigues, R., Roque, L., Espadinha, C., Pinto, A., Domingues, R., Dinis, J., Catarino, A., Pereira, T. & Leite, V. (2007). Comparative genomic hybridization, BRAF, RAS, RET, and oligo-array analysis in aneuploid papillary thyroid carcinomas. *Oncol.Rep.*, 18, 917-926.

Rousset, B., Ziercher, L. & Borson-Chazot, F. (2011). Molecular analyses of thyroid tumors for diagnosis of malignancy on fine-needle aspiration biopsies and for prognosis of invasiveness on surgical specimens. *Ann.Endocrinol.(Paris).*

Rusk, N. (2009). Cheap third-generation sequencing. *Nat Meth,* 6, 244.

Russo, D., Damante, G., Puxeddu, E., Durante, C. & Filetti, S. (2011). Epigenetics of thyroid cancer and novel therapeutic targets. *J.Mol.Endocrinol.,* 46, R73-R81.

Sahin, U., Tureci, O., Schmitt, H., Cochlovius, B., Johannes, T., Schmits, R., Stenner, F., Luo, G., Schobert, I. & Pfreundschuh, M. (1995). Human neoplasms elicit multiple specific immune responses in the autologous host. *Proc.Natl.Acad.Sci.U.S.A,* 92, 11810-11813.

Sandoval, J., Heyn, H. A., Moran, S., Serra-Musach, J., Pujana, M. A., Bibikova, M. & Esteller, M. (2011). Validation of a DNA methylation microarray for 450,000 CpG sites in the human genome. *Epigenetics.,* 6.

Sanger, F. & Coulson, A. R. (1975). A rapid method for determining sequences in DNA by primed synthesis with DNA polymerase. *J.Mol.Biol.,* 94, 441-448.

Sanger, F., Nicklen, S. & Coulson, A. R. (1977). DNA sequencing with chain-terminating inhibitors. *Proc.Natl.Acad.Sci.U.S.A,* 74, 5463-5467.

Schadt, E. E., Turner, S. & Kasarskis, A. (2010). A window into third-generation sequencing. *Hum.Mol.Genet.,* 19, R227-R240.

Schaferling, M. & Nagl, S. (2006). Optical technologies for the read out and quality control of DNA and protein microarrays. *Anal.Bioanal.Chem.,* 385, 500-517.

Schena, M., Shalon, D., Davis, R. W. & Brown, P. O. (1995). Quantitative monitoring of gene expression patterns with a complementary DNA microarray. *Science,* 270, 467-470.

Senner, C. E. (2011). The role of DNA methylation in mammalian development. *Reprod.Biomed.Online..*

Shinawi, M. & Cheung, S. W. (2008). The array CGH and its clinical applications. *Drug Discov.Today,* 13, 760-770.

Simon, R. (2009). Analysis of DNA microarray expression data. *Best Pract.Res.Clin.Haematol.,* 22, 271-282.

Simon, R., Korn, E. L., McShane, L. M., Radmacher, M. D., Wright, G. W. & Zhao, Y. (2004). *Design and analysis of DNA microarray investigations.* (1st edition), Springer Verlag, ISBN 978-0-387-00135-7, New York

Southern, E. M. (1975). Detection of specific sequences among DNA fragments separated by gel electrophoresis. *Journal of Molecular Biology,* 98, 503-517.

Stein, L., Rothschild, J., Luce, J., Cowell, J. K., Thomas, G., Bogdanova, T. I., Tronko, M. D. & Hawthorn, L. (2010). Copy number and gene expression alterations in radiation-induced papillary thyroid carcinoma from chernobyl pediatric patients. *Thyroid.,* 20, 475-487.

Stekel, D. (2003). *Microarray Bioinformatics* (1st edition), Cambridge University Press, ISBN 0-521-52587-X, United Kinddom

Stempfer, R., Syed, P., Vierlinger, K., Pichler, R., Meese, E., Leidinger, P., Ludwig, N., Kriegner, A., Nohammer, C. & Weinhausel, A. (2010). Tumour auto-antibody screening: performance of protein microarrays using SEREX derived antigens. *BMC.Cancer,* 10, 627.

Tan, H. T., Low, J., Lim, S. G. & Chung, M. C. (2009). Serum autoantibodies as biomarkers for early cancer detection. *FEBS J.,* 276, 6880-6904.

Thirlwell, C., Eymard, M., Feber, A., Teschendorff, A., Pearce, K., Lechner, M., Widschwendter, M. & Beck, S. (2010). Genome-wide DNA methylation analysis of archival formalin-fixed paraffin-embedded tissue using the Illumina Infinium HumanMethylation27 BeadChip. *Methods,* 52, 248-254.

Uhlenhopp, E. L. & Krasna, A. I. (1969). Denaturation of DNA at pH 7.0 by acid and alkali. *Nature,* 223, 1267-1269.

Urban, A. E., Korbel, J. O., Selzer, R., Richmond, T., Hacker, A., Popescu, G. V., Cubells, J. F., Green, R., Emanuel, B. S., Gerstein, M. B., Weissman, S. M. & Snyder, M. (2006). High-resolution mapping of DNA copy alterations in human chromosome 22 using high-density tiling oligonucleotide arrays. *Proc.Natl.Acad.Sci.U.S.A,* 103, 4534-4539.

Vierlinger, K., Mansfeld, M. H., Koperek, O., Nohammer, C., Kaserer, K. & Leisch, F. (2011). Identification of SERPINA1 as single marker for papillary thyroid carcinoma through microarray meta analysis and quantification of its discriminatory power in independent validation. *BMC.Med.Genomics,* 4, 30.

Watson, J. D. & Crick, F. H. (1953). Molecular structure of nucleic acids; a structure for deoxyribose nucleic acid. *Nature,* 171, 737-738.

Wheelan, S. J., Martinez, M. F. & Boeke, J. D. (2008). The incredible shrinking world of DNA microarrays. *Mol.Biosyst.,* 4, 726-732.

Williams, M. D., Zhang, L., Elliott, D. D., Perrier, N. D., Lozano, G., Clayman, G. L. & El-Naggar, A. K. (2011). Differential gene expression profiling of aggressive and nonaggressive follicular carcinomas. *Hum.Pathol.*.

Xing, M., Cohen, Y., Mambo, E., Tallini, G., Udelsman, R., Ladenson, P. W. & Sidransky, D. (2004). Early occurrence of RASSF1A hypermethylation and its mutual exclusion with BRAF mutation in thyroid tumorigenesis. *Cancer Res.,* 64, 1664-1668.

Zuo, H., Gandhi, M., Edreira, M. M., Hochbaum, D., Nimgaonkar, V. L., Zhang, P., Dipaola, J., Evdokimova, V., Altschuler, D. L. & Nikiforov, Y. E. (2010). Downregulation of Rap1GAP through epigenetic silencing and loss of heterozygosity promotes invasion and progression of thyroid tumors. *Cancer Res.,* 70, 1389-1397.

6

Evaluation and Management of Pediatric Thyroid Nodules

Melanie Goldfarb[1,2] and John I. Lew[1]
[1]*University of Miami Leonard M. Miller School of Medicine*
[2]*University of Southern California Keck School of Medicine*
USA

1. Introduction

The prevalence of palpable thyroid nodules in patients less than 21 years of age is only .05-1.8% (American Cancer Society [ACS], 2009; Dinauer & Francis, 2007; Dinauer et al, 2008; Gosepath et al, 2007; Halac & Zimmerman, 2005, Niedziela, 2006; Ortel & Klinck 1965; Rallison et al 1991; Wartofsky, 2000; Wiersinga, 2007). However, the true incidence of incidental nodules may be higher than 13% in the pediatric and adolescent group based on autopsy studies. This is in comparison to the adult population where the rate of palpable thyroid nodules approaches 5% with autopsy studies showing up to 70% of adults harboring incidental thyroid nodules (Ezzat S et al, 1994; Guth et al, 2009). Risk factors for the development of malignant thyroid nodules in pediatric patients include female sex, puberty, family history of thyroid cancer, head and neck radiation exposure, and iodine-deficiency (Crom et al, 1997; Fleming, 1984; Fowler et al, 1989; Josephson & Zimmerman, 2008; Samaan, 1987; Solt et al, 2001).

Close to ten percent of all thyroid carcinomas occur in patients less than 21 years of age (Machens, 2010). Differentiated thyroid carcinoma (DTC) constitutes 3-8% of all childhood malignancies depending on the age group, and the numbers are thought to be increasing (ACS, 2009; Hameed & Zacharin, 2005; Hogan et al, 2009; Horner et al, 2010; Pacini, 2002; Ries et al, 2003; Waguespack et al, 2006). The majority of patients are adolescents between the ages of 15-19 with only 5% of cancers occurring in patients less than ten years of age (Hogan et al, 2009; Steliarova-Foucher et al, 2006). Familial thyroid carcinoma comprises 5% of all pediatric thyroid cancer, most commonly of the medullary subtype as part of the Multiple Endocrine Neoplasia 2 (MEN2) syndrome (Halac & Zimmerman, 2005; Loh, 1997; Nose, 2001). About 25% of pediatric thyroid nodules are malignant which is four- to five-fold the incidence compared to adults, and up to 30-50% in strictly surgical series (Canadian pediatric thyroid nodule study group [Canadian], 2008; Corrias et al, 2010; Dinauer et al, 2001; Hung, 1999; Lafferty & batch, 1997; Niedziela, 2006; Wiersinga, 2007; Yip et al, 1994).

Patients less than 21 years of age can present with a palpable thyroid nodule discovered on physical examination. More recently, however, more thyroid nodules are discovered as incidental findings by ultrasound or other imaging studies performed for other reasons (Corrias et al, 2008 % 2010, Canadian, 2008). The main risk factor for thyroid malignancy in these patients is a history of head and neck radiation therapy or exposure that is dose and age dependent, which carries a relative risk of 6-18.3 (Ceccarelli et al, 1988; Crom, 1997; Duffy & Fitzgerald, 1950; Faggiano, et al 2004; Gharib et al 2006; Goepfert et al, 1984; Harness et al, 1992; Pacini, 2002; Sklar et al, 2000; Tucker et al, 1991; Viswanathan et al, 1994, Winship & Rosvoll, 1970). Other risk factors consist of a history of bone marrow transplant preceded by radiation therapy, family history of MEN2, Cowden's disease, Carney's complex, and Familial Adenomatous Polyposis (FAP) (Brignardello et al, 2008; Camiel et al, 1968; Halac & Zimmerman, 2005; Smith & Kerr, 1973).

2. Clinical evaluation

2.1 History

There are important questions the clinician should ask when evaluating a thyroid nodule in a pediatric patient. The most important risk factor for DTC is a history of head and neck radiation therapy or exposure (Harness, 1992). Radiation is a known risk factor for developing papillary thyroid cancer (PTC) (DeGroot & Paloyan, 1973; Sigurdson 1985). Today, many PTC patients are cancer survivors, having received internal γ radiation as part of a treatment protocol for lymphoma, especially Mantle radiation for Hodgkin's disease (HD), non-Hodgkin's lymphoma (NHL), leukemia, in preparation for a bone marrow transplant, or retinoblastoma. In a study of 16,500 leukemia survivors, thyroid carcinoma was the most common second malignancy in patients with a history of HD and NHL and the third most common after leukemia (Maule et al, 2007). High risk patients with thyroid nodules may have also received radiation forty to fifty years ago at very young ages for an enlarged thymus, acne, enlarged tonsils and adenoids, tinea capitis, or shoe size measurement (Mehta et al, 1989). Another type of high dose exposure that should be considered is external β radiation seen secondarily from such nuclear accidents as Chernobyl in 1986 and Japan in 2011. As a consequence, Japanese clinicians may see an increase in the number of pediatric thyroid cancers in the next three to ten years. These cancers are exclusively of the papillary subtype, have different RET/PTC rearrangements, and behave somewhat differently than sporadic tumors (Demidchik et al, 2006; Dinauer et al, 2008; Pacini, 2002).

An equally important risk factor for pediatric thyroid cancer is a family history of MEN2 or medullary thyroid cancer (MTC). An inquiry about family history of pheochromocytoma or a family member that may have had an unexpected complication during an operation of an unknown cause should also be performed. Penetrance of MTC is 100% in patients that have any of the responsible genes, and all of these patients will need, at a minimum, total thyroidectomy with central compartment lymph node dissection.

For solitary thyroid nodules, duration, growth and/or previous signs of infection such as erythema, pain or swelling are important. A thyroid nodule that varies in size over a period of time may be indicative of a cyst, and a thyroid cyst that has been previously drained or infected should make the clinician think of a thyroglossal duct cyst. The significance of nodular growth has been debated in the literature with some studies reporting that it is a risk factor for thyroid carcinoma (Canadian, 2008; Corrias et al, 2001; Degroot & Paloyan, 1973; O'Kane, 2010). Nevertheless, a thyroid nodule that has enlarged requires further diagnostic evaluation.

For both solitary thyroid nodules and multinodular goiters, symptoms of compression, including shortness of breath or coughing while lying down in the supine position and/or dysphagia are indications for surgical resection. Additionally, one must ask about a permanent change in voice, which, although rare, may indicate recurrent laryngeal nerve compression or involvement by a thyroid cancer.

The clinician should also inquire about symptoms of hypo- or hyperthyroidism such as weight loss or gain, palpitations, nervousness, excitability, or fatigue. Additionally, male gender itself is a risk factor for thyroid cancer, although less so in those patients less than ten years of age (Harach & Williams, 1985).

2.2 Physical exam

When evaluating any child or adolescent with thyroid nodules, a complete head and neck physical examination should be performed. This clinical exam entails palpating the thyroid gland for the presence of multiple nodules and/or diffuse glandular enlargement as well as the cervical lymph node basins for adenopathy. Any thyroid nodule or lymph node should be characterized as soft or firm, mobile or fixed, and for any tenderness to palpation. While soft and mobile thyroid nodules are usually associated with benignity, firm and fixed thyroid nodules are usually associated with malignancy. Although there is some controversy over whether solitary palpable nodules have an increased risk for cancer compared to those nodules that are discovered incidentally or part of a multinodular goiter, most studies in both adult and pediatric populations report similar rates of thyroid malignancy regardless of clinical presentation (AACE/AME, 2006; Cooper et al, 2009; Corrias et al, 2001; Frates et al, 2006; Gandolfi et al, 2004; Gharib, 2007; Leenhardt et al, 1999; Papini, 2002). Similar to nodular growth, tenderness is a finding with conflicting reports in the literature as to its significance in predicting thyroid cancer (Canadian, 2008; Lugo-Vicente, 1998).

For the rare patient with or a family history of MEN2, an examination for marfanoid habitus, pectus excavatum, mucosal neuromas and skin lesions should also be performed.

3. Diagnostic procedures

3.1 Neck ultrasound

Neck ultrasound has become an extension of the physical exam for many clinicians. This imaging modality has been shown to be cost-effective and accurate in the evaluation of thyroid nodules in adult patients (Milas et al, 2005; Solorzano et al, 2004). Neck ultrasound provides information on the size, shape, and composition of thyroid nodules, evaluates the contralateral thyroid lobe for additional nodules, and allows the clinician to examine the cervical lymph node chains for suspicious adenopathy. This is especially important in the pediatric age group since up to 50% of these thyroid cancer patients in contemporary series present with positive lymph nodes (Hay et al, 2008; Hogan et al, 2009; Pacini, 2002). Since the 1980s, neck ultrasound has been used to evaluate thyroid nodules in pediatric and adolescent patients with a history of head and neck radiation therapy or exposure (Corrias et al, 2001; Crom et al, 1997; Dorzd et al, 2009; O'Kane, 2010; Poyhonen & Lenko, 1986; Solt et al, 2001). In the past decade, the use of ultrasound in guiding FNA biopsy has also led to a decreased rate of insufficient samples (Danese et al, 1998; Izquierdo et al, 2009, Kim MJ et al, 2008).

To evaluate the thyroid gland and surrounding lymph nodes, a 10-14 MHz linear array transducer is used. Appropriate technique entails examination of the thyroid gland and any nodules in both the transverse and longitudinal view, and identifying landmarks such as the trachea, internal jugular vein and carotid artery. Each thyroid nodule should be measured in three dimensions and individual characteristics documented including regular vs. irregular borders, solid vs. cystic architecture, hypo-, iso- or hyperechogenicity, presence of microcalcifications, and the presence of taller greater than wider dimensions. Cervical lymph nodes should similarly be evaluated for elongated vs. rounded shape, regular vs. irregular borders, absence of a fatty echogenic hila, heterogeneous echogenicity, calcifications, and irregular blood flow throughout the node vs. normal central hilar vessels.

Although individual ultrasound characteristics are not reliable in predicting benignity or malignancy of thyroid nodules, certain combinations of ultrasound features do have a predictive value. One study demonstrated that hypoechoic thyroid nodules with irregular borders and microcalcifications carry a 30X risk for malignancy (Jabiev et al, 2009). (Figure 1) Other studies have shown similar ultrasound features predict thyroid malignancy in addition to intrinsic vascularity, taller greater than wider dimension (Figure 2), irregular halo, and elastography (Moon et al, 2011; Chan et al, 2003). Conversely, thyroid nodules with regular borders, cystic component, iso- or hyperechogenicity and no

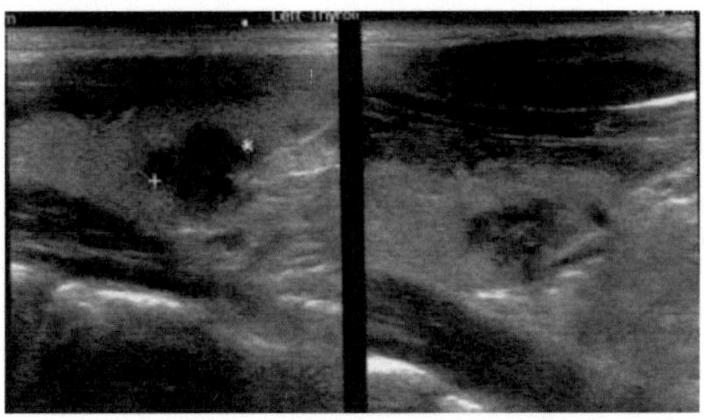

A

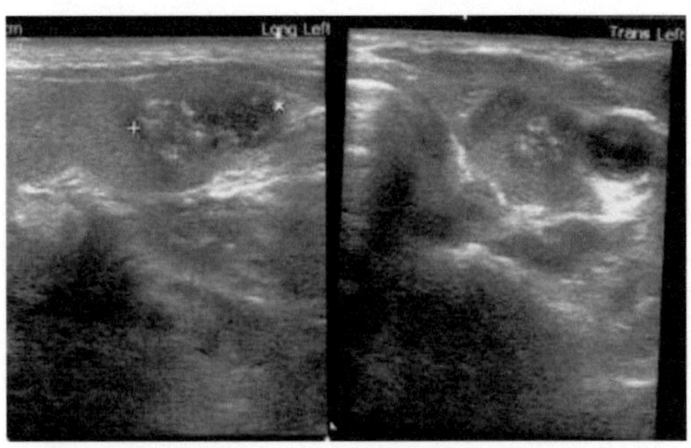

B

Fig. 1. Ultrasound features of malignant thyroid nodules. **Figures 1A & B** Ultrasound nodule characteristics include irregular borders, hypoechoic echogenicity, and microcalcifications

microcalcifications can predict benignity in patients without a history of radiation or thyroid cancer (Figure 3) (Goldfarb et al, 2011). In one study of pediatric patients, malignant thyroid nodules were more likely to have microcalcifications, lymphadenopathy and altered nodular vascular pattern, although each characteristic was only present in 47-73% of patients. Furthermore, a subset of patients deemed to have benign ultrasound findings, namely nodules with regular borders, normal vasculature, no calcifications, and no suspicious lymph nodes were followed without any change in exam for at least one year (Corrias et al, 2010).

Neck ultrasound showing a hypervascular nodule in a patient with biochemical hyperthyroidism is consistent with a toxic thyroid nodule. On a comparable note, a diffusely enlarged hypervascular and hypoechoic gland, especially in a patient with ophthalmopathy and biochemical hyperthyroidism, is consistent with Graves' disease. Additionally, multiple nodules in a hyperthyroid patient suggest a toxic multinodular goiter.

An important component of the information obtained with ultrasound is the evaluation of the contralateral thyroid lobe and the surrounding lymph nodes. (Figure 4) Multiple studies have shown that ultrasound allows the surgeon to plan for extent of thyroidectomy (Mazzaglia, 2010; Papini, 2002; Park et al, 2009; Stulak et al, 2006). The authors (M.G and J.I.L) believe that ultrasound should be used routinely in the evaluation of thyroid nodules in pediatric patients with reports in the literature suggesting its advantage for this specific purpose (Corrias et al, 2008; Stulak et al, 2006; Wada et al, 2009).

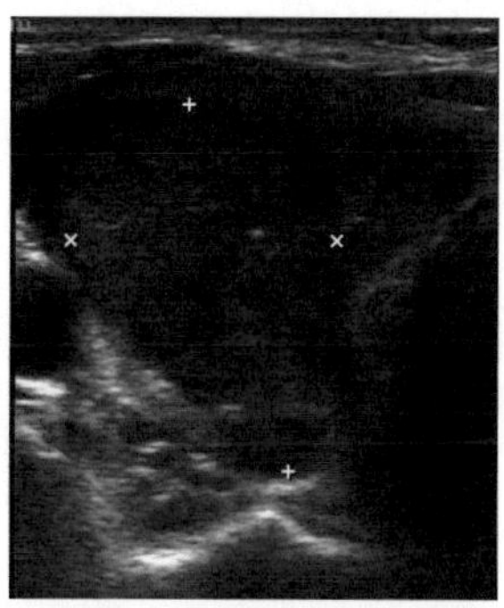

Fig. 2. Thyroid nodule with taller > wider dimensions

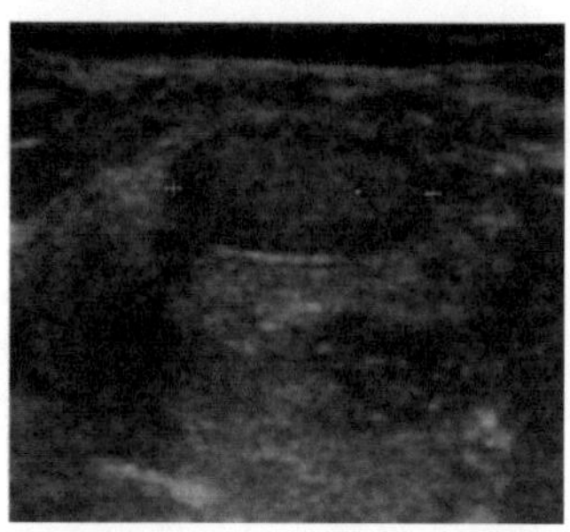

Fig. 3. Example of thyroid nodule with benign ultrasound features
Ultrasound nodule characteristics include regular borders, solid and cystic components, and no microcalcifications

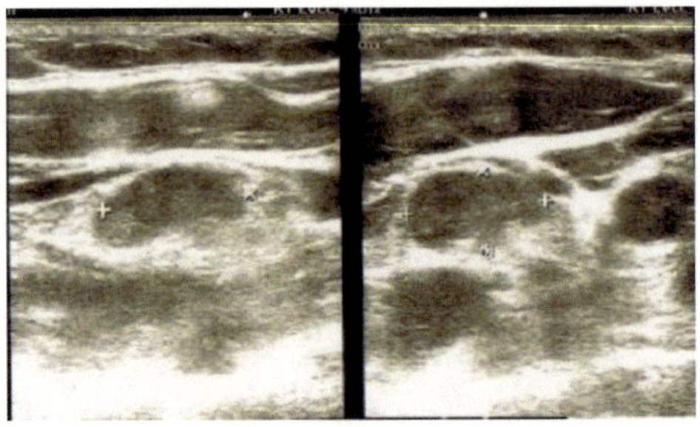

A

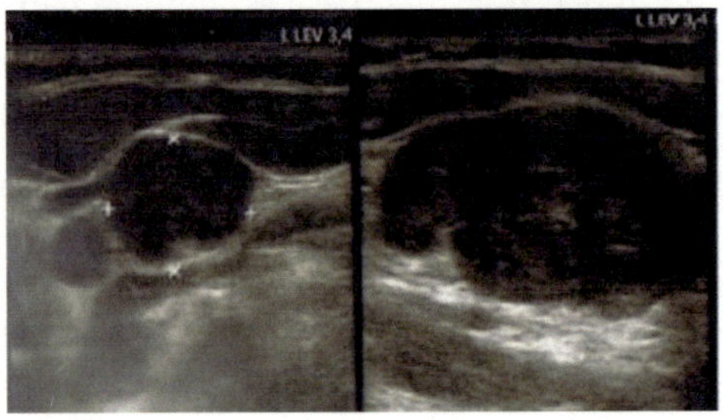

B

Fig. 4. **Ultrasound features of abnormal lymph nodes**
Figure 4A &B Abnormal lymph nodes demonstrate an enlarged size, microcalcifications, irregular borders, and a solid component

3.2 Scintigraphy

Thyroid scintigraphy is mentioned mainly for historic purposes. Before ultrasound, radioisotope scans were utilized for evaluating thyroid nodules. "Hot" nodules were indicative of hyperfunctioning thyroid nodules or, if diffuse activity, Graves' disease, and unlikely to be malignant. Conversely, "cold" nodules were thought to be highly suspicious for thyroid malignancy (Corrias et al, 2001; Scholtz et al, 2011). Aside from its inaccuracy, patients who undergo thyroid scintigraphy are subjected to radiation that may be of concern in pediatric patients. As such, there are very few, if any, indications for routine thyroid scintigraphy in these younger patients with thyroid nodules.

3.3 Fine Needle Aspiration (FNA)

Fine needle aspiration (FNA) has been extensively studied in adults. In general, FNA is a safe, cost-effective procedure that can be performed in the office or clinic setting. When positive for cancer, FNA is 90-98% sensitive for predicting thyroid cancer depending on institution (Tee et al, 2007). With an FNA diagnosis of malignancy, the appropriate surgical procedure can be performed that usually involves total thyroidectomy for all nodules greater than one cm, and central and/or lateral neck dissection when involved lymph nodes are identified either preoperatively and/or intraoperatively. In pediatric patients, however, there remains disagreement over the accuracy of FNA with some groups reporting high sensitivity and specificity whereas others suggesting the opposite; one group reported a sensitivity as low as 70% (Amriki et al, 2005; Arda et al, 2001; Bargen et al, 2010; Canadian, 2008; Corrias et al, 2001; Hosler et al, 2006; Izquierdo et al, 2009; Lugo-Vicente, 1998; Willgerodt et al, 2006). Additionally, "indeterminate" FNA biopsies may have up to a 50% chance of malignancy in multiple series with their malignant potential determined only on final pathology (Bargen et al, 2010; Brooks, 2001; Gharib, 2007; Kim E et al, 2003; Mandell, 2001; Raab, 1995). In one surgical series, benign FNA biopsy carried up to a 17% risk of thyroid malignancy (Tee, 2007).

The imprecision of FNA, seemingly equal to ultrasound evaluation, becomes more important when considering FNA in pediatric patients. While FNA is safe and easily accomplished in pediatric patients, other factors should be taken into account (Willgerodt et al, 2006). For those patients, especially in the younger age groups, clinicians must take into consideration the potential inability or maturity for such patients to sit still for the procedure, an increased sensitivity to or fear of needle sticks, and a smaller space to maneuver both the ultrasound and FNA needle with precision.

As such, the authors suggest a more selective use of FNA in pediatric patients, and ultrasound may be used to identify those patients who require further FNA diagnosis. The main role for FNA is making a definitive diagnosis of cancer in a thyroid nodule or lymph node with very suspicious ultrasound characteristics for preoperative planning (Lugo-Vicente, 1998).

FNA is performed with a 22-25 gauge needle in young adult and pediatric patients. Local anesthetic can be used at the discretion of the clinician. Studies have shown that multiple passes at different areas within the nodules as well as multiple slides give the most accurate biopsy results (Alexander et al, 2002). Aspirated contents should immediately be placed in fixative, and in an ideal setting, reviewed immediately by a cytopathologist for adequacy of sample. In general, thyroid nodules in the superior pole and/or anteriorly located are most easily biopsied in the office setting, whereas those nodules residing in a posterior location are more easily biopsied by interventional radiology.

3.4 Other imaging

In patients with a diagnosis of thyroid cancer, many advocate a preoperative chest X-ray to exclude for obvious pulmonary metastases (Hung, 1999; Waugepack et al, 2006). Another consideration is a non-contrast CT or MRI to identify pathologic lymphadenopathy or extensive thyroid disease preoperatively. Care must be taken not to order an intravenous contrast scan so as not to interfere with postoperative radioactive iodine scanning and treatment.

3.5 Laboratory testing

If not done already, laboratory evaluation should include thyroid-stimulating hormone (TSH) to determine if patients are euthyroid, hypothyroid or hyperthyroid. In patients that are suspected to have medullary thyroid carcinoma, calcitonin, CEA, and calcium levels should be obtained, and urine or plasma free metanephrines and normetanephrines to exclude underlying pheochromocytoma associated with MEN2.

4. Initial management

4.1 Cystic nodules

Whereas cystic thyroid nodules in adults are generally thought to be benign, there is some evidence to suggest the same does not hold true in pediatric patients (Yastovich et al, 1998). In adults, thyroid nodules with a cystic component can have a malignancy rate of at least 13% (Chan et al, 2003). For purely cystic thyroid nodules with regular borders, a reasonable initial management approach is FNA under ultrasound guidance. The fluid should be sent for cytology and the patient should be monitored with serial ultrasound exam at six months and then yearly thereafter for three years. Although FNA may be repeated a second time, the patient should be advised to undergo surgical resection, usually diagnostic thyroid lobectomy with isthmusectomy if the thyroid cyst recurs. Thyroid lesions with mixed solid and cystic components should be evaluated based on a combination of ultrasound characteristics as outlined below.

4.2 Toxic nodules

Thyroid lobectomy with isthmusectomy for a solitary toxic nodule in pediatric patients is currently performed (Astl et al, 2004; Canadian, 2008). Although radioactive iodine therapy and anti-thyroid medications are efficacious in a certain percentage of patients, many pediatricians believe that the benefits of surgical resection outweigh the risks of receiving radioactive iodine therapy (RAI), the substantial rate of permanent hypothyroidism, noncompliance with medication, and need for immediate relief of hyperthyroid symptoms (school and social performance) in this particular age group (Sherman et al, 2006). Thyroidectomy for benign disease can be performed by an experienced thyroid surgeon with minimal complications (Raval et al, 2009). When only removing half of a patient's thyroid gland, there is no risk of permanent hypoparathyroidism and rendering a patient hypothyroid is much abated. For toxic multinodular goiters, similar risks of non-surgical therapy apply with an even higher rate of failure for both RAI and medical therapy, as well as a greater chance for permanent hypothyroidism. These patients typically undergo total thyroidectomy due to bilateral thyroid nodules. While a risk for permanent hypoparathyroidism exists, the rate is very low in the hands of an experienced thyroid surgeon.

4.3 Solitary thyroid nodules

In the pediatric population, a significant number of patients will be referred for surgical consultation with clinical indications that necessitate thyroidectomy. These surgical indications include (but are not limited to) a history of head and neck radiation, history of MEN2, toxic nodule or multinodular goiter, obstructive symptoms, and fixed or firm nodule. In a pediatric patient with no evaluation, ultrasound examination should be performed based on the following recommendations.

4.3.1 Benign ultrasound features

Although large clinical studies with surgical cohorts have not been performed in the pediatric population, some clinicians have reported successful monitoring of pediatric patients with serial ultrasound exams based on benign features alone (Corrias et al, 2010). Such benign thyroid nodules are iso- or hyperechoic, have regular borders, no microcalcifications, and no suspicious lymphadenopathy. Such nodules can be safely monitored with a neck ultrasound exam at six months and then yearly thereafter for three to five years as recommended by current ATA guidelines, or every two years by Korean consensus guidelines (Cooper et al, 2009; Moon et al, 2011). If thyroid nodule ultrasound characteristics change or new clinical factors develop that warrant surgical resection, FNA or diagnostic thyroid lobectomy with isthmusectomy should be considered. One long term study of 56 patients who were originally thought to have benign disease based on ultrasound and/or FNA were later found to have PTC (Ito et al, 2007). Only 5.3% of these patients developed recurrent disease and none died, suggesting that such thyroid cancers have an indolent course.

4.3.2 Malignant ultrasound features

Thyroid nodules that present with suspicious features such as irregular borders, microcalcifications, corresponding suspicious lymph nodes and hypoechogenicity may require surgical resection regardless of FNA results. Either diagnostic thyroid lobectomy with isthmusectomy and frozen section or total thyroidectomy depending on patient preference may be performed.

4.3.3 Equivocal ultrasound features

Since there are no large surgical series characterizing combinations of ultrasound features in the pediatric age group, nodules that have a mix of both benign and malignant features should be biopsied. Any FNA result other than benign should be regarded with suspicion since a 25% malignancy rate exists in such thyroid nodules of this pediatric age group. Benign FNA results in a patient with equivocal ultrasound features should at minimum receive close follow-up, and surgical resection should be considered for definitive diagnosis.

For pediatric patients with FNA results, subsequent management and following recommendations are made.

4.3.4 Benign FNA results

In patients with benign FNA results, benign ultrasound features, no worrisome aspect of the history or physical exam, and no indication for surgical resection, thyroid nodules can be safely monitored with serial ultrasound exams for the next three to five years. However, benign FNA results may have up to a 17% false negative rate. If there are other clinical indications for surgical resection, such as obstructive symptoms, fixed nodule, or a history of head/neck radiation therapy or exposure, thyroid lobectomy with isthmusectomy should be performed. For benign FNA results in a thyroid nodule with suspicious ultrasound characteristics and no other clinical indications for surgical resection, either diagnostic thyroid lobectomy and isthmusectomy or close monitoring with serial ultrasound exams may be indicated. In such situations, the patient should be counseled that thyroid malignancy cannot be entirely excluded, and surgical resection may be required for definitive diagnosis.

4.3.5 Indeterminate FNA results (Bethesda III-Atypical cells and Bethesda IV-Follicular neoplasm

Current ATA guidelines recommend surgical resection for any Bethesda IV follicular neoplasm (Cooper et al, 2009). For Bethesda III lesions, the current recommendation is repeat FNA. However, in pediatric patients, the next course of action should also be based on thyroid nodule ultrasound features and other risk factors. In the absence of any definite risk factors, management options include close monitoring with serial ultrasound exams if the nodule has benign features or diagnostic thyroid lobectomy with isthmusectomy for thyroid nodules with suspicious ultrasound characteristics or patient preference.

4.3.6 Suspicious/malignant FNA results (Bethesda V and VI)

Any thyroid nodule with an FNA diagnosis of cancer (Bethesda VI) requires surgical resection that usually consists of total thyroidectomy with or without neck dissection. Pediatric patients have a high rate of multifocality and a higher risk of recurrent disease if a lesser operation is performed (Cooper et al, 2009; Demidchik et al, 2006; Hay et al, 2010; Hung, 1999; Jarzab et al, 2000; Thompson & Hay, 2004; Welsh-Danaher et al, 1998). In addition, total thyroidectomy allows for the potential use of RAI therapy to treat metastatic disease. Total thyroidectomy also allows patients to be monitored with serum TG and TG antibodies for recurrent disease. Careful examination of the central and lateral neck compartment lymph nodes should be undertaken with preoperative ultrasound for potential neck dissection. Suspicious appearing lymph nodes associated with malignant thyroid nodules confirmed by FNA are considered cancerous until proven otherwise. Such suspicious lymph nodes may warrant FNA preoperatively for surgical planning or frozen section in the operating room.

The sensitivity of "suspicious" or Bethesda V FNA results is somewhat institutional dependent. Rate of malignancy can be upward of 95% for such FNA biopsies. If, however, the clinician's respective institution has a lower rate of malignancy in Bethesda V specimens, an approach with diagnostic thyroid lobectomy with isthmusectomy may be undertaken. Frozen section may play a role in determining a definitive diagnosis of thyroid cancer in the operating room, allowing for total thyroidectomy at the first operation.

4.4 Multinodular goiter

Multiple thyroid nodules discovered on ultrasound examination in pediatric patients is important for surgical planning. Ultrasound features for each thyroid nodule should be evaluated, and further management undertaken as outlined for solitary thyroid nodules. If there is an indication for surgical resection for any single nodule based on risk factors, ultrasound features or FNA results, the presence of bilateral thyroid nodules should prompt consideration for total thyroidectomy. Small and less than one cm thyroid nodules with benign features can usually be monitored with serial ultrasound exams. An informed discussion should be carried out with the pediatric patient and parents.

5. Conclusion

Thyroid nodules in the pediatric patient require careful and vigilant evaluation. Since elements of a patient's history, physical exam, or risk factors may be indications for surgical resection, ultrasound should be further utilized as a key diagnostic tool to help evaluate any thyroid nodule in the pediatric population.

6. References

AACE/AME Task Force on thyroid nodules. American Association of Clinical Endocrinologists and Associazione Medici Endocrinologi medical guidelines for clinical practice for the diagnosis and management of thyroid nodules. Endocr Pract 2006; 12: 63-102

Alexander EK, Heering JP, Benson CB etal. Assessment of nondiagnostic ultrasound-guided fine needle aspirations of thyroid nodules. J Clin Endocrinol Metab 2002; 87: 4924-4927

American Cancer Society. Cancer facts and figures 2009. American Cancer Society, Atlanta, GA, USA 2009

Amrikachi M, Ponder TB, Wheeler TM, etal. Thyroid fine-needle aspiration biopsy in children and adolescents: experience with 218 aspirates. Diagn Cytopathol 2005; 32(4): 189-92

Arda IS, Yildirim S, Demirhan B, etal. Fine needle aspiration biopsy of thyroid nodules. Arch Dis Child 2001;85(4):313-7

Astl J, Dvorakova M, Vlck P, etal. Thyroid surgery in children and adolescents. International J Pediatr Otorhinolaryngol 2004; 68: 1273-8

Bargren AE, Meyer-Rochow GY, Sywak MS, etal. Diagnostic utility of fine-needle aspiration cytology in pediatric differentiated thyroid cancer. World J. Surg 2010; 34(6): 1254–1260

Brignardello E, Corrias A, Isolato G, etal. Ultrasound screening for thyroid carcinoma in childhood cancer survivors: a case series. J Clin Endocrinol Metab 2008; 93: 4840-4843

Brooks AD, Shaha AR, DuMornay W, etal. Role of fine-needle aspiration biopsy and frozen section analysis in the surgical management of thyroid tumors. Ann Surg Oncol 2001; 8: 92-10001

The Canadian pediatric thyroid nodule study group. The Canadian pediatric nodule study: an evaluation of current management practices. J Pediatric Surg 2008; 43:826-30

Camiel MR, Mulé JE, Alexander LL, etal. Thyroid carcinoma with Gardner's syndrome._N Engl J Med 1968; 279(6):326

Chan BK, Desser TS, McDougall IR, Weigel RJ, Jeffrey RB., Jr Common and uncommon sonographic features of papillary thyroid carcinoma. J Ultrasound Med. 2003;22:1083–1090

Ceccarelli C, Pacini F, Lippi F, etal. Thyroid cancer in children and adolescents. Surgery 1988;104(6):1143-8

Cooper DS, Doherty GM, Haugen BR, etal. American Thyroid Association (ATA) guidelines taskforce on thyroid nodules and differentiated thyroid cancer. Revised American thyroid association management guidelines for patients with thyroid nodules and differentiated thyroid cancer. Thyroid 2009; 19(11): 1167-1214

Corrias A, Cassio A, Weber G, etal. Thyroid nodules and cancer in children and adolescents affected by autoimmune thyroiditis. Arch Pediatr adolesc med 2008; 162(6): 526-531

Corrias A, Einaudi S, Chioboli E, etal. Accuracy of fine needle aspiration biopsy of thyroid nodules in detecting malignancy in childhood: comparison with conventional clinical, laboratory, and imaging approaches. J Clin Endocrinol Metab 2001; 86(10): 4644-4648

Corrias A, Mussa A, Baronio F, etal. Diagnostic features of thyroid nodules in pediatrics. Arch Pediatr Adolesc Med 2010; 164(8): 714-719

Crom DB, Kaste SC, Tubergen DG, etal. Ultrasonography for thyroid screening after head and neck irradiation in childhood cancer survivors. Med Pediatr Oncol 1997; 28(`):15-21

Danese D, Sciacchitano, S, Farsetti A, etal. Diagnostic accuracy of conventional versus sonography-guided fine-needle aspiration biopsy of thyroid nodules. Thyroid 1998; 8: 15-21

Dinauer CA, Breuer C, Rivkees SA. Differentiated thyroid cancer in children: diagnosis and management. Curr Opin Oncol 2008; 20(1): 59-65

Dinauer C, Francis GL. Thyroid cancer in children. Endocrinol Metab Clin North Am 2007; 36(3): 779-806

DeGroot L, Paloyan E. Thyroid carcinoma and radiation, A Chicago endemic. JAMA 1973; 225:487-491

Demidchik YE, Demidchik EP, Reiners C, etal. Comprehensive clinical assessment of 740 cases of surgically treated thyroid cancer in children of Belarus. Ann Surgery 2006; 243(4): 525-532

Dorzd VM, Lushchik ML, Polyanskaya ON, etal. The usual ultrasonographic features of thyroid cancer are less frequent in small tumors that develop after a long latent period after the Chernobyl radiation release accident. Thyroid 2009; 19: 725-734

Duffy BJ, Fitzgerald PJ. Thyroid cancer in childhood and adolescence; a report on 28 cases. Cancer 1950 ; 3(6):1018-32

Ezzat S, Sarti DA, Cain DR, Braunstein GD. Thyroid incidentalomas. Prevalence by palpation and ultrasonography. Arch Intern Med 1994; 154(16):1838-40

Faggiano A, Coulot J, Bellon N, etal. Age-dependent variation of follicular size and expression of iodine transporters in human thyroid tissue. J Nucl Med 2004; 45:232-7

Fleming ID, Black TL, Thompson EI etal. Thyroid dysfunction and neoplasia in children receiving neck irradiation for cancer. Cancer 1984; 55: 1190-1194

Fowler CL, Pokorny WJ, Harberg FJ. Thyroid nodules in children: current profile of a changing disease. South Med J 1989;82(12):1472-8

Frates MC, Benson CB, Doubilet PM, etal. Prevalence and distribution of carcinoma in patients with solitary and multiple thyroid nodules on sonography. J Clin Endocrinol Metab 2006; 91:3411–3417

Gandolfi PP, Frisina A, Raffa M, etal. The incidence of thyroid carcinoma in multinodular goiter: retrospective analysis. Acta Biomed 2004; 75(2):114-7

Gharib H, Papini E, Valcavi R, etal. American Association of Clinical Endocrinologists and Associazione Medici Endocrinologi medical guidelines for clinical practice for the diagnosis and management of thyroid nodules. Endocr Pract 2006; 12(1): 63-102

Gharib H, Papini E. Thyroid nodules: clinical importance, assessment, and treatment. Endocrinol Metab Clin North Am 2007; 36: 707-735

Goepfert H, Dichtel WJ, Samaan NA.. Thyroid cancer in children and teenagers. Arch Otolaryngol 1984;110(2):72-5

Goldfarb M, Gondek SS, Solorzano C, etal. Surgeon performed ultrasound can predict benignity in thyroid nodules. Surgery 2011; In Press

Gosepath J, Spix C, Talebloo B, etal. Incidence of childhood cancer of the head and neck in Germany._Ann Oncol 2007;18(10):1716-21

Guth S, Theune U, Aberle J, etal. Very high prevalence of thyroid nodules detected by high frequency (13MHz) ultrasound examination. Eur J Clin Invest 2009; 39(8): 699-706

Halac I, Zimmerman D. Thyroid nodules and cancers in children. Endocrinol Metab Clin North Am 2005; 34: 725-44

Hameed R, Zacharin MR. Changing face of paediatric and adolescent thyroid cancer. Paediatr Child Health 2005;41(11):572-4

Harach HR, Williams ED. Childhood thyroid cancer in England and Wales. Br. J. Cancer 72(3), 777–783 (1995)

Harness JK, Thompson NW, McLeod MK,etal. Differentiated thyroid carcinoma in children and adolescents. World J Surg 1992;16(4):547-53

Hay ID, Gonzalez-Losada T, Reinalda MS, etal. Long-term outcome in 215 children and adolescents with papillary thyroid cancer treated during 1940 through 2008. World J Surg 2010; 34: 1192-1202

Hogan AR, Zhuge Y, Perez EA,etal. Pediatric thyroid carcinoma: Incidence and outcomes in 1753 patients. J Surg Research 2009; 156: 167-172

Horner MJ, Ries LAG, Krapcho M etal. SEER Cancer Statistics Review, 1975–2006. National Cancer Institute, Bethesda, MD, USA 2010

Hosler GA, Clark I, Zakowski MF, etal. Cytopathologic analysis of thyroid lesions in the pediatric population. Diagn Cytopathol 2006

Hung W. Solitary thyroid nodules in 93 children and adolescents: a 35-years experience. Horm Res 1999; 52(1): 15-18

Ito Y, Higashiyama T, Takamura Y etal. Long-term follow-up for patients with papillary thyroid carcinoma treated as benign nodules. Anticancer Res 2007; 27(2): 1039–1043

Izquierdo R, Shankar R, Kort K, Khurana K. Ultrasound-guided fine-needle aspiration in the management of thyroid nodules in children and adolescents. Thyroid 2009; 19(7): 703–705

Jabiev AA, Ikeda MH, Reis IM, et al. Surgeon-Performed Ultrasound can Predict Differentiated Thyroid Cancer in Patients with Solitary Thyroid Nodules. Ann Surg Oncol 2009; 16: 3140-3145

Jarzab B, Handkiewicz Junak D, Wloch J etal. Multivariate analysis of prognostic factors for differentiated thyroid carcinoma in children. Eur. J. Nucl. Med 2000; 27(7): 833–841

Josefson J, Zimmerman D. Thyroid nodules and cancers in children. Pediatr Endocrinol Rev 2008;6:14–23

Kim ES, Nam-Goong IS, Gong GY, etal. Postoperative findings and risk for malignancy in thyroid nodules with cytological diagnosis of the so-called "follicular neoplasm". Korean J Intern Med 2003; 18:94-7

Kim MJ, Kim EK, Park SI, etal. US-guided fine needle aspiration of thyroid nodules: indications, techniques, results. Radiograph 2008; 28(7): 1869-86

Lafferty AR, Batch JA. Thyroid nodules in childhood and adolescence-thirty years of experience. J Pediatr Endocrinol Metab 1997; 10: 479-86

Leenhardt L, Hejblum G, Franc B, etal. Indications and limits of ultrasound-guided cytology in the management of nonpalpable thyroid nodules. J Clin Endocrinol Metab 1999; 84: 24-28

Loh KC. Familial nonmedullary thyroid carcinoma: a meta-review of case series. Thyroid 1997; 7:107–113

Lugo-Vicente H, Ortiz VN, Irizarry H, etal. Pediatric thyroid nodules: management in the era of fine needle aspiration. J Pediatr Surg 1998; 33(8): 1302-5

Machens A, Lorenz K, Thanh PN, etal. Papillary thyroid cancer in children and adolescents does not differ in growth pattern and metastatic behavior. J Pediatrics 2010; 157(4): 648-652

Mandell DL, Genden EM, Mechanick JI, etal. Diagnostic accuracy of fine-needle aspiration and frozen section in nodular thyroid disease. Otolaryngol Head Neck Surg 2001; 124: 531-536

Maule M, Scelo G, Pastore G, etal. Risk of second malignant neoplasms after childhood leukemia and lymphoma: an international study. J Natl Cancer Inst 2007; 99: 790-800

Mazzaglia, P. Surgeon-Performed Ultrasound in Patients Referred for Thyroid Disease Improves Patient Case by Minimizing Performance of Unnecessary Procedures and Optimizing Surgical Treatment. WJS 2010; 34: 1164-1170

Mehta MP, Goetowski PG, Kinsella TJ. Radiation induced thyroid neoplasms 1920 to 1987: A vanishing problem? Int J Rad Oncol Biol Physics 1989; 16(6):1471-1475

Milas M, Stephen A, Berber E, etal. Ultrasonography for the endocrine surgeon: a valuable clinical tool that enhances diagnostic and therapeutic outcomes. Surgery 2005; 138(6): 1193-1200

Moon WJ, Baek JH, Jung SL, etal. Ultrasonography and the ultrasound-based management of thyroid nodules: consensus statement and recommendations. Korean J Radiol 2011; 12(1): 1-14

Niedziela M. Pathogenesis, diagnosis, and management of thyroid nodules in children. Endocr Relat Cancer 2006; 13(2): 427-453

Nose V. Familial Thyroid cancer: A review. Mod Pathol 2011; 24 Suppl 2:S19-33

O'Kane P, Shelkovoy E, McConnell RJ, etal. Frequency of undetected thyroid nodules in a large I-131-exposed population repeatedly screened by ultrasonography: results from the ukranian-american cohort study of thyroid cancer and other thyroid disease following the Chernobyl accident. Thyroid 2010; 20(9): 959-964

Ortel JE, Klinck GH. Structural changes in the thyroid glands of healthy young men. Med Ann DC 1965; 34:75-77

Pacini F. Thyroid cancer in children and adolescents. J Endocrinol invest 2002; 25:572-73

Papini E, Guglielmi R, Bianchini A, etal. Risk of malignancy in nonpalpable thyroid nodules: predictive value of ultrasound and color-Doppler features. J Clin Endocrinol Metab 2002;87(5):1941-6

Park JS, Son KR, Na DG, Kim E, Kim S. Performance of preoperative sonographic staging of papillary thyroid carcinoma based on sixth edition of the AJCC/UICC TNM classification system. AJR 2009; 192:66-72

Poyhonen L, Lenko HL. Ultrasound imaging in diffuse thyroid disorders of children. Acta Paediatr Scand 1986; 75: 272-278

Raab SS, Silverman JF, Elsheikh TM, etal. Pediatric thyroid nodules: disease demographics and clinical management as determined by fine needle aspiration. Pediatrics 1995; 95: 46-49

Rallison ML, Dobyns BM, Meikle AW, etal. Natural history of thyroid abnormalities: prevalence, incidence, and regression of thyroid disease in adolescents and young adults. Am J Med 1991; 91(4): 363-70

Raval MV, Browne M, Chin AC, eta al. Total thyroidectomy for benign disease in the pediatric patient-feasible and safe. J Ped Surg 2009; 44:1529-1533

Ries LAG, Harkins D, Krapcho M, etal (eds) SEER Cancer statistic review, 1975-2003, NCI, Bethesda, MD. http://seer.cancer.gov/csr/1975-2003

Samaan NA, Schultz PN, Ordonez HG, etal. A comparison of thyroid carcinoma in those who have and have not had head and neck irradiation in childhood. J Clin Endocrinol Metab 2007; 64: 219-223

Scholz S, Smith JR, Chaignaud B, etal. Thyroid surgery at Children's Hospital Boston: a 35-year single-institution experience. J Pediatr Surg 2011; 46(3): 437-42

Sherman J, Thompson GB, Lteif A, etal. Surgical management of Graves' disease in childhood and adolescence: an institutional experience. Surgery 2006; 140: 1056-62

Sklar C, Whitton J, Mertens A, etal. Abnormalities of the thyroid in survivors of Hodgkin's disease: data from the childhood cancer survivor study. J Clin Endocrinol Metab 2000; 85: 3227-3232

Smith WG, Kern BB. The nature of the mutation in familial multiple polyposis: papillary carcinoma of the thyroid, brain tumors, and familial multiple polyposis. Dis Colon Rectum 1973; 16(4):264-71

Sigurdson AJ, Ronckers CM, Mertens AC, etal. Primary thyroid cancer after a first tumour in childhood (the childhood cancer survivor study): a nested case-control study. Lancet 2005; 365: 2014-2023

Solorzano CC, Carneiro DM, Ramirez M, etal. Surgeon-performed ultrasound in the management of thyroid malignancy. Am Surg 2004; 70(7): 576-580

Solt I, Gaitini D, Pery M, etal. Comparing thyroid ultrasonography to thyroid function in long-term survivors of childhood lymphoma. Med Pediatr Oncol 20001;35(1):35-40

Steliarova-Foucher E, Stiller CA, Pukkala E, etal. Thyroid cancer incidence and survival among European children and adolescents (1978–1997): Report from the Automated Childhood Cancer Information System project. Eur J Cancer 2006; 42(13): 2150-2169

Stevens C, Lee JKP, Sadatsafavi M, Blair G. pediatric thyroid fine-needle aspiration cytology: a meta-analysis. J Ped Surg 2009; 44: 2184-2191

Stulak JM, Grant CS, Farley DR, etal. Value of preoperative ultrasonography in the surgical management of initial and reoperative papillary thyroid cancer. Arch Surg 2006; 141:489-94

Tee YY, Lowe AJ, Brand CA, Judson RT, Fine-needle aspiration may miss a third of all malignancy in palpable thyroid nodules: a comprehensive literature review, Ann Surg 2007; 246: 714–720

Thompson GB, Hay ID. Current strategies for surgical management and adjuvant treatment of childhood papillary thyroid carcinoma. World J. Surg 2004; 28(12): 1187–1198

Tucker MA, Jones PH, Boice JD Jr, etal. Therapeutic radiation at a young age is linked to secondary thyroid cancer. The Late Effects Study Group._Cancer Res 1991; 51(11): 2885-8

Viswanathan K, Gierlowski TC, Schneider AB. Childhood thyroid cancer. Characteristics and long-term outcome in children irradiated for benign conditions of the head and neck. Arch Pediatr Adol Med 1994;148(3): 260-5

Wada, N, Sugino K, Mimura T, etal. Treatment strategy of papillary thyroid carcinoma in children and adolescents: clinical significance of the initial nodal manifestation. Ann Surg Oncol 2009; 16: 3442-2449

Waguespack S, Wells S, Ross J, etal. Thyroid cancer. SEER AYA monograph, in Bleyer A, O'Leary M, Barr R etal (eds): Cancer Epidemiology in Older adolescents and young adults 15-29 years of age, Including SEER Incidence and Survival 1975-2000. NIH Pub NOO. 06-5767, Bethesda, MD, NCI, 2006

Wartofsky L. The thyroid nodule. In: Wartofsky L (ed) Thyroid cancer: a comprehensive guide to clinical management 2000. Uhmana Press, Totawa, NJ p3-7

Welch Dinauer CA, Tuttle RM, Robie DK, McClellan DR, Francis GL. Extensive surgery improves recurrence-free survival for children and young patients with class I papillary thyroid carcinoma. J Pediatr Surg 1999; 34(12): 1799–1804

Wiersinga WM. Management of thyroid nodules in children and adolescents. Hormones 2007; 6(3): 194-199

Willgerodt H, Keller E, Bennek J, etal. Diagnostic value of fine-needle aspiration biopsy of thyroid nodules in children and adolescents. J Pediatr Endocrinol Metab 2006; 19(4): 507-15

Winship T, Rosvoll RV. Cancer of the thyroid in children. Proc Natl Cancer Conf 1970; 6: 677-81

Yastovich A, Laberge JM, Rodd C, etal. Cystic thyroid lesions in children. J Pediatr Surg 1998; 33:866-70

Yip FW, Reeve TS, Poole AG, etal. Thyroid nodules in childhood and adolescence. Aust N Z J Surg 1994; 64: 676-8

7

Papillary Thyroid Cancer in Childhood and Adolescence with Specific Consideration of Patients After Radiation Exposure

Yuri Demidchik[1], Mikhail Fridman[1], Kurt Werner Schmid[3], Christoph Reiners[2], Johannes Biko[2] and Svetlana Mankovskaya[1]

[1]Belarusian Medical Academy for Postgraduate Education,
[2]Institute of Pathology and Neuropathology, University Hospital of Essen, University of Duisburg-Essen,
[3]University of Wuerzburg,
[1]Belarus
[2,3]Germany

1. Introduction

Papillary thyroid carcinoma (PTC) in children and adolescents is a medical problem that attracts attention of investigators and clinicians primarily because of the high incidence of this malignancy in individuals exposed to radioactive isotopes of iodine in case of nuclear reactor emergencies. New facts uncovered by various research groups make it possible to see the clinical and pathological peculiarities of these tumours in a new light and suggest that the aetiology can modify the biological behaviour of PTC. In particular, relative monomorphism of the structure of post-Chernobyl cancers was detected and morphology varies depending on the patients' age and the time of radiation exposure (LiVolsi et al., 2011).

For 25 years now child and adolescent thyroid cancer patients with and without a history of radiation exposure were concentrated in the Republican Thyroid Cancer Centre in Minsk where they undergo diagnostics, treatment and follow-up (Demidchik et al., 2006). This presents a unique opportunity to compare cases depending on the presumed cancer aetiology and to analyze similarities and differences in the molecular-genetic background of carcinogenesis, morphological structure and extension of these tumours.

The purpose of this study was to look into PTC in childhood and adolescence. We analyzed children between 1 and 14 years of age and adolescents between 15 and 18 years of age who were not exposed to known carcinogenic risks such as irradiation and did not have any indications of hereditary thyroid cancers (e.g. specifically cribriform-morular architecture). The second group consisted of patients of the same age in whom second primary papillary cancers of thyroid developed during the surveillance for primary malignancies in other organs or systems that were treated with external irradiation and/or chemotherapy. The third group, containing the largest number of PTC cases, consisted of children and adolescents with the history of exposure to radioactive isotopes of iodine in the framework of the Chernobyl Reactor Accident in 1986.

1.1 Epidemiology

Thyroid cancer is uncommon in childhood and adolescence. The incidence of all thyroid cancer types in children and adolescents varies from 0.04-0.17 per 100 000 in Ukraine, Germany, and Russia up to 0.54 in the USA (Hogan et al., 2009; Machens et al., 2010; Romanchishen et al., 2008; Tronko et al., 1999). The age-specific rates differ in paediatric age subgroups, for example, in Canada it is 0.2 per 100 000 children at the age of 5-9 years and 0.4 at the age of 10-14 years (O'Gorman et al., 2009), in USA 0.09 and 0.44 correspondingly (Hogan et al., 2009).

In Belarus, the incidence of thyroid carcinoma in children has been increasing since 1990 and a case-control study established a connection between this raise and the effect of the radioiodine that was released as a result of the Chernobyl accident (Astakhova et al., 1998; Kazakov et al., 1992; E.P. Demidchik et al., 1994, 2002; Yu.E. Demidchik et al., 2007). The highest rate of paediatric thyroid cancer was registered in 1995 at 3.29 per 100 000 for the whole country and 10.5 per 100 000 in southern regions of Belarus (e.g. Gomel). This was followed later by a marked decline of the age-standardized rate and was 0.14 per 100,000 (Savva et al., 2008). The proportion of PTC amid thyroid malignancies in the childhood population of Belarus was 87% in 1989-1997 (Steliarova-Foucher et al., 2006). It need to be clarified that after the demise of follicular carcinoma (major revision was done as the criteria that were used in soviet pathology practice since 1960es were abandoned after the training under supervision of leading westerner thyropathologists at the beginning of 1990es) the real numbers of PTC is close to 100%.

However, even more recently (2005-2008) the thyroid carcinoma incidence rate (IR) in patients under 18 in Belarus amounts to 1.29 per 100 000. Thus, paediatric thyroid cancer incidence is still high in Belarus among radiation-exposed and unexposed patients (Fig.1).

The majority of studies addressing the clinical and pathological characteristics of childhood thyroid carcinoma have reported on less than 100 cases, even if all types of thyroid cancer (sporadic, radiogenic and genetically determined) were included (Dinauer et al., 1998; Grigsby et al., 2002; Machens et al., 2010; O'Gorman et al., 2010). Moreover, some studies extended the patients' age to 19 and 20 (Dinauer et al., 1998; Romanchishen et al., 2008) and thus only partially meet the criteria of childhood thyroid cancer.

2. Diagnostics

In Belarus, mass screening using mobile teams and prophylactic examinations in schools and outpatient clinics was started in 1987. Prior to 1987 the diagnosis of thyroid disease was based primarily on clinical evaluation with particular attention to risk factors, which clinicians took into account: the history of radiation exposure, genetic predisposition, age, gender, lymph nodes status, tracheal or vascular pressure symptoms, recurrent nerve palsy and thyroid nodule features (size, consistency and fixation). Currently in Belarus, thyroid carcinomas in the exposed population are frequently diagnosed using screening by ultrasound and fine needle aspiration biopsy. This method allows detection of small thyroid

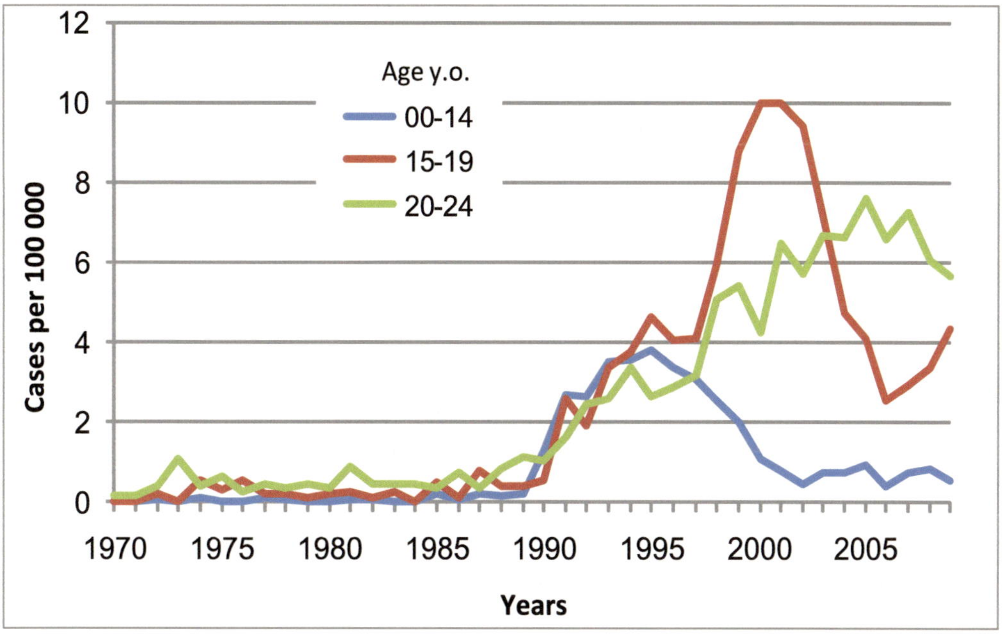

Fig. 1. Annual incidence (per 100 000) of thyroid cancer in Belarus

nodules, including microcarcinomas. Reported sensitivity, accuracy and specificity of this approach are equal to 90-100%, 80-95% and 80-100% respectively in cases of papillary carcinomas. Follicular carcinomas can rarely be diagnosed outright by ultrasound-guided fine needle aspiration biopsy as even positive data are reliable in less than 10% of cases (Chang et al., 2006; Sangalli et al., 2006; Florentine et al., 2006)

The evaluation of patients with thyroid nodules included determining possible predisposing factors, evaluation of present complaints, clinical findings, thyroid function tests, thyroglobulin (Tg) levels, anti-TPO, anti-microsomal and anti-Tg antibodies, imaging procedures (cervical ultrasound scan, chest radiograph, computed tomography scan), and the cytological findings yielded with fine needle aspiration cytology. One diagnostic problem was determining the presence of thyroid cancer in the presence of coexisting multinodular goiter. These patients usually received TSH suppressive therapy with levothyroxine. Dynamic ultrasound examination permitted recognizing structural changes such as enlargement of thyroid nodules or enlarged neck lymph nodes. These signs were suspicious of malignancy. Symptomatic patients usually complained of a neck mass (12.3%). Less commonly (2.8%) there were signs of hypothyroidism. In only 0.5% of cases were symptoms of advanced carcinoma (as e.g. hoarseness or problems with swallowing) recorded.

Preoperative work-up of patients suspected to have thyroid cancer included staging by computed tomography, MRI, thyroid scintigraphy with ^{131}I and serum thyroglobulin measurements. Typically, intraoperative frozen sections made it possible to diagnose the majority of papillary carcinomas.

PTC got its name because of its peculiarity to build papillary structures like cauliflower vegetations, connective tissue stalks which have small blood and lymphatic vessels. There is also frequent connection of classic papillary formations with zones of follicular and solid structures, besides there are some carcinomas in which there are no papillas at all.

Classification of PTC is made up taking into consideration various principles. Due to the peculiarities of tumour architecture investigators point out papillary, follicular, solid (solid-alveolar) and combined variants of structure. If we delved deeply from tissue to cell level, PTC can be classified according to the ability of cytoplasm stained by hematoxylin and eosin (common, clear and oxyphilic variants) and according to nuclear - cytoplasmic correlation (tall and columnar cell variants). At last, PTC can be divided according to the size (microcarcinoma) and growth essentials (solitary, multifocal and diffuse forms).

Many investigators tried to correlate clinical and morphological signs taking into consideration variants of PTC according to the WHO histological classification. For instance, the thyroid tumours that were discovered after the Chernobyl nuclear accident were virtually all of the papillary type (95%). Within the papillary group several subtypes were noted including classical or usual type, follicular and solid variants and mixed patterns. Diffuse sclerosing distribution, cribriform/morular type and Warthin-like variant were rare. No tall cell or columnar cell forms were identified (LiVolsi, 2011). To our opinion a potential bias of this conclusion lays in interobserver variability and lack of distinct borders for designation of this or that PTC variant. Thus, before comparing different forms of thyroid cancer in children and adolescents, it is necessary to dwell on definitions which were used in reports and subsequent analysis of the material.

Classical PTC is characterized by the formation of papillae made up of fibrovascular cores lined by one or two layers of neoplastic cells with a distinctive set of nuclear features which includes enlargement, elongation, clearing, thickened nuclear membranes, intranuclear cytoplasmic pseudoinclusions, nuclear grooves and small nucleoli closely opposed to the nuclear membrane. This pattern was usually mixed with the solid and follicular areas (DeLellies, R.A. & Williams, 2004).

The follicular variant of papillary thyroid carcinoma is almost exclusively arranged in follicles (without papillae formation but small solid areas are not unusual) lined by cells with characteristic PTC nuclei and usually presents as an encapsulated or circumscribed tumour with pushing borders and less commonly as a partially/non-encapsulated infiltrative neoplasm.

The solid variant is recognized by predominantly solid areas or a nested pattern of growth with prominent intratumoural capillary networks. These represent more than 50% of the tumour mass and can be associated with the follicular structures and even classic papillary vegetations.

Tall-cell variant (TCV) of papillary thyroid carcinoma is defined as being composed largely of tall cells with height at least twice the width and eosinophilic cytoplasm as well as basally oriented nuclei (many of them contain large intranuclear cytoplasmic eosinophilic pseudoinclusions). These cells represent 50% or more of the papillary carcinoma cells to make the diagnosis of tall cell variant (Morris et al., 2010). In paediatric cases we have seen predominantly follicular and solid areas composed of tall-cell PTC nuclei.

Diffuse sclerosing variant of PTC (DSV) is characterized by diffuse involvement of one or both lobes, extensive sclerosis, numerous psammoma bodies, typical papillary carcinoma elements, widespread squamous metaplastic changes and dense lymphocytic infiltration. Some cases had dominant tumour mass of conventional papillary carcinoma with prominent fibrosis. We observed formed lymphoid follicles, intensive lymphoplasmacytic infiltration, diffuse scattered psammoma bodies and tumour emboli in lymphatic channels and in surrounding normal-looking thyroid gland. These particular tumours more likely represent the early phase of classical DSV. In our investigation we define such designation as 'beginning'DSV or monofocal PTC with DSV-like intrathyroidal dissemination.

Diagnostic criteria for extrathyroidal extension and multifocal growth are important for staging of the disease. Some pathologists believe that the presence of adipose tissue within the normal thyroid gland and its pseudocapsule implies that thyroid carcinoma complexes within fat tissue cannot be accepted as a criterion of extrathyroidal extension (Mete O. et al., 2010). To skip controversies surrounding diagnostic criteria we divided extrathyroidal extension in tables as in a case of invasion of skeletal muscle and fat tissue as well. The differences in estimation of the prevalence of multifocality across studies may be explained by the conflicting definitions used for multifocality and multicentricity. This inconsistency makes it difficult to analyze the literature on the subject. Some professionals consider tumour emboli in lymphatic channels as 'multifocality'. To our opinion, this phenomenon should be diagnosed only in true multicentric transformation of the follicular epithelium (in case of independent clonal proliferations). Some situations are difficult to interpret without molecular investigation but tumours that differ from each other by anatomical sites and/or morphological structure and accompanied by fibrosis we define as multifocal. On the other hand, glands with a large clinical papillary cancer and multiple small intrathyroidal foci are 'lymphatic spread'.

3. Treatment

Optimal treatment of thyroid cancer in patients of any age includes surgery, radioiodine therapy for ablation of the thyroid remnant or treatment of distant metastases and levothyroxine suppressive therapy (Reiners & Demidchik, 2003; Luster et al., 2007; Reiners et al., 2008, 2009).

Patients with the history of exposure to radiation are considered as a high risk group (Clark, 2005). This point of view is based on the assumption that radionuclides of iodine affect the whole thyroid gland with an increased risk of multifocality. Therefore, the risk of tumour relapse in the thyroid remnant after partial resection is theoretically higher than in patients with sporadic carcinomas. There are many studies about the technique of operative intervention in patients with thyroid cancer. Today, prognostic factors for this disease have been carefully studied and treatment methods have been improved. Total thyroidectomy is considered the procedure of choice in patients with multifocal cancers, large tumour size, extrathyroidal extension and regional or distant metastasis. One important reason for recommending a total thyroidectomy is to faciliatate the ablation of the thyroid remnant and treatment of local or distant metastases with radioiodine (Luster et al., 2007; Reiners, 2009). Survival rates and quality of life of patients after surgical treatment remain high even in those cases when the findings at surgery reveal invasive carcinomas with involvement of adjacent organs and tissue structures of the neck (Gilliland et al., 1997, Lerch et al., 1997, Schlumberger, 2001, Shaha et al., 1997).

4. Comparative clinical and morphological analysis of sporadic papillary thyroid cancer, PTC as second malignancy and post-Chernobyl PTC

We define cancers as possibly radiation induced that developed in patients exposed to radioiodine in the context of the Chernobyl accident (this process was completed by June 1986). Therefore, for all patients in the sporadic group born after February 1987 (the eldest of which was 18 in 2005), the fall-out from Chernobyl likely did not play a role in thyroid carcinogenesis (LiVolsi et al., 2011). As a third group, we consider patients with second primaries of the thyroid that developed after treatment for another preceding primary malignancy. In the context of thyroid cancer external irradiation and probably the effect of chemotherapeutic agents for the combined therapy of hemoblastosis and other neoplasms in childhood have to be taken into consideration (Acharya et al., 2003; LiVolsi et al., 2011; Naing et al., 2009; Seaberg et al., 2005; Taylor et al., 2009).

4.1 Sporadic cancer

We analyzed 150 children and adolescents who had sporadic PTC (118 girls and 32 boys - 3.7:1 - aged from 4 to 18 years inclusively). Most patients underwent total thyroidectomy (126; 84.0%) or lobectomy (21; 14.0%) with simultaneous lymph node removal (133; 88.7%) on one or both sides of the neck. Lymph node central neck dissection included excision of level VI; bilateral selective or modified radical neck dissection was also performed (levels II – V). The number of removed lymph nodes varied from 1 to 87. In the latter part of the study the majority of patients (83; 55.3%) received radioiodine therapy for thyroid remnant ablation (75; 50.0%) with an average activity of 3.7 (0.31-9.44) GBq. In patients with lung metastases (8; 5.3%) a higher average activity of 7.42 (5.5-12.89) GBq of radioiodine was delivered. In all children and adolescents, TSH suppressive therapy was used as part of the treatment. The average follow-up time for patients in this group was 66.0 months (29.7-303.3).

Clinical and pathologic data on 150 patients with sporadic PTC is presented in Table 1.

The median size of sporadic carcinoma tumour nodules was 12 (1-100) mm both for children and adolescents. Total involvement of thyroid gland was observed among the patients that suffered from diffuse sclerosing PTC and the maximum tumour size made up 100 mm. The tumour dimension surpassed 10 mm in 49 (62.8%) of children and 43 (59.7%) adolescents. Lung metastases (children; 8 cases, 10.3%) and multifocal growth (children and adolescents, 5 cases, 3.3%) were rare.

Classical type of PTC that included pure papillary or mixture of patterns dominated both in children (25; 32.1%) and adolescents (36; 50.0%) followed by follicular and tall cell variants. Extrathyroidal extension took place in one of every three patients (children and adolescents, 49; 32.7%). PTC involved veins (29; 19.3%) and lymph vessels (120; 80.0%) in one of every five children and adolescents (tumour complexes and/or psammoma bodies, 4 of 5 cases).

PTC was more likely to develop in the background of asymptomatic autoimmune thyroiditis that was evenly distributed in all age groups (21 of 78 children, 26.9%; 17 of 72 adolescents, 26.4%).

	Age groups, years at presentation		Total (n=150)
	4-14 years (n=78)	15-18 years (n=72)	
Age at diagnosis, mean± SD	11.8±2.2	16.1±1.0	13.8±2.8
Gender (girls: boys)	2.5:1	6.2:1	3.7:1
girls	56 (71.8%)	62 (86.1%)	118 (78.7%)
boys	22 (28.2%)	10 (13.9%)	32 (21.3%)
Tumour size, mm median (range)	12.0 (1-100)	11.5 (3-58)	12.0 (1-100)
≤10 mm	29 (37.2%)	29 (40.3%)	58 (38.7%)
1-5 mm	5(6.4%)	12 (16.7%)	17 (11.4%)
6-10 mm	24 (30.8%)	17 (23.6%)	41 (27.3%)
≥11 mm	49(62.8%)	43(59.7%)	92(61.3%)
Localization			
Subcapsular	36 (46.2%)	18 (25.0%)	54 (36.0%)
Inside lobe	37 (47.4%)	46 (63.8%)	83 (55.4%)
Isthmus	5 (6.4%)	8 (11.2%)	13 (8.6%)
Local spreading, N0:	19(24.3%)	23 (31.5%)	42 (28.0%)
intrathyroidal	10 (12.8%)	15 (20.8%)	25 (16.7%)
extrathyroidal	4 (5.1%)	4 (5.6%)	8 (5.3%)
not reported, pTx	5 (6.4%)	4 (5.6%)	9 (6.0%)
Regional spreading, N+:	59(75.7%)	49 (68.0%)	108 (72.0%)
N1a	10 (12.8%)	17 (23.6%)	27 (18.0%)
N1b	49 (62.8%)	32 (44.4%)	81 (54.0%)
N1b unilateral	31(39.7%)	28 (38.9%)	59 (39.3%)
N1b bilateral	18(23.1%)	4 (5.6%)	19 (12.7%)
Distant metastases, M1 (lungs)	8 (10.3%)	0	8 (5.3%)
Tumour histology (predominant architecture):			
Papillary	28 (35.9%)	31 (43.0%)	59 (39.3%)
Follicular	29 (37.2%)	28 (38.9%)	57 (38.0%)
Solid	21 (26.9%)	13 (18.1%)	34 (22.7%)
Histological types:			
Classical PTC	25 (32.1%)	36 (50%)	61 (40.7%)
Follicular	16 (20.5%)	15 (20.9%)	31 (20.7%)
Diffuse sclerosing (DSV)	5 (6.4%)	4 (5.5%)	9 (6.0%)
Monofocal with diffuse sclerosing involvement (DSV-like)	10 (12.8%)	2 (2.8%)	12 (8.0%)
Tall cell	11 (14.1%)	8 (11.1%)	19 (12.6%)
Solid	11 (14.1%)	7 (9.7%)	18 (12.0%)
Multifocal growth	3 (3.9%)	2 (2.8%)	5 (3.3%)
Morphological specifications:			
Infiltrative growth	57 (73.1%)	54 (75.0%)	111 (74.0%)
1. Intrathyroidal (pT1-T2)	17 (21.8%)	20 (27.8%)	37 (24.7%)
2. Extrathyroidal extension (pT3)	31 (39.7%)	18 (25.0%)	49 (32.7%)
in fat tissue	29 (37.2%)	16 (22.2%)	45 (30.0%)
in muscle	2 (2.5%)	2 (2.8%)	4 (2.7%)
3. pTx	9 (11.5%)	16 (22.2%)	25 (16.7%)

circumscribed/encapsulated growth (pT1, pT2, pTx)	7 (9.0%)	11 (15.3%)	18 (12.0%)
Diffuse involvement (DSV and DSV-like - pT1-pTx)	14 (17.9%)	7 (9.7%)	21 (14.0%)
Intratumoural fibrosis:			
Focal	48 (52.0%)	37 (51.4%)	85 (56.7%)
Septal	6 (8.0%)	13 (18.1%)	19 (12.7%)
Massive (central scarring)	25 (32.0%)	19 (26.4%)	44 (29.3%)
Blood vessels involvement	20 (25.6%)	9 (12.5%)	29 (19.3%)
Lymph vessels involvement	66 (84.6%)	54 (75%)	120 (80%)
Nodular type of mononuclear infiltration	20 (25.6%)	13 (18.0%)	33 (22.0%)
Sparse mononuclear infiltration	35 (44.9%)	39 (54.2%)	74 (49.3%)
Comorbidity:			
Autoimmune thyroiditis	21 (26.9%)	17 (26.4%)	38 (25.3%)
Follicular adenoma	0	3 (4.2%)	3 (2.0 %)
Nodular goitre	0	4 (5.5%)	4 (2.7%)
Treatment:			
Surgical:			
Total thyroidectomy	65 (83.3%)	61 (84.7%)	126 (84.0%)
Lobectomy	13 (16.7%)	8 (11.1%)	21 (14.0%)
Resection	0	3 (4.2%)	3 (2.0%)
Neck dissection	67(85.9%)	66(91.7%)	133(88.7%)
Number of dissected cervical lymph nodes /N+ median (range)	26 (2-87)/4 (1-77)	22 (1-65)/1 (1-18)	24 (1-87)/3 (1-77)
I-131 therapy:			
ablation (GBq) median (range)	n=41 4.0 (0.61-9.44)	n=34 3.48 (0.31-6.7)	n=75 3.7 (0.31-9.44)
treatment for lung metastases (GBq), median (range)	n=8 7.42 (5.5-12.89)	-	n=8 7.42 (5.5-12.89)
Follow-up, months median (range)	79.35 (29.72-303.25)	57.22 (29.69-102.9)	66.03 (29.69-303.25)

Table 1. Clinical and pathologic features of sporadic PTC

The distribution of TNM tumour stages according to tumour size of sporadic PTC is shown in Table 2.

The most striking feature of this comparison is the high rate of extrathyroidal extension (patients in pT3 stage observed in 40.0%) and lymph node metastases (N1 discovered in 72.0%). However, it is easy to understand that even small tumours within the size of up to 10 mm corresponding to a volume of 0.5 ml which is too large to be harboured in the small thyroid lobe of a young child with a volume of less than 2 ml (Farahati et al., 1999).

The inability to define the T-category (pTx observed in 36 patients. 24.0%) can largely be attributed to surgeons or pathologists sectioning the specimen prior to it being properly processed. This fact draws attention to the necessity to follow strict rules while dealing with thyroid carcinomas and illustrates the need for standardization of sampling: removed parts

pT/tumour size	N0	N1a	N1b	Total	M0	M1
T1a (1-10mm)	14 (9.3%)	10 (6.7%)	9 (6.0%)	33 (22.0%)	33 (22.0%)	0
1-5mm	6 (4.0%)	5 (3.3%)	2 (1.0%)	13 (8.7%)	13 (8.7%)	0
6-10mm	8 (5.3%)	5 (3.3%)	7 (4.7%)	20 (13.3%)	20 (13.3%)	0
pT1b(11-20mm)	9 (6.0%)	2 (1.0%)	8 (5.3%)	19 (13.0%)	19 (13.0%)	0
pT2 (21-40mm)	2 (1.0%)	0	0	2 (1.0%)	2 (1.0%)	0
pT3	8 (5.3%)	8 (5.3%)	44 (29.3%)	60 (40.0%)	52 (34.7%)	8 (5.3%)
1-10mm	3 (2.0%)	5 (3.3%)	9 (6.0%)	17 (11.3%)	16 (10.7%)	1 (0.6%)
≥11 mm	5 (3.3%)	3 (2.0%)	35 (23.3%)	43 (28.7%)	36 (24.0%)	7 (4.7%)
pTx	9 (6.0%)	7 (4.7%)	20 (13.3%)	36 (24.0%)	36 (24.0%)	0
1-10mm	3 (2.0%)	2 (1.0%)	4 (2.7%)	9 (6.0%)	9 (6.0%)	0
≥11 mm	6 (4.0%)	5 (3.3%)	16 (10.7%)	27 (18.0%)	27 (18.0%)	0
n (%)	42 (28.0%)	27 (18.0%)	81 (54.0%)	150 (100%)	142 (94.7%)	8 (5.3%)

Table 2. Tumour size, lymph node and distant metastases in children and adolescence with sporadic PTC (according to AJCC/UICC TNM. 7th edition)

of the thyroid gland should be sectioned by the pathologist only along cephalocaudal axis (from the upper to the lower pole in vertical plane).

4.2 Second primary thyroid cancer

There were 34 patients with the second primary malignant thyroid tumour in the follow-up period from 1995 to 2010, where PTC was detected in 32 individuals (94.1%). One person had medullary carcinoma and the other one suffered from poorly differentiated cancer.

Only 23 from 32 cases of PTC (10 girls and 13 boys) were enrolled into the study because the tumour in the thyroid gland was diagnosed at the age of 8-18 years. In seven cases primary metachronous papillary cancer developed when the patients were aged 19-32 years. Finally, two adolescents underwent treatment for brain neoplasms (astrocytoma and medulloblastoma) at the age of 4-8 and were excluded from the study due to the fact that thyroid tumours had cribriform morular structures (generative mutation of APC-gene, Turcot syndrome, was detected in 1 case).

The first primary malignancy was detected in the patients at a median age of 4.7 years (1-12 years). Median latent period till the second tumour (thyroid cancer) was 9.2 years (4-16 years).

Treatment for the first malignant neoplasm (hemoblastosis, sarcoma, medulloblastoma) was provided in accordance with the standard protocols. External irradiation was used in all the cases (the total absorbed doses for the primary tumour varied from 12 to 54 Gy). Surgical and postoperative treatment of thyroid carcinomas was also standardized: as a rule, total thyroidectomy (21; 91.4%) with bilateral neck dissection (in 21 of 23 patients. 91.3%) was performed. Thirteen patients underwent from 1 to 4 ablative courses of radioiodine therapy (average activity 4.36 GBq, 0.3-7.8 GBq). In one case a patient who was previously treated for Hodgkin's lymphoma at the age of 3.6, five years later the diffuse sclerosing variant of PTC (pT3N1bM1) with distant metastases to lungs was diagnosed and treated with 4 courses of radioiodine therapy (13.6 GBq) after surgery.

Eleven of 23 patients with secondary papillary cancer had been treated previously for malignant lymphoma (9 patients with Hodgkin's disease). In seven patients leukaemia was the primary malignancy (acute myeloblastic leukaemia was diagnosed in one patient who died of sepsis which was in progress while treating the third recurrence of hemoblastosis). Acute lymphoblastic leukemia was diagnosed in six patients. These data are in accordance with the observation that the risk of second primary malignancy in the thyroid is much higher if Hodgkin disease, non-Hodgkins lymphoma or leukemia has been the primary malignancy (Meadows et al., 2009). One patient with medulloblastoma was cured. Three more girls and one boy had soft tissue malignancies of the head, neck and urinary bladder. The last patient was diagnosed with embryonal rhabdomyosarcoma of the urinary bladder which was detected at the age of 1.4. He then developed an astrocytoma of the brainstem 14 years later and PTC was detected two years after brain tumour at the age of 17.

For patients who developed PTC after treatment for lymphoma, the latent period from completion of lymphoma treatment till verification of papillary thyroid cancer was 8.6 years (5 to 13 years). The median period until the development of PTC for the patients with leukemia was 6.9 years (4 to 12 years) and for patients with soft tissue tumours the latency was a median of 14.0 years (10 to 16 years).

As a rule, thyroid malignancies are likely to develop after irradiation of the neck. However, combined treatment was carried out in the case of embryonal rhabdomyosarcoma of urinary bladder (according to the protocol CWS-91), which consisted of irradiation of the suprapubic area with a total absorbed dose of 40 Gy and chemotherapy with vincristine, doxorubicin, cyclophosphamide, actinomycin D and ifosfamide. In 1992 it may have been impossible to provide complete protection of the neck while irradiating a one-year old child, and this may have contributed to the development of papillary thyroid carcinoma after 16 years, though alternative hypotheses must also be considered.

It should be noted that one patient was subjected to unusual aggressive external irradiation. This female was diagnosed to have aggressive fibromatosis involving soft tissues around right scapulae in May 1985 that was removed. Then, from January to March 1986, the patient was treated for tumour relapse (three lumps 5x4, 6x6 and 4x3cm) which required removal of the medial part and lower corner of the right scapular bone, right sided VI-VIII ribs and adjacent soft tissues. In addition, postoperative irradiation was carried out with 40 Gy at the right scapula and 16 Gy at the left supraclavicular area (February-March 1986). In April 1986, new nodule of irregular shape in soft tissues of lumbar spine was detected with the size of 8x1.5 cm. After radiation therapy with the dose of 60 Gy (15/04-19/05 1986) the tumour became 5x3.5 cm. In July of the same year besides a paravertebral tumour located in soft tissues at level D10-D11 another tumour 6x5.5 cm appeared in the area of medial side of the left scapula. The patient was exposed to irradiation again with the dose of 46 Gy. In November 1996, a tumour in the right lobe of thyroid gland was detected and lobectomy with isthmus resection was carried out (follicular thyroid cancer with minimal invasion of the capsule was diagnosed; later it was reclassified as a follicular variant of PTC).

A few relapses of desmoid tumour still took place: nodules in gluteus on the right and left sides (removed and irradiated with a dose of 60 Gy), a lump in the right thigh treated with hyper fractionated external beam therapy with a total absorbed dose of 25 Gy. The area of the right thigh and iliac nodes additionally were irradiated with 60 Gy. The patient then got chemotherapy with cyclophosphamide (1500 mg) and cisplatin (120 mg) from October 1998 to March 1999 (4 courses). The treatment failed to stabilize the progress, and there were further relapses in 2001 and 2006 that led to surgical excision of the long head of the right side biceps (nodule 7.5x6.0x2.8 cm) and consecutive radiotherapy with 40 Gy again. At present, there is no progression of both tumours and the patient gets substitutive hormonal treatment for thyroid carcinoma.

Clinical and pathologic data for the 23 patients with PTC as a second primary malignancy are presented in Table 3.

Characteristics	Age groups, years at presentation		Total (n=23)
	4-14 years (n=10)	15-18 years (n=13)	
Age at diagnosis.			
mean± SD	11.0±2.0	16.3±1.2	14.0±3.1
Sex (girls: boys)	1:1	1:1.6	1:1.3
girls	5 (50%)	5 (38.5%)	10 (43.5%)
boys	5 (50%)	8 (61.5%)	13 (56.5%)
Tumour size, mm			
median (range)	10 (8-50)	10 (3-45)	10 (3-50)
≤10 mm	6 (60%)	8 (61.5%)	14 (60.9%)
1-5 mm	0	2 (15.4%)	2 (8.7%)
6-10 mm	6 (60%)	6 (46.1%)	12 (52.2%)
≥11 mm	4 (40%)	5 (38.5%)	9 (39.1%)
Localization:			
Subcapsular	6 (60%)	8 (61.5%)	14 (60.9%)
Inside lobe	2 (20%)	5 (38.5%)	7 (30.4%)
Isthmus	2 (20%)	0	2 (8.7%)
Local spreading, N0:	1 (10%)	5 (38.5%)	6 (26.1%)
intrathyroidal	1 (10%)	3 (23.1%)	4 (17.4%)
extrathyroidal	0	2 (15.4%)	2 (8.7%)
not-reported, pTx	0	0	0
Regional spreading, N+:	9 (90%)	8 (61.5%)	17 (73.9%)
N1a	5 (50%)	5 (38.5%)	10 (43.5%)
N1b	4 (40%)	3 (23.1%)	7 (30.4%)
N1b unilateral	3 (30%)	3 (23.1%)	6 (26.1%)
N1b bilateral	1 (10%)	0	1 (4.3%)
Distant metastases, M1 (lungs)	1 (10%)	0	1 (4.3%)
Tumour histology (predominant architecture):			
Papillary	3 (30%)	6 (46.2%)	9 (39.1%)
Follicular	5 (50%)	6 (46.2%)	11 (47.8%)
Solid	2 (20%)	1 (7.7%)	3 (13.1%)
Histological types:			
Classical PTC	4 (40%)	4 (30.8%)	8 (34.8%)
Follicular	2 (20%)	3 (23.1%)	5 (21.7%)
Diffuse sclerosing (DSV)	1 (10%)	1 (7.7%)	2 (8.6%)
Monofocal with diffuse sclerosing involvement	1 (10%)	1 (7.7%)	2 (8.6%)

Characteristics	Age groups, years at presentation		Total (n=23)
	4-14 years (n=10)	15-18 years (n=13)	
(DSV-like)			
Tall cell	0	3 (23.1%)	3 (13%)
Solid	2 (20%)	1 (7.7%)	3 (13%)
Multifocal growth	0	0	0
Morphological specifications:			
Infiltrative growth	8 (80%)	8 (61.5%)	16 (69.8%)
1. Intrathyroidal (pT1-T2)	2 (20%)	1 (7.7%)	3 (13%)
	6 (60%)	7 (53.9%)	13 (56.8%)
2. extrathyroidal extension (pT3)	6 (60%)	7 (53.9%)	13 (56.8%)
in fat tissue	0	0	0
in muscle			
circumscribed/encapsulated growth	0	3 (23.1%)	3 (13%)
Diffuse involvement (DSV and DSV-like)	2 (20%)	2 (15.4%)	4 (17.2%)
Intratumoural fibrosis:			
Focal	4 (40%)	7 (53.9%)	11 (47.8%)
Septal	3 (30%)	3 (23.1%)	6 (26.1%)
Massive (central scarring)	3 (30%)	1 (7.7%)	4 (17.2%)
Blood vessel involvement	5 (50%)	3 (23.1%)	8 (34.8%)
Lymph vessel involvement	9 (90%)	9 (69.3%)	18 (78.3%)
Nodular type of mononuclear infiltration	2 (20%)	2 (15.4%)	4 (17.2%)
Sparse mononuclear infiltration	6 (60%)	11 (84.7%)	17 (73.9%)
Comorbidity:			
Autoimmune thyroiditis	0	0	0
Follicular adenoma	0	0	0
Nodular goitre	0	1 (7.7%)	1 (4.3%)
Treatment			
Surgical:			
Total thyroidectomy	10 (100%)	11 (84.7%)	21 (91.4%)
Lobectomy	0	1 (7.7%)	1 (4.3%)
Resection	0	1 (7.7%)	1 (4.3%)
neck dissection	10 (100%)	10 (77%)	20 (87%)
number of dissected cervical lymph nodes /N+ median (range)	21 (6-64)/5 (1-18)	13 (3-39)/1 (1-18)	19 (3-64)/3 (1-18)
Ablation (GBq) median (range)	n=7 4.36 (2.1-7.805)	n=6 4.59 (0.307-7.696)	n=13 4.36 (0.307-7.805)
Treatment for lung metastases (GBq), median (range)	13.352±NA	-	13.352±NA
Follow-up, months from the end of treatment for PTC median (range)	104.99 (84.2-171.85)	68.38 (18.15-186.64)	99.35 (18.15-186.54)

Table 3. Clinical and pathologic features of PTC as second primary malignancy

In sporadic cases of PTC (Table 1) the gender rate was different between children and adolescents with an increasing preponderance of females (from 2.5:1 to 6.2:1 accordingly). However, in second primary malignancies (females) these differences were not detected (1:1 in children, 1:1.6 in adolescents). Another divergence with sporadic PTC was the complete absence of autoimmune thyroiditis in second primary thyroid cancers. With respect to the other characteristics, PTC as a second primary malignancy presented very similar to sporadic PTC.

The distribution of TNM tumour stages according to tumour size of PTC as second primary malignancy is shown in Table 4.

pT/tumour size	N0	N1a	N1b	Total	M0	M1
T1a (1-10mm)	1 (4.3%)	2 (8.7%)	0	3 (13.0%)	3 (13.0%)	0
1-5mm	1 (4.3%)	1 (4.3%)	0	2 (8.7%)	2 (8.7%)	0
6-10mm	0	1 (4.3%)	0	1 (4.3%)	1 (4.3%)	0
pT1b (11-20mm)	3 (13.0%)	0	0	3 (13.0%)	3 (13.0%)	0
pT2 (21-40mm)	0	0	0	0	0	0
pT3	2 (8.7%)	8 (34.7%)	7 (30.4%)	17 (73.9%)	16 (69.6%)	1 (4.3%)
1-10mm	1 (4.3%)	6 (26.0%)	4 (17.4%)	11 (47.8%)	11 (47.8%)	0
≥11 mm	1 (4.3%)	2 (8.7%)	3 (13.0%)	6 (26.1%)	5 (21.7%)	1 (4.3%)
Total (%)	6 (26.0%)	10 (43.6%)	7 (30.4%)	23 (100.0%)	22 (95.7%)	1 (4.3%)

Table 4. Tumour size, lymph nodes and distant metastases in children and adolescents with PTC as second primary malignancy according to AJCC/UICC TNM. 7th edition

When comparing the extension of tumour disease in two groups (table 2 and 4) it should be noted that the majority of patients (74%) operated for sporadic PTC showed minimal extrathyroidal extension. The rate of local metastases was similar in both groups (72% vs. 74%). Organ metastases were only observed in cases with extracapsular spread of thyroid carcinoma.

4.3 Post-Chernobyl PTC

The victims of the Chernobyl disaster represent a quite homogenous cohort. There is a general agreement now that the minimal latent period for the development of radiation-induced thyroid cancer is approximately 4 years. The incidence of radiogenic thyroid carcinoma is higher in females (1.6:1). European findings also indicate that the number of cases of thyroid carcinoma in males is lower than in females (Farahati et al., 1997). The vast majority of radiation-associated thyroid cancers are PTC with a high incidence of extrathyroidal extension and lymph node metastases (49.1% and 64.6%, respectively). (Pacini et al., 1997; Williams et al., 2004; Williams et al.; 2008; Reiners et al. 2008).

Clinical and pathologic data of 908 patients with post-Chernobyl PTC are presented in Table 5.

As in the two previous groups, post-Chernobyl PTC cases are characterized by infiltrative growth (82.6%), a high rate of extrathyroidal extension (37.0%) and nodal metastases (74.4%). Multifocal growth was detected much more frequently (6.2%) than in children and adolescents with sporadic (3.3%) or second primary (0) carcinomas.

Characteristics	Age groups, years at presentation		Total (n=908)
	4-14 years (n=508)	15-18 years (n=400)	
Demographics Age at diagnosis, mean± SD	12.0±2.4	16.8±1.1	14.1±3.1
Gender (girls: boys)	1.6:1	2.0:1	1.88:1
girls	314 (61.8%)	266 (66.5%)	580 (63.9%)
boys	194 (38.2%)	134 (33.5%)	328 (36.1%)
Tumour size. mm median (range)	12 (1-85)	12 (1-124)	12 (1-124)
≤10 mm	199 (39.2%)	178 (44.5%)	377 (41.5%)
1-5 mm	16 (3.2%)	43 (10.7%)	59 (6.5%)
6-10 mm	183 (36.0%)	135 (33.8%)	318 (35.0%)
≥11 mm	309 (60.8%)	222 (55.5%)	531 (58.5%)
Localization:			
Subcapsular	245 (48.2%)	198 (49.5%)	443 (48.8%)
Inside lobe	239 (47.0%)	177 (44.3%)	416 (45.8%)
Isthmus	24 (4.8%)	25 (6.2%)	49 (5.4%)
Local spreading, N0:	124 (24.4%)	109 (27.2%)	233 (25.7%)
intrathyroidal	53 (10.4%)	73 (18.3%)	126 (13.9%)
extrathyroidal	22 (4.3%)	15 (3.7%)	37 (4.1%)
non-detected pTx	49 (9.6%)	21 (5.2%)	70 (7.7%)
Regional spreading. N+:	384 (75.6%)	291 (72.8%)	675 (74.4%)
N1a	217 (42.7%)	104 (26.0%)	321 (35.3%)
N1b	167 (32.9%)	187 (46.8%)	354 (39.1%)
N1b unilateral	137 (27.0%)	158 (39.5%)	295 (32.5%)
N1b bilateral	30 (5.9%)	29 (7.3%)	59 (6.5%)
Distant metastases, M1 (lungs)	75 (14.8%)	28 (7.0%)	103 (11.3%)
Tumour histology (predominant architecture):			
Papillary	138 (27.2%)	154 (38.5%)	292 (32.2%)
Follicular	253 (49.8%)	191 (47.8%)	444 (48.9%)
Solid	117 (23.0%)	55 (13.7%)	172 (18.9%)
Histological types:			
Classical PTC	200 (39.4%)	151 (37.8%)	351 (38.7%)
Follicular	158 (31.1%)	126 (31.5%)	284 (31.3%)
Diffuse sclerosing (DSV)	13 (2.6%)	13 (3.3%)	26 (2.9%)
Monofocal with diffuse sclerosing involvement (DSV-like)	26 (5.1%)	18 (4.5%)	44 (4.8%)
Tall cell	23 (4.5%)	45 (11.3%)	68 (7.5%)
Solid	88 (17.3%)	40 (10.0%)	128 (14.1%)
Clear cell	0	2 (0.5%)	2 (0.2%)
Oncocytic	0	5 (1.1%)	5 (0.6%)
Multifocal growth	22 (4.3%)	34 (8.5%)	56 (6.2%)

Characteristics	Age groups, years at presentation		Total (n=908)
	4-14 years (n=508)	15-18 years (n=400)	
Morphological specifications:			
Infiltrative growth	440 (86.6%)	310 (77.5%)	750 (82.6%)
1. Intrathyroidal (pT1-T2)	91 (17.9%)	106 (26.5%)	197 (21.7%)
2. extrathyroidal extension (pT3)	195 (38.4%)	141 (35.3%)	336 (37.0%)
in fat tissue	173 (34.1%)	136 (34.0%)	309 (34.0%)
in muscle	22 (4.3%)	5 (1.3%)	27 (3.0%)
3. pTx	154 (30.3%)	62 (15.5%)	216 (23.8%)
4. pT4	0	1 (0.2%)	1 (0.1%)
circumscribed/encapsulated growth (pT1, pT2, pTx)	29 (5.7%)	59 (14.8%)	88 (9.7%)
Diffuse involvement DSV and DSV-like (pT1-pTx)	39 (7.7%)	31 (7.7%)	70 (7.7%)
Intratumoural fibrosis:			
Focal	217 (42.7%)	188 (47.0%)	405 (44.6%)
Septal	86 (16.9%)	69 (17.3%)	155 (17.1%)
Massive (central scarring)	190 (37.4%)	128 (32.0%)	318 (35.0%)
Blood vessel involvement	105 (20.7%)	62 (15.5%)	167 (18.4%)
Lymph vessel involvement	442 (87.0%)	316 (79.0%)	758 (83.5%)
Nodular type of mononuclear infiltration	76 (15.0%)	63 (15.8%)	139 (15.3%)
Sparse mononuclear infiltration	394 (77.6%)	286 (71.5%)	680 (74.9%)
Comorbidity:			
Autoimmune thyroiditis	25 (4.9%)	43 (10.8%)	68 (7.5%)
Follicular adenoma	9 (1.8%)	10 (2.5%)	19 (2.1%)
Nodular goitre	16 (3.1%)	32 (8.0%)	48 (5.3%)
Surgical treatment:			
Total thyroidectomy	306 (60.2%)	315 (78.8%)	621 (68.4%)
Lobectomy	182 (35.9%)	76 (19.0%)	258 (28.4%)
Resection	20 (3.9%)	9 (2.3)	29 (3.2%)
Neck dissection	435 (85.6%)	349 (87.3%)	784 (86.3%)
Number of dissected cervical lymph nodes/N+ median	8 (1-61)/3 (1-44)	19 (1-95)/3 (1-46)	12 (1-95)/ 5 (1-46)
Ablation (GBq) median (range)	n=259 5.2 (0.4-28.1)	n=228 4.9 (0.3-40.4)	n=487 5.1 (0.3-40.4)
Treatment for lung metastases (GBq), median (range)	n=95 16.3 (1.2-52.9)	n=33 21.9 (2.4-60.5)	n=128 17.2 (1.2-60.5)
Follow-up, months median (range)	184.8 (122.5-270.0)	131.6 (68.1-253.9)	165.4 (68.1-270.0)

Table 5. Clinical and pathologic features of post-Chernobyl PTC

The distribution of TNM tumour stage according to tumour size of post-Chernobyl PTC is shown in the table 6.

pT/tumour size	N0	N1a	N1b	Total	M0	M1
T1a (1-10mm)	99 (10.9%)	46 (5.1%)	34 (3.8%)	179 (19.7)	178 (19.6%)	1 (0.1%)
1-5mm	47 (5.2%)	11 (1.2%)	5 (0.6%)	63 (6.9%)	63 (6.9%)	0
6-10mm 116	52 (5.7%)	35 (3.9%)	29 (3.2%)	116 (12.8%)	115 (12.7%)	1 (0.1%)
pT1b (11-20mm)	27 (3.0%)	30 (3.3%)	29 (3.2%)	86 (9.5%)	86 (9.5%)	0
pT2 (21-40mm)	1 (0.1%)	2 (0.2%)	3 (0.3%)	6 (0.7%)	6 (0.7%)	0
pT3-4	39 (4.3%)	136 (15.0%)	205 (22.6%)	380 (40.9%)	303 (33.3%)	77 (8.5%)
1-10mm	23 (2.5%)	48 (5.3%)	37 (4.1%)	108 (11.9%)	101 (11.1%)	7 (0.8%)
≥11 mm	16 (1.8%)	88 (9.7%)	168 (18.5%)	272 (29.0%)	202 (22.2%)	70 (7.7%)
pTx	67 (7.4%)	107 (11.8%)	83 (9.1%)	257 (28.3%)	232 (25.6%)	25 (2.8%)
1-10mm	36 (4.0%)	32 (3.5%)	22 (2.4%)	90 (9.9%)	85 (9.4%)	5 (0.6%)
≥11 mm	31 (3.4%)	75 (8.3%)	61 (6.7%)	167 (18.4%)	147(16.2%)	20 (2.2%)
n (%)	233 (25.7%)	321 (35.4%)	354 (39.0%)	908 (100%)	805 (88.7%)	103 (11.3%)

Table 6. Tumour size, lymph nodes and distant metastases in children and adolescents with post-Chernobyl PTC according to AJCC/UICC TNM. 7th edition

According to our data, 22.6% of our patients with post-Chernobyl PTC were treated in stage pT3N1b and nearly all cases with associated distant metastases belonged to this group.

4.4 Comparison of sporadic PTC, PTC as second primary cancer and post-chernobyl PTC

We analyzed pathologic peculiarities, associated with local carcinoma spread (Table 7) and metastases in lymph nodes (Table 8).

Thus, high risk of extrathyroidal extension in patients with sporadic PTC is associated with several morphological peculiarities:

1. Tumour size≥11 mm
2. Subcapsular localization
3. Diffuse sclerosing variant (classical)
4. Massive intratumoural fibrosis (central scarring)
5. Blood or/and lymph vessel involvement

In PTC as second primary malignancy, only lymph vessel involvement seems to be a predictor of the risk for extrathyroidal extension (however, we must bear in mind the small number of patients in this group). On the other hand, for post-Chernobyl PTC, extrathyroidal extension is correlated to many features:

1. Tumour size≥11 mm
2. Subcapsular or isthmus localization
3. Predominance of follicular structures
4. Diffuse sclerosing variant and monofocal papillary carcinoma with diffuse sclerosing involvement of the thyroid gland (DSV-like) as well
5. Infiltrative growth and/or diffuse involvement (DSV and DSV-like)
6. Massive intratumoural fibrosis (central scarring)

Pathology	sporadic PTC			second primary PTC			post-Chernobyl PTC		
	pT-stage			pT-stage			pT-stage		
	T1&T2 (n=54)	T3&T4 (n=60)	P value	T1&T2 (n=6)	T3&T4 (n=17)	P value	T1&T2 (n=271)	T3&T4 (n=380)	P value
Tumour size:									
≥11 mm	22 (40.7%)	43 (71.7%)	0.0012	3 (50.0%)	6 (35.3%)	NS	92 (33.9%)	272 (71.6%)	< 0.0001
Localization (dominant):									
Subcapsular	11 (20.4%)	31 (51.7%)	0.0008	3 (50.0%)	11 (64.7%)	NS	74 (27.3%)	270 (71.1%)	< 0.0001
Inside lobe	40 (74.1%)	21 (35.0%)	< 0.0001	3 (50.0%)	4 (23.4%)	NS	188 (69.4%)	82 (21.5%)	< 0.0001
Isthmus	3 (5.5%)	8 (13.3%)	NS	0	2 (11.8%)	NS	9 (3.3%)	28 (7.4%)	0.0380
Tumour histology, dominate architecture:									
Papillary	25 (46.3%)	20 (33.3%)	NS	3 (50.0%)	6 (35.3%)	NS	109 (40.2%)	102 (26.8%)	0.0004
Follicular	22 (40.7%)	25 (41.7%)	NS	3 (50.0%)	8 (47.0%)	NS	121 (44.7%)	204 (53.7%)	0.0260
Solid	7 (13.0%)	15 (25.0%)	NS	0	3 (17.7%)	NS	41 (15.1%)	74 (19.5%)	NS
Histological types:									
Classical	27 (50.0%)	20 (33.3%)	NS	3 (50.0%)	5 (29.2%)	NS	110 (40.6%)	127 (33.4%)	NS
Follicular	13 (24.1%)	12 (20.0%)	NS	3 (50.0%)	2 (11.8%)	NS	91 (33.6%)	127 (33.4%)	NS
Diffuse sclerosing(DSV)	0	9 (15.0%)	0.0030	0	2 (11.8%)	NS	0	18 (4.7%)	< 0.0001
Monofocal with diffuse sclerosing involvement (DSV-like)	3 (5.5%)	2 (3.4%)	NS	0	2 (11.8%)	NS	5 (1.8%)	20 (5.3%)	0.0365
Tall cell	6 (11.1%)	9 (15.0%)	NS	0	3 (17.7%)	NS	30 (11.1%)	27 (7.1%)	NS
Solid	5 (9.3%)	8 (13.3%)	NS	0	3 (17.7%)	NS	33 (12.2%)	59 (15.5%)	NS
Oncocytic	0	0	NS	0	0		2 (0.7%)	1 (0.3%)	NS
Clear cell	0	0	NS	0	0		0	1 (0.3%)	NS
Pathological specifications:									
Infiltrative growth	37 (68.5%)	49 (81.7%)	NS	3 (50.0%)	13 (76.5%)	NS	197 (72.7%)	337 (88.7%)	< 0.0001
circumscribed/ encapsulated growth	14 (26.0%)	0	< 0.0001	3 (50.0%)	0	0.0113	69 (25.5%)	5 (1.3%)	< 0.0001

Pathology	sporadic PTC			second primary PTC			post-Chernobyl PTC		
	pT-stage			pT-stage			pT-stage		
	T1&T2 (n=54)	T3&T4 (n=60)	P value	T1&T2 (n=6)	T3&T4 (n=17)	P value	T1&T2 (n=271)	T3&T4 (n=380)	P value
diffuse involvement (DSV and DSV-like)	3 (5.5%)	11 (18.3%)	NS	0	4 (23.5%)	NS	5 (1.8%)	38 (10.0%)	< 0.0001
Fibrosis									
focal intratumoural fibrosis	34 (63.0%)	27 (45.0%)	NS	1 (16.7%)	10 (58.8%)	NS	152 (56.1%)	145 (38.2%)	< 0.0001
septal	10 (18.5%)	3 (5.0%)	0.0365	2 (33.3%)	4 (23.5%)	NS	58 (21.4%)	54 (14.2%)	0.0203
massive (central scarring)	9 (16.7%)	29 (48.3%)	0.0004	1 (16.7%)	3 (17.7%)	NS	41 (15.1%)	173 (45.5%)	< 0.0001
Blood vessel involvement	5 (9.3%)	22 (36.7%)	0.0008	2 (33.3%)	6 (35.3%)	NS	22 (8.1%)	114 (30.0%)	< 0.0001
Lymph vessel involvement	31 (57.4%)	60 (100%)	< 0.0001	2 (33.3%)	16 (94.1%)	0.0078	169 (62.4%)	359 (94.5%)	< 0.0001
Mononuclear infiltration									
nodular type	9 (16.7%)	15 (25.0%)	NS	0	4 (23.5%)	NS	22 (8.1%)	76 (20.0%)	< 0.0001
sparse	32 (59.3%)	32 (53.3%)	NS	5 (83.3%)	12 (70.6%)	NS	213 (78.6%)	268 (70.5%)	0.0223
Autoimmune thyroiditis comorbidity	12 (22.2%)	10 (16.7%)	NS	0	0		26 (9.6%)	23 (6.1%)	NS

Table 7. The relationship between characteristics of the primary tumour and spread of sporadic, second-primary and post-Chernobyl PTC beyond the thyroid gland capsule (Note: N.S. - not significant)

7. Blood or/and lymph vessel involvement
8. Nodular type of mononuclear infiltration

In our opinion, the most intriguing finding is the association between radiogenic PTC and a predominantly follicular architecture with extrathyroidal extension. It should be mentioned that tumours with pure follicular, papillary or solid pattern had no preponderance for local spread beyond the thyroid gland but carcinomas of mixed structure did ($p<0.001$). In addition, if any follicular or solid formation was identified in the post-Chernobyl PTCs, it was also commonly associated with extrathyroidal extension ($p<0.001$ if solid structures appeared and $p=0.03$ for whichever size of follicular pattern). These differences may be explained by the molecular features of PTC in children and adolescents, as well as by peculiarities of tumour growth in young individuals.

High risk of metastases in regional lymph nodes in patients with sporadic PTC is associated with several morphological peculiarities:

1. Largely subcapsular localization
2. Diffuse sclerosing variant (classical)

Pathology	sporadic PTC			second-primary PTC			post-Chernobyl PTC		
	pN-stage			pN-stage			pN-stage		
	N0 (n=42)	N1 (n=108)	P value	N0 (n=6)	N1 (n=17)	P value	N0 (n=233)	N1 (n=675)	P value
Tumour size:									
≥11 mm	22 (52.4%)	70 (64.8%)	NS	4 (66.7%)	5 (29.4%)	NS	75 (32.2%)	456 (67.6%)	< 0.0001
Localization (dominant):									
Subcapsular	10 (23.8%)	44 (40.7%)	0.0008	3 (50.0%)	11 (64.7%)	NS	79 (33.9%)	364 (53.9%)	< 0.0001
Inside lobe	31 (73.8%)	52 (48.1%)	< 0.0001	3 (50.0%)	4 (23.4%)	NS	146 (62.7%)	270 (40.0%)	< 0.0001
Isthmus	1 (2.4%)	12 (11.2%)	NS	0	2 (11.8%)	NS	8 (3.4%)	41 (6.1%)	0.0380
Tumour histology/ dominate architecture:									
Papillary	9 (21.4%)	50 (46.3%)	NS	3 (50.0%)	6 (35.3%)	NS	52 (22.3%)	240 (35.5%)	0.0004
Follicular	24 (57.2%)	33 (30.6%)	NS	3 (50.0%)	8 (47.0%)	NS	137 (58.8%)	307 (45.5%)	0.0260
Solid	9 (21.4%)	25 (23.1%)	NS	0	3 (17.7%)	NS	44 (18.9%)	128 (19.0%)	NS
Histological types:									
Classical	13 (31.0%)	48 (44.4%)	NS	3 (50.0%)	5 (29.2%)	NS	73 (31.3%)	278 (41.2%)	NS
Follicular	16 (38.1%)	15 (13.9%)	NS	3 (50.0%)	2 (11.8%)	NS	104 (44.6%)	180 (26.7%)	NS
Diffuse sclerosing (DSV)	0	9 (8.3%)	0.0030	0	2 (11.8%)	NS	0	26 (3.9%)	< 0.0001
Monofocal with diffuse sclerosing involvement (DSV-like)	1 (2.4%)	11 (10.2%)	NS	0	2 (11.8%)	NS	3 (1.3%)	41 (6.1%)	0.0365
Tall cell	7 (16.7%)	12 (11.1%)	NS	0	3 (17.7%)	NS	14 (6.0%)	54 (8.0%)	NS
Solid	5 (11.8%)	13 (12.1%)	NS	0	3 (17.7%)	NS	36 (15.5%)	92 (13.6%)	NS
Oncocytic	0	0	NS	0	0		2 (0.9%)	3 (0.4%)	NS
Clear cell	0	0	NS	0	0		1 (0.4%)	1 (0.1%)	NS
Morphological specifications:									
Infiltrative growth	25 (59.5%)	86 (79.6%)	NS	3 (50.0%)	13 (76.5%)	NS	158 (67.8%)	592 (87.7%)	< 0.0001
circumscribed/ encapsulated growth	16 (38.1%)	2 (1.9%)	< 0.0001	3 (50.0%)	0	0.0113	72 (30.9%)	16 (2.4%)	< 0.0001

Pathology	sporadic PTC			second-primary PTC			post-Chernobyl PTC		
	pN-stage			pN-stage			pN-stage		
	N0 (n=42)	N1 (n=108)	P value	N0 (n=6)	N1 (n=17)	P value	N0 (n=233)	N1 (n=675)	P value
Diffuse involvement (DSV and DSV-like)	1 (2.4%)	20 (18.5%)	NS	0	4 (23.5%)	NS	5 (1.8%)	67 (9.9%)	< 0.0001
Fibrosis									
Focal	26 (61.9%)	59 (54.6%)	NS	1 (16.7%)	10 (58.8%)	NS	111 (47.6%)	296 (43.8%)	NS
Septal	5 (11.9%)	14 (13.0%)	NS	2 (33.3%)	4 (23.5%)	NS	57 (24.5%)	96 (14.2%)	0.0005
Massive (central scarring)	11 (26.3%)	33 (30.6%)	NS	1 (16.7%)	3 (17.7%)	NS	45 (19.7%)	269 (39.9%)	< 0.0001
Blood vessels involvement	3 (7.1%)	26 (24.1%)	0.0206	2 (33.3%)	6 (35.3%)	NS	26 (11.2%)	146 (21.6%)	< 0.0001
Lymph vessels involvement	14 (33.3%)	106 (98.1%)	< 0.0001	2 (33.3)	16 (94.1)	0.0078	104 (44.6)	649 (96.2)	< 0.0001
Mononuclear infiltration									
Nodular type	1 (2.4%)	32 (29.6%)	< 0.0001	0	4 (23.5%)	NS	15 (6.4%)	123 (18.2%)	< 0.0001
Sparse	26 (61.9%)	48 (44.4%)	NS	5 (83.3%)	12 (70.6%)	NS	184 (79.0%)	489 (72.4%)	0.0223
Autoimmune thyroiditis comorbidity	13 (30.9%)	25 (23.1%)	NS	0	0		18 (7.7%)	49 (7.3%)	NS

Table 8. The relationship between tumour characteristics and nodal involvement of sporadic, second-primary and post-Chernobyl PTC (Note: N.S. – not significant)

3. Blood or/and lymph vessel involvement
4. Nodular type of mononuclear infiltration

High risk of nodal disease in patients with PTC as second primary malignancy ("iatrogenic") is associated with only morphological detail: lymph vessel involvement. As for post-Chernobyl PTC it has the same characteristics for N1 as in a case of extrathyroidal spread excluding predominance of follicular architecture:

1. Tumour size≥11 mm
2. Subcapsular or isthmus localization
3. Predominance of papillary structures
4. Diffuse sclerosing variant and monofocal PTC with diffuse sclerosing involvement of the thyroid gland (DSV-like) as well
5. Infiltrative growth and/or diffuse involvement (DSV and DSV-like)
6. Massive intratumoural fibrosis (central scarring)
7. Blood or/and lymph vessel involvement
8. Nodular type of mononuclear infiltration

Comparing morphological specifications which are rather important for nodal disease and extrathyroidal spread it should be noted that many features are intermixed. Association of the nodular type of productive inflammation with increased risk of expansion of metastases in lymph nodes ($p<0.001$) may have several explanations. First, cytokines and chemokines produced by mononuclear cells promote the survival of tumors, especially clones that developed as a result of activation of the RET proto-oncogene (e.g. mainly observed in the papillary phenotype). Variants of papillary carcinoma with remarkable ability for invasion of lymphatic vessels and metastatic dissemination can appear as a result of such clone selection (lymphogenous, intrathyroidal and regional). Secondly, extended antigen stimulation by autoimmune thyroiditis (Hashimoto thyroiditis) may lead to emergence of papillary carcinoma through activation of ERK-kinase in epithelial cells (Guarino V. et al., 2010).

Tumour histoarchitectonics probably play an important role in pathological and clinical behaviour of thyroid cancer but our current knowledge does not always permit a full understanding of the observations we have made. For example, why is a high proportion of follicular structures associated with stage pT3? And why is a largely papillary pattern associated with an elevated risk of N1 disease? Additionally, why do carcinomas of "pure" architecture appear less aggressive than PTC with mixed patterns?

5. Conclusion

Early assessment of post-Chernobyl thyroid carcinoma and sporadic thyroid carcinomas indicated that irradiation does not discriminate between genders; the female-to-male ratio was significantly higher in Italy and France (2.5/1), compared to the ratio of patients from post-Chernobyl Belarus (1.6/1). The overwhelming majority of the post-Chernobyl thyroid malignancies were PTC compared to a relatively high percentage of follicular carcinomas that was found in Italy/France (15.2%). This disproportion could be more likely explained by direct radiation-induced double-strand DNA breaks which preferentially lead to deletions and rearrangements. This mechanism is a characteristic for PTC but not for follicular carcinomas (DeLellies R.A. & Williams E.D., 2004), therefore predominance of PTC is non-directly supported radiation as a source for thyroid malignancies.

While comparing the pathology of malignant thyroid tumors of pediatric Belarusian patients with naturally-occurring thyroid carcinomas from patients from Italy and France it was identified that extrathyroidal extension and lymph node metastases were significantly more frequent in thyroid cancers in Belarus (49.1%, 64.6% respectively) compared to thyroid cancers in Italy/France, where it was 24.9% and 53.9%, respectively. It was hypothesized that these differences depend on the age at presentation: mean age at diagnosis in radiation-induced cases was 11 years in children and 15 years in adolescents while naturally-occurring thyroid carcinomas were diagnosed after 14 years of age (Pacini F. et al., 1997). Our research group and others documented that patient age did not have any influence on the tumors' ability to grow beyond the thyroid capsule and /or metastasize to lymph nodes or internal organs (Machens A. et al., 2010). Moreover, based on the rate of thyroid lymphocytic infiltration and circulating antithyroperoxidase antibody it was suggested that thyroid autoimmunity could be an additional consequence of the Chernobyl accident (Pacini F. et al., 1997). However, it is quite normal for us to see full-blown mononuclear infiltration in patients with sporadic PTC as well (autoimmune thyroiditis plays the leading role in the background pathology (n=38, 25.3%)).

It seems to be logical that sporadic PTC in children and adolescents from Belarus show few differences in comparison with the well-known clinical and morphological features of non-radiation induced thyroid cancers in other countries. For example, the female to male ratio is the same as in the rest of the world (3.7:1 in our own material, 4:1 for all histological variants of carcinoma according to long-term USA statistical data (Hogan et al., 2009). The lymph node metastases (72%) are as widespread as extrathyroidal extension (32.7%). In other countries the frequency of lymphatic nodes' involvement in children and adolescents appears to be also at a high level - from 40.7% in Canada up to 84.3% in Germany (Machens et al., 2010; O'Gorman et al., 2010). The data concerning extrathyroidal extent also varies considerably: from 9.6% in Russia up to 67.6% in South Korea (Koo J. et al., 2009, Romanchishen et al., 2008).

There are other nontrivial differences. In the period between 1986 and 2008 there were 150 sporadic papillary carcinoma patients and 42 cases of other malignant tumours composed of follicular cells—well differentiated carcinoma, no other specified (as it was defined by international group of pathologists (LiVolsi et al., 2011) who participated in Chernobyl tissue bank project), n=22, follicular thyroid carcinoma (FTC, n=4), collision carcinomas such as PTC and FTC (n=3), poorly differentiated carcinoma (4) and cribriform morular variant of PTC (n=9). This contradicts the worldwide data that put follicular carcinoma in much significant place after papillary carcinoma (its frequency varies from 6.1% in Russia up to 10-11% in Great Britain, Canada and the USA) (Romanchishen A.F. et al., 2008; Harach H.R. & Williams E.D., 1995; O'Gorman C.S. et al., 2010; Hogan et al., 2009). Besides, in our research primary tumor size (mean 15.8±14.3 mm, median 12 mm) was smaller than in German (median 31 mm) and Canadian (mean 23±15 mm) children and adolescents (Machens A. et al., 2010; O'Gorman C.S. et al., 2010). Moreover, multifocal growth was observed rarely, though other reports indicate that childhood thyroid cancers are typically not multifocal (Grigsby P.W. et al., 2002; DeLellies, R.A. & Williams, 2004). Finally, though prior reports have indicated that PTC in children and adolescents is prone to relapse (Demidchik Y.E. et al., 2006; Grigsby P.W. et al., 2002; Naing S. et al., 2009), with one report indicating a recurrence rate of up to 34% (Grigsby P.W. et al., 2002), here we observed a recurrence in only one case.

A notion prevails that radiogenic and sporadic papillary cancers do not differ in phenotype, but the distribution of variants of papillary carcinoma in both groups are a little different. For example, Ukrainian and Russian reports of post-Chernobyl cancer in children and adolescents indicate that the follicular (follicular-solid) variant occurs much more often than others types (Tronko M.D. et al., 1999; Williams E.D. et al., 2004). On the contrary, carcinoma of classical structure dominates in paediatric sporadic carcinomas (Harach H.R. & Williams E.D., 1995). Some researchers state that DSV appears in children and adolescents more often. However, as shown in tables 1, 3 and 5, regardless of the aetiology, the most frequent variant of carcinoma in children and adolescents in Belarus is the classical variant of papillary carcinoma.

Patients who received treatment for Hodgkin's lymphoma comprised 40.1% of all thyroid cancers that occurred as second primary malignancies. Children fell ill at an average age of 7. Such tumors appear in boys more often than in girls (6 boys and three girls in our own material). Moreover, in both cases of non-Hodgkins lymphoma, male patients were affected. As a result, gender proportion typical for the first cancer determined the ultimate predominance of boys in the group of patients with second primary cancers. However, in the work of Acharya et al. (2003), out of 33 patients with confirmed history of therapeutic irradiation, 18 were diagnosed with Hodgkin's disease. Ten others had non-Hodgkin's lymphoma and 3 had acute leukemia, but the gender proportion was 2.3:1 girls:boys. The exact age when the first malignant tumour grew is not given (the median is given - 12 years and interval - from 3.7 to 18.3 years) and in the quoted research thyroid cancer appeared in the interval from 6.2 to 30.1 years.

Other features that indicate a difference between the variants of PTC of different aetiology are directly connected with the parameters of pathological aggressiveness. Ability to spread into surrounding tissues (pT3) is to a greater degree characteristic for second-primary carcinoma (73.9% of all observations). High frequency of autoimmune thyroiditis again brings up the question of what comes first: cancer in the background of a chronic inflammatory process or changes observed by the pathologist in surgical material that indicate a tumour-associated immunoreaction. It may also be theorized that long existing inflammatory responses with associated tissue renewal and repair leads to lower degrees of aggressiveness of thyroid carcinoma since it is connected to both upregulation of molecules of major histocompatibility complex (for example, HLA-Dr) or direct cytotoxic action of lymphocytes and macrophages on tumour cells (Guarino V. et al., 2010), with structural reorganization of thyroid gland tissue. Sclerosis, hyalinosis and mechanical compression of lymphatic vessels or compensatory-adaptive node of vascular walls as a response to local anoxia should have considerably impeded tumour cell embolism. Nevertheless, in our research autoimmune thyroiditis was identified in patients from both the sporadic and post-Chernobyl carcinoma groups and did not influence the invasive or metastatic potential.

Ultimately, tumour aetiology has no real impact on the clinical course and on the overall favourable prognosis of thyroid carcinoma, and the age of patients (children as compared to adolescents) is not essential for treatment planning or for disease outcome (Machens et al., 2010). On the other hand, observations show that the exposure to irradiation potentially induces clinicopathological characteristics of high-grade thyroid carcinomas, e.g. potential for multifocal growth, lymphovascular invasion, extrathyroidal spread, regional and distant metastasis, or recurrences (Naing et al., 2009). With the help of various statistical methods our own research discovered some characteristics which indicate clinical courses of papillary carcinomas in patients with the history of irradiation somewhat differ from the one of sporadic carcinomas, but the prognostic significance of this fact is not yet clear in spite of our large cohort of post-Chernobyl cancers. We believe that a more extended observation period and addition of new cases of sporadic and second-primary papillary carcinomas to the cohorts described here will give the possibility to define more precisely the role that aetiology plays for prognosis and treatment planning in children and adolescents.

6. References

Acharya, S.; Sarafoglou, K.; LaQuaglia, M.; et al. (2003) Thyroid neoplasms after therapeutic radiation for malignancies during childhood or adolescence. *Cancer*, 97, 10, 2397–2403, ISSN 0008-543X

Astakhova, L.; Anspaugh, L., Beebe, G.; et al. (1998) Chernobyl-related thyroid cancer in children of Belarus: a case-control study. *Radiat Res,* 150, 349–356, ISSN 0033-7587

Beasley, N.J.; Walfish, P.G.; Witterick, I.; Freeman, J.L. (2001) Cause of death in patients with well-differentiated thyroid carcinoma. *Laryngoscope,* 111, 6, 989-991 ISSN 1531-4995

Chang, S.H., Joo, M., Kim, H. (2006) Fine Needle Aspiration Biopsy of Thyroid Nodules in Children and Adolescents. *J Korean Med Sci,* 21, 469-73, ISSN 1011-8934

Clark, O.H. (2005) Papillary Thyroid Carcinoma: Rationale for Total Thyroidectomy. In: *Textbook of Endocrine Surgery.* Orlo H. Clark, Quang-Yang Duh and Electron Kebebew. Elsevier Saunders, 110-113, ISBN 0-7216-0139-1, Philadelphia, USA

DeLellies, R.A. & Williams E.D. (2004) *World Health organization classification of tumours. Pathology and genetics of tumours of endocrine organs.* Ronald A. DeLellies, Ricardo V. Lloyd, Philipp U. Heitz, Charis Eng. IACR Press, Lyon, France, ISBN 92 832 2416 7

Demidchik, E.P., Demidchik, Yu.E., Gedrevich, Z.E., et al. (2002) Thyroid Cancer in Belarus. In: *Chernobyl: Message for the 21th Century.* Shunichi Yamashita, Yoshisada Shibata, Masaharu Hoshi and Kingo Fujimura, 69-75, Elsevier, ISBN 0-444-50869-4, Amsterdam, The Netherlands

Demidchik, E.P., Kazakov, V.S., Astakhova, L.N., et al. (1994) Thyroid Cancer in Children After the Chernobyl Accident: Clinical and Epidemiological Evaluation of 251 Cases in the Republic of Belarus. In: *Nagasaki Symposium on Chernobyl: Update and Future.* Shigenobu Nagataki, 21-30, Elsevier, ISBN 0-444-81953-3, Amsterdam, The Netherlands

Demidchik, Yu.E., Demidchik, E.P., Saenko, V.A., et al. (2007) Childhood Thyroid Cancer in Belarus. In: *Radiation Risk Perspertives.* Yoshisada Shibata, Hiroyuki Namba, Keiji Suzuki and Masao Tomonaga, 32-38, Elsevier, ISBN 978-0-444-52888-9, Amsterdam, The Netherlands

Demidchik, Yu.E., Saenko, V.A., Yamashita, S.(2007) Childhood Thyroid Cancer in Belarus, Russia, and Ukraine after Chernobyl and at Present, Arq Bras Endocrinol Metab, 51, 5, 748-762, ISSN 0004-2730

Demidchik, Y.E.; Demidchik, E.P.; Reiners, C.; et al. (2006) Comprehensive clinical assessment of 740 cases of surgically treated thyroid cancer in children of Belarus. *Annals of surgery,* 243, 4, 525-532, ISSN 0003-4932

Dinauer, C.A. (1998) Clinical features associated with metastasis and recurrence of differentiated thyroid cancer in children, adolescents and young adults. *Clinical Endocrinology,* 49, 619–628, ISSN 0300-0664

Farahati, J.; Bucsky, P.; Parlowsky, T.; et al., (1997) Characteristics of differentiated thyroid carcinoma in children and adolescents with respect to age, gender, and histology. *Cancer,* 80, 11, 2156-2162, ISSN 0008-543X

Farahati, J.; Reiners, C.; Demidchik, E.P.; (1999) Is the UICC/AJCC classification of primary tumor in childhood thyroid carcinoma valid? *J. Nucl. Med.,* 40, 12, 2125, ISSN 0161-5505

Florentine, B.D., Staymates, B., Rabadi, M., et al. (2006) The reliability of fine-needle aspiration biopsy as the initial diagnostic procedure for palpable masses: a 4-year experience of 730 patients from a community hospital-based outpatient aspiration biopsy clinic. *Cancer,* 107, 2, 406-16, ISSN 0008-543X

Harrah, H.R. & Williams, E.D. (1995) Childhood thyroid cancer in England and Wales. *Br J Cancer,* 72, 777-783, ISSN 0007-0920

Hogan, A.R.; Zhuge, Y.; Perez, E.A.; et al. (2009) Pediatric thyroid carcinoma: incidence and outcomes in 1753 patients. *J Surg Res*, 156, 167-172, ISSN 0022-4804

Gemsenjager, E.; Heitz, P.U.; Martina B. (1997) Selective treatment of differentiated thyroid carcinoma. *World J Surg.*, 21,5, 546-51; discussion 551-552, ISSN 0364-2313

Gilliland, F.D.; Hunt, W.C.; Morris D.M.; Key C.R. (1997) Prognostic factors for thyroid carcinoma. A population-based study of 15,698 cases from the Surveillance, Epidemiology and End Results (SEER) program 1973-1991. *Cancer*, 79, 3, 564-573 ISSN 0008-543X

Gimm, O. & Dralle, H. (2001) The current surgical approach to non-medullary thyroid cancer. *Thyroid cancer.* H.-J.Biersack, F.Grunwald. Springer, 81-89, ISBN 3-540-22309-6

Grigsby, P.W.; Gal-or, A.; Michalski, J.; Doherty, G.M. (2002) Childhood and adolescent thyroid carcinoma. *Cancer*, 95, 724-729, ISSN 0004-2730

Groot, G.; Colquhoun, B.P.; Murphy, F.A. (1992) Unilateral versus bilateral thyroid resection in differentiated thyroid carcinoma. *Can J Surg*, 35, 5, 517-520, ISSN 0008-428X

Guarino, V.; Castellone, M.D.; Avilla, E.; Melillo, R.M. (2010) Thyroid cancer and inflammation. *Molecular and Cellular Endocrinology*, 321, 94–102, ISSN 0303-7207

Kazakov, V.S.; Demidchik, E.P.; Astakhova, L.N. (1992) Thyroid cancer after Chernobyl. *Nature*, 359, 21, ISSN 0028-0836

Koo, J.; Hong, S.; Park, C. (2009) Diffuse sclerosing variant is a major subtype of papillary thyroid carcinoma in the young. *Thyroid*, 19, 1225-1231, ISSN 1557-9077

Lerch, H.; Schober, O.; Kuwert,T.; Saur, H.B. (1997) Survival of differentiated thyroid carcinoma studied in 500 patients. *J. Clin. Oncol.*, 15, 5, 2067-2075, ISSN 0732-183X

LiVolsi, V.A.; Abrosimov, A.A.; Bogdanova, T.; et al. (2011) The Chernobyl Thyroid Cancer Experience: Pathology. *Clinical Oncology*, 23, 261-267, ISSN 1433-2981

LiVolsi, V.A. (2011) Papillary thyroid carcinoma: an update. *Modern Pathology*, 24, S1-S9, ISSN 0893-3952

Luster, M.; Lassmann, M.; Freudenberg, L.S.; et al. (2007) Thyroid cancer in childhood: management strategy, including dosimetry and long-term results. *Hormones (Athenes)*, 6, 4, 269-278, ISSN 1109-3099

Machens, A.; Lorenz, K.; Nguyen, T.; et al. (2010) Papillary thyroid cancer in children and adolescents does not differ in growth pattern and metastatic behavior. *J Pediatr*, 157, 648-652, ISSN 0022-3476

Meadows, A.T.; Friedman, D.L.; Neglia, J.P.; et al. (2009) Inskip Second Neoplasms in Survivors of Childhood Cancer:

Findings From the Childhood Cancer Survivor Study Cohort. *J Clin Oncol*, 27, 14, 2356-2362, ISSN 0732-183X

Mete, O.; Rotstein, L.; Asa, S.L. (2010) Controversies in thyroid pathology: thyroid capsule invasion and extrathyroidal Extension. *Ann Surg Oncology*, 17, 386–391, ISSN 1068-9265

Morris, L.G.T.; Shaha, A.R.; Tuttle, R.M.; et al. (2010) Tall-Cell Variant of Papillary Thyroid Carcinoma: a matched pair analysis of survival. *Thyroid*, 20, 2, 153-158, ISSN 1557-9077

Naing, S.; Collins, B.J.; Schneider, A.B. (2009) Clinical behavior of radiation-induced thyroid cancer: factors related to recurrence. *Thyroid*, 19, 5, 479-485, ISSN 1557-9077

O'Gorman, C.S.; Hamilton, J.; Rachmiel, M.; et al. (2010) Thyroid cancer in childhood: a retrospective review of childhood course. *Thyroid,* 20, 375-380, ISSN 1050-7256

Pacini, F.; Vorontsova, T.; Demidchik, E.P.; et al. (1997) Post-Chernobyl thyroid carcinoma in Belarus children and adolescents: comparison with naturally occurring thyroid carcinoma in Italy and France. *J Clin Endocrinol Metab,* 82, 3563- 3569 ISSN 0021-972X

Reiners, C.; Demidchik, Y.E. (2003) Differentiated thyroid cancer in childhood: pathology, diagnosis, therapy. *Pediatr. Endocrinol. Rev.,* 1 suppl. 2, 230-236, ISSN 1565-4753

Reiners, C.; Demidchik, Y.E.; Drozd, V.M.; et al. (2008) Thyroid cancer in infants and adolescents after Chernobyl. *Minerva Endocrinol.,* 33, 4, 381-395, ISSN 0391-1977

Reiners, C.; (2009) Radioactivity and thyroid cancer. *Hormones (Athens),* 8, 3, 185-191, ISSN 1109-3099

Romanchishen, A.F.; Thompson, D.B.; Gostimskiy, A.V. (2008) Surgical and postsurgical treatment for childhood and adolescent thyroid carcinoma. *Vestnik Chirurgii,* 67, 55-58 (in Russian), ISSN 0042-4625 2009

Sangalli, G. Serio, G., Zampatti, C., Bellotti, M., Lomuscio, G.(2006) Fine needle aspiration cytology of the thyroid: a comparison of 5469 cytological and final histological diagnoses. *Cytopathology,* 17, 245–250, ISSN 1365-2303

Savva, N.N.; Zborovskaya, A.A.; Aleynikova, O.V. (2008) Childhood malignancies in Belarus: incidence, survival, mortality, palliative care. Minsk: RNMB (in Russian), ISBN 978-985-6846-27-7

Seaberg, R.M.; Eski, S.; Freeman J.L. (2009) Influence of previous radiation exposure on pathologic features and clinical outcome in patients with thyroid cancer. Archives of otolaryngology, head & neck surgery, 135, 4, 355-359, ISSN 0886-4470

Shaha, A.R.; Shah, J.P.; Loree, T.R. (1997) Differentiated thyroid cancer presenting initially with distant metastasis. *Am. J. Surg,* 174, 5, 474-476, ISSN 0002-9610

Steliarova-Foucher, E.; Stiller, C.A.; Pukkala, E.; et al. (2006) Thyroid cancer incidence and survival among European children and adolescents (1978-1997): report from the Automated Childhood Cancer Information System project. *Eur J Cancer,* 42, 2150-69, ISSN 0959-8049

Taylor, A.J.; Croft, A.P.; Palace, A.M.; et al. (2009) Risk of thyroid cancer in survivors of childhood cancer: results from the British Childhood Cancer Survivor Study, *Int.J.Cancer,* 125, ISSN 1097-0215

Tronko, M.D.; Bogdanova, T.I.; Komissarenko, I.V.; et al. (1999) Thyroid carcinoma in children and adolescents in Ukraine after the Chernobyl nuclear accident: statistical data and clinicomorphologic characteristics. *Cancer* 86, 149-156, ISSN 0008-543X

Williams, E.D.; Abrosimov, A.; Bogdanova, T.; et al., (2004) Thyroid carcinoma after Chernobyl: latent period, morphology and aggressiveness. *Br J Cancer 90,* 2219-2224, ISSN 0007-0920

Williams, E.D.; Abrosimov, A.; Bogdanova, T.; et al. (2008) Morphologic characteristics of Chernobyl-related childhood papillary thyroid carcinomas are independent of radiation exposure but vary with iodine intake. *Thyroid,* 18, 847-852, ISSN1050-7256

8

Thyroid Cancer in the Pediatric Population

Silva Frieda, Nieves-Rivera Francisco and Laguna Reinaldo
University of Puerto Rico, School of Medicine, San Juan, Puerto Rico

1. Introduction

Thyroid Cancer is the third most common solid tumor in children, accounting for 35% of the carcinomas in pediatric populations. The reported incidence in the United States is relatively low compared to other tumors (approximately 0.2-0.5 per 100,000/year) with a reported age adjusted incidence of 8.5 per 100,000. As in adults, the tumors are more frequent in females. The female to male incidence ratios vary with age. In children under the age of 10 the ratio is 1.2:1, in the 10-21 year old group it is 3.6:1(Shapiro, 2005). Overall, 10% of all cases occur in patients younger than 21 years and the reported average age at presentation is 11-19 years (Shapiro, 2005, Parisi, 2007).

The initial clinical presentation of pediatric thyroid cancer is usually an asymptomatic mass in the neck. Thirty three to fifty percent of those identified neck masses are subsequently diagnosed as malignant. Certain characteristic features, such as firmness of the mass and the degree of fixation to surrounding tissues, as well as lymphadenopathy and/or vocal cord paralysis are associated with an increased probability of malignancy. Pain, tenderness, difficulty swallowing and respiratory problems are not typically reported in the majority of pediatric patients (Jarzab, 2005). Important risk factors for the development of thyroid cancer in children include exposure to external radiation, congenital hypothyroidism and a history of prior malignancies (Parisi, 2007, Niedziela, 2006).

The location of well-differentiated tumors *(WDTC)* in the gland is variable; however the majority (68%) of the reported malignancies are localized in the right lobe. Children with thyroid tumors are generally clinically euthyroid (Jarzab, 2005).

The four main histologic types of pediatric thyroid cancers are papillary, papillary-follicular variant, follicular (FTC), and medullary carcinoma. The majority of the tumors (90-95%) are classified as well differentiated type, *i.e.*, papillary and follicular type (Niedziela, 2006). Medullary tumors are diagnosed in 5-8% of the patients and produce calcitonin. Medullary carcinomas arise from the parafollicular cells or C cells while the papillary and follicular tumors originate from the follicular epithelium. Medullary tumors will be discussed later in the chapter.

Papillary thyroid tumors (PTC) are larger in pediatric patients as compared to tumors in adults at presentation. Capsular invasion is seen in 67% of the pediatric patients (Parisi, 2007, Niedziela, 2006). Unlike adults, pediatric patients often present with extensive regional nodal disease and distant metastasis at diagnosis. Cervical nodal disease ranges from 60-

90%; distant metastasis occurs in 13-23%, most commonly to the lung (Parisi, 2007, Jarzab, 2005). Tracheoesophageal nodes are the ones most frequently involved, followed by the mid jugular and the lower deep jugular group. Bulky nodal metastasis may be associated with small tumors, 1cm or less. Lung metastasis occurs more frequently in patients with extra capsular invasion, bilateral tumors and patients below age 7 at diagnosis. Pulmonary metastases in children are typically miliary and rarely nodular as opposed to adults. Metastases to the lungs are functional in 95% of the cases (Luster, 2007, Mitsutake, 2005). This is related to greater expression of the sodium iodide symporter (NIS) in pediatric thyroid cancers. The increased expression of NIS in pediatric tumors implies a greater degree of differentiation compared to adult papillary cancers. Long-term survival is also poorer; however the reported difference in survival is narrow (Shapiro, 2005).

2. Diagnosis

Thyroid tumors are suspected by a history of an anterior neck palpable mass with or without hoarsenes . Further imaging evaluation studies should include thyroid ultrasound which is the method of choice for the assessment of nodular disease. It is a rapid, safe, noninvasive, and readily available technique. In addition, sonographic evaluation helps to distinguish cystic from solid lesions and allows guidance for fine needle aspiration biopsy (FNA). The sonographic appearance of thyroid cancer varies with the histologic type. PTC lesions are usually solid and hypoechoic with (i.e., 70% of the affected) increased vascularity and micro calcifications. The presence of microcalcifications is highly specific for PTC. On the other hand, FTC is more frequently iso- or hyperechoic with a thick and irregular halo. The latter appearance associated with the presence of suspicious regional lymph nodes increases the risk of malignancy in pediatric thyroid nodules. However, the presence of cystic lesions should not be ignored since 50% of all malignant thyroid lesions have a cystic component and 8% of sonographic cystic lesions represent neoplasia (Niedziela, 2006,Jarzab, 2005,Luster, 2007).

Presently ultrasound-guided fine needle aspiration (FNA) is the most reliable and cost effective method to establish a cytologic diagnosis in up to 73% of lesions prior to surgery. Specifically, a true positive diagnosis can be obtained in up to 90% of the lesions with PTC. However, in children FNA accuracy may be less than in adults as reported by Parisi & Niedziela. Therefore, a negative FNA must be interpreted with caution and it should not be used as the sole predictor of malignancy.

Nuclear thyroid scintigraphy with 99mTc-pertechentate or 123-Iodine may be used in the initial evaluation. It helps in the identification of the "cold nodule", a lesion described as a well-defined area with less radiotracer uptake as compared to normal tissue. It must be remember that only 10-15% of cold lesions in a thyroid scintiscan are malignant, meaning that sonographic guided FNA is needed for a definite diagnosis. In addition, lesions less than 1 cm may be missed, an important limitation of nuclear thyroid imaging to bear in mind.

Immunocytochemical studies are used to further improve the diagnosis. Several tumor markers have been studied in an attempt to enhance diagnosis. Among these are telomerase, galactin-3 and cytokeratin-19. Unfortunately, none have been able to distinguish benign from malignant lesions in children, particularly in cases of follicular tumors or follicular variant of papillary thyroid cancer (Xu, 2003, Mitsutake, 2005).

Recently, interest has focused on genetic markers as a diagnostic tool since they might have a role in terms of tumor behavior. Kimura et al (2003) studied 177 cases of PTC and found RET, NTRK, BRAF and/or RAS mutations in 70% of the tumors. Namba et. al. (2003) reported that papillary lesions with BRAF gene mutation have more aggressive extrathyroidal invasion with less favorable prognosis. This is more frequently seen in the columnar type and the classic PTC variant (Xu, 2003, Mitsutake, 2005). It leads to the origin of oncogene BRAF which activates MAPK kinase. Activation of this cascade has the effect of inappropriate cell proliferation and differentiation into neoplasia.

Other investigators have reported over expression of MET in papillary cancers. Together with the tyrosine kinase receptor ligand it is associated to a higher recurrence risk in children. Gupta (2001) et al found that patients with PTC with the greatest number of proliferating lymphocytes in thyroid infiltrates have the longest disease free survival (Jarzab, 2005, Griffith 2006). On the other hand, patients with intense expression of B7-2 antigen had a greater propensity for recurrence (Jarzab, 2005). Kroll et. al. identified a mutation in follicular thyroid cancers - twenty to fifty percent of them harbor an interchromosomal translocation that fuses PAX8 to PPARγ. This acts as an oncoprotein. FTC that do not have PAX8 / PPARγ recombination are often associated with RAS mutations (Xu, 2003,Mitzutake, 2005,Griffith, 2006).

3. Tumor staging

The American Thyroid Association (ATA) published in 2009 the guidelines for the management of thyroid nodes and differentiated thyroid cancer. Using the TNM classification pediatric thyroid cancer is classified as a TNM stage I or II, according to the presence or absence of distant metastasis regardless of the existence of lymph node metastases.

It is recognized that pediatric thyroid cancer at diagnosis often involves spread to lymph nodes as well as distant metastasis. Based on these characteristics at diagnosis, some authors have recommended the use of a sub stage classification that takes into consideration major risk factors such as gender, multifocality, lymph node invasion, distant metastasis and young age. Based on the frequency of extensive disease, lymph node and the presence of distant metastasis and the high recurrence rate, most children should be included in the high risk group, even when most staging systems classify them in Stage 1 or Stage 2 (Wada, 2009).

4. Surgical treatment

Treatment of WDTC is intended to eradicate disease and improve recurrence free survival. The primary treatment modality remains surgical excision followed by radioiodine ablation and thyroid hormone suppression therapy; a paradigm followed in many institutions.

The extent of surgical removal is still a matter of debate in many places. The ATA and the American Association of Clinical Endocrinologists have recommended a total or near total thyroidectomy if feasible in most of the cases (Cooper, 2009). Total thyroidectomy remains the preferred operation in tumors greater than T1a (>1cm). It is generally accompanied by dissection of the central lymphatic compartment since local lymph node disease increases the risk of local and regional recurrence (Parisi, 2007, Niedziela, 2006, Handkiewicz, 2007). Patients who undergo total thyroidectomy have a higher rate of recurrence-free survival. Patients with intrathyroidal lesions less than 1cm can be considered candidates for less than total thyroidectomy if the lesion is unifocal, there is no previous history of radiation exposure, and there is no evidence for either lymph node or distant metastasis at diagnosis.

Complications of surgery are rare in the hands of experienced surgeons. The most common complication is parathyroid dysfunction, resulting in hypocalcemia and low serum PTH concentrations. The hypoparathyrodism is usually transient and resolves in several weeks with some patients requiring temporary treatment. A more serious complication is the irreversible damage to the recurrent laryngeal nerve causing permanent vocal cord paralysis and hoarseness; however, in our practice we have never seen such a case. Nowadays the use of intraoperative probe reduces surgical time and complications.

4.1 Post-surgical evaluation and radioiodine treatment

A sonographic evaluation is advisable to assess the size of the thyroid remnant and determine the adequacy of excision after surgery. Images should depict a volume of less than 2 ml of thyroid tissue at approximately 1 month after its removal.

Thyroid ablation with radioiodine (RAI) is routinely recommended to destroy any residual tissue after surgery. The goal of the postsurgical treatment is to ablate the thyroid remnant and evaluate the extent of functional thyroid tissue and/or metastatic disease. The radioiodine dose should be individualized and is often empirically adjusted to tumor size and disease extension. Therefore, RAI doses ranging from 30-200 mCi (1.1-7.4 GBq) have been employed. The use of low dose vs. high dose treatments is still a debated issue, since some authors claim there is little difference in efficacy between the 30mCi and the 100 mCi. The higher activity is more effective in detecting and treating metastatic disease. In our practice we use doses in the pediatric population similar to those in adults. For patients with disease extension to neck nodes we recommend 100mCi (3.7 GBq) and for patients with distant metastasis we have used 150-200 mCi (5.6-7.4 GBq). We pursue Whole Body Scan (WBS) post therapy usually 5-7 days after the therapeutic radioiodine dose. In most patients, the WBS demonstrates post surgical residual functioning tissue in the thyroid bed, additional loco-regional nodes or distant metastases. Post therapy scintigraphy may detect new lesions in up to 46% of the cases (Silva, 2010) .

Thyroid ablation therapy reduces the risk of recurrence in the thyroid bed and neck lymph nodes, independent of the extent of the surgical procedure. Both treatment modalities (surgery and RAI ablation) are independent predictors of recurrence free survival. Local relapse is reduced to 6.3% when 131-I is administered after surgery. Recurrence rate in the thyroid bed and local lymph nodes is also reduced when total thyroidectomy and ablation therapy are given. This is especially important in the pediatric population given their longer life expectancy. It has been found that sex, age and histology do not correlate with thyroid bed recurrence free survival. Nodal recurrences are more frequent in patients with the histologic subtype of papillary carcinoma, classical variant as compared to the follicular variant. Specifically, the 10 year nodal recurrence free survival has been reported at 83% for papillary carcinoma, classic type vs. 95% for the follicular variant type (Parisi, 2006, Luster, 2007, Handkiewicz, 2007).

In patients with lung metastasis, there is often incomplete post therapy remission. Several authors have reported a high incidence of persistent disease after therapeutic iodine in patients with lung metastasis. Repeated courses of ablation therapy is often needed. Since ablation therapy could have adverse effects on the lungs (i.e., pneumonitis with fibrosis), it is important to monitor pulmonary function in this population.

The tumor response to RAI therapy is related to the size of the residual tissue or tumor burden. Tumoral masses with small volume (i.e., less than 1 mm) in children results in poorer therapeutic response. This is related to the effect of the iodine beta radiation range, as established in the Monte Carlo simulation test published by Reynolds, Robbins and Maxon. Approximately 90% of the ionizing radiation emitted by the 131-iodine decay will be absorbed outside the tumor range (Silva, 2010).

Juvenile thyroid cancer is known to have a high recurrence rate. The rate may be as high as 40% in patients less than 20 years of age and higher within the first 7 years of diagnosis. Twenty year recurrence free survival is about 10% in patients diagnosed at age 10 or less. In fact, age is a major determinant of risk of recurrence, particularly in those younger than 10 years (Niedziela, 2006, Jarzab, 2005). Overall younger patients have a poorer prognosis than those diagnosed later in life. In spite of these data, it should be emphasized that prognosis is still excellent with an overall survival rate of 95% for over a 12.9 years of follow up in large series (Shapiro, 2005, Parisi, 2007).

Five and ten year survival rates in pediatric patients with thyroid cancer have been reported as high as 98-99%. However, the mortality rate may become significant in cases with distant metastasis or recurrent disease. In the latter, the cumulative mortality rate varies from 30-58% in a period of 12-20 years.

Over the last several years, FDG-PET studies have been included in the armamentarium of diagnostic tests in the follow up of patients with thyroid cancer. PET imaging is recommended in selected cases only, specifically those with negative iodine WBS and positive or rising thyroglobulin levels. FDG uptake can identify recurrent disease in up to 70-80% of those cases; uptake is associated with a poor outcome and decreased survival (Parisi, 2007).

5. Risks of radioiodine therapy in the pediatric population

Radioiodine therapy can have complications, both in the short and in the long term. Short term complications include nausea, sialadenitis, pain and swelling in the neck. The frequency of these varies from 10-50%. Long term effects are related to the radiation-induced mutations (i.e., radiation carcinogenesis). These are of utmost importance given the long life expectancy the pediatric group has at the time of diagnosis.

In terms of the gonadal axis, RAI therapy is associated with an earlier menopause compared with the general female population. In males azoospermia and oligospermia have been described. Increased risks of secondary malignancies, mainly solid tumors and leukemias, have also been reported. Pulmonary fibrosis has been reported in patients with extensive pulmonary metastasis; in fact up to 10% of pediatric patients can develop pulmonary fibrosis. All of the above complications are dose dependent (Parisi, 2007).

6. Follow up

Hormonal suppressive therapy follows the ablation therapy and is aimed at reducing the risk of tumor re growth and recurrences. The recommended TSH suppression level may be in the range of 0.1-0.5 mU/L and should be dependent on the presence or absence of persistent disease.

Serum thyroglobulin (Tg), a tumor specific marker, is a valuable assay during follow up. Tg is only produced by the follicular cells. After thyroidectomy, Tg should be undetectable. The assay of thyroglobulin is recommended before ablation therapy (under TSH stimulation) and 6-12 months after therapy (on suppression). The predictive value for disease progression is well established in the literature.

Stimulated levels of serum thyroglobulin more than 2 or 3 ng/ml after recombinant TSH are considered diagnostic of tumor recurrences. A rising value of Tg alerts the clinician to the presence of active disease and is more sensitive if the sample is measured after TSH stimulation. It is recommended to have the samples analyzed in the same laboratory using the same assay method. Thyroglobulin antibodies (TgAb) must be determined in the same serum sample since the presence of TgAb invalidates the thyroglobulin results. (Goldsmith, 2011).

Some authors have reported that Tg use is not completely reliable for follow up purposes. Specifically, they do not advocate the sole use of Tg as a method for follow up in affected patients when screening for persistent or recurrent disease. False negative Tg values have been reported in 4-35% of the patients with evidence of local or metastatic disease. Undetectable serum Tg has been reported in patients treated with RAI, with small volumes of disease. Other reasons associated with the low or undetectable Tg levels are the presence of TgAb, immunologically inactive Tg or technical limitations of the assay method. Thus, relying on Tg values as a single criterion in the long term follow up of thyroid cancer should be exercised with caution. In our center, pediatric patients are evaluated annually for at least three consecutive years and thereafter every two or three years depending on the clinical follow up evaluation. All patients are evaluated withTg and Tg Ab levels as well as a neck ultrasound. Neck ultrasound is an excellent tool for the early detection of neck nodal metastasis and should be used in conjunction with the Tg measurement in the follow up of patients whenever possible (Parisi, 2007, Niedziela, 2006, Jarzab, 2005). In our clinic, patients with initial distant metastasis, 131-I Whole body scan is done one year after the therapeutic dose to determine if an adittional therapeutic doses is necessary. Clinical follow up is recommended until adulthood.

7. Medullary Thyroid Carcinoma

Medullary thyroid carcinoma (MTC) originates in calcitonin-producing cells (C-cells) of the thyroid gland and accounts for 3% to 9% of thyroid cancers. MTC is diagnosed histologically when nests of C-cells appear to extend beyond the basement membrane and infiltrate and destroy thyroid follicles. At least half occur in kindreds and are apparently inherited as an autosomal dominant trait. It may be part of multiple endocrine neoplasia type 2 (MEN 2) including the phenotypes MEN 2A, familial medullary thyroid carcinoma (FMTC), and MEN 2B.

MTC in persons with MEN 2 typically present at a younger age than sporadic MTC and is more often associated with C-cell hyperplasia as well as multifocality or bilaterality. Symptoms of MTC include neck pain, a palpable neck mass, and/or diarrhea resulting from hypercalcitoninemia [Callender et al 2008]. Metastatic spread to cervical and regional lymph nodes (i.e., parathyroid, paratracheal, jugular chain, and upper mediastinum) or to distant sites including the liver, lungs, or bone is common and is frequently present in individuals with a palpable thyroid mass or diarrhea [Cohen & Moley 2003].

The responsible mutated gene causing inherited MTC is the ret tyrosine kinase which has been mapped to 10q11.2.

The FMTC subtype constitutes approximately 10%-20% of cases of MEN 2. By operational definition MTC is the only clinical manifestation of FMTC. The age of onset of MTC is later in FMTC and the penetrance of MTC is lower than that observed in MEN 2A and MEN 2B [Eng et al 1996, Machens et al 2001, Machens & Dralle 2006, Zbuk & Eng 2007, American Thyroid Association Guidelines Task Force 2009].

The MEN 2B subtype accounts for approximately 5% of cases of MEN 2. MEN 2B is characterized by the early development of an aggressive form of MTC in all affected individuals [Skinner et al 1996]. Individuals with MEN 2B who do not undergo thyroidectomy at an early age (age <1 year) are likely to develop metastatic MTC at an early age. Prior to intervention with early prophylactic thyroidectomy, the average age of death in individuals with MEN 2B was 21 years.

The American Thyroid Association Guidelines Task Force has classified mutations based on their risk for aggressive MTC [American Thyroid Association Guidelines Task Force 2009]. The classification may be used in (1) predicting phenotype and in (2) recommendations regarding the ages at which to (a) perform prophylactic thyroidectomy and (b) begin biochemical screening for pheochromocytoma and hyperparathyroidism. Annual biochemical screening for MEN 2A beginning at age eight years has been recommended for individuals with mutations of codons 630 and 634 and at age 20 years for mutations in all other codons [American Thyroid Association Guidelines Task Force 2009]. Screening for FMTC is indicated just as for patients in kindreds with MEN 2. MEN 2B patients identified by genetic screening should undergo thyroidectomy at 6 months of age. However screening should not be precluded and still be pursued early in life in children at risk of carrying MEN 2B genes since disease manifestation could be aggressive and devastating. The best time for surgery should be individualized (author personal experience). A basal or stimulated calcitonin level of ≥100 pg/ml is an indication for surgery [Costante et al 2007, American Thyroid Association Guidelines Task Force 2009].

The standard treatment for MTC is surgical removal of the thyroid and lymph node dissection [American Thyroid Association Guidelines Task Force 2009]. Chemotherapy and radiation are less effective in the treatment of MTC than surgical removal [Moley et al 1998, Cohen & Moley 2003]. All individuals who have undergone thyroidectomy need thyroid hormone replacement therapy. Autotransplantation of parathyroid tissue is not typically performed at the time of thyroidectomy unless there is evidence of hyperparathyroidism [American Thyroid Association Guidelines Task Force 2009]. Prophylactic thyroidectomy is the primary preventive measure for individuals with an identified germline *RET* mutation [American Thyroid Association Guidelines Task Force 2009]. Prophylactic thyroidectomy is safe for all age groups; however, the timing of the surgery is controversial. According to the consensus statement from the American Thyroid Association Guidelines Task Force, the age at which prophylactic thyroidectomy is performed can be guided by the codon position of the *RET* mutation. These guidelines continue to be modified as more data becomes available.

For all individuals with a *RET* mutation who have not had a thyroidectomy, annual biochemical screening with calcitonin is recommended with immediate thyroidectomy if results are abnormal [Szinnai et al 2003]. Annual serum calcitonin screening [American Thyroid Association Guidelines Task Force 2009] should begin for children with: MEN 2B at age six months and MEN 2A or FMTC at age three to five years. Caution should be used in interpreting calcitonin results for children younger than age three years, especially those younger than age six months. Prophylactic thyroidectomy should not be offered routinely to at-risk individuals in whom the disorder has not been confirmed. *RET* gene molecular genetic testing should be offered to probands with any of the MEN 2 subtypes and to all at-risk members of kindreds in which a germline *RET* mutation has been identified in an affected family member.

Alternate therapies are still under investigation with potential benefits in the near future. Among these: Adenoviral vectors expressing a dominant-negative truncated form of *RET*, DeltaTK; potential of tyrosine kinase inhibitors, such as vandetanib.

8. Conclusion

Well differentiated is the most common pediatric thyroid cancer and usually presents as a solitary mass. The disease is frequently extensive at diagnosis. Surgical management is important for the initial control of the disease, follow by radioiodine therapy. High therapeutic radioiodine doses are required in the majority of the cases. Long term follow up with hormonal suppressive therapy is recommended. Neck sonogram and serum thyroglobulin level is recommended for the first 3 consecutive years. In spite of the extensive disease, overall long term survival in these patients is excellent.

9. References

American Thyroid Association Guidelines Task Force; Medullary thyroid cancer: management guidelines of the American Thyroid Association. *Thyroid.* 2009;19:565–612.

Cooper D, Doherty G, Haugen B, et al. Revised American Thyroid Association management guidelines for patients with thyroid nodules and differentiated thyroid cancer. *Thyroid*: 19 No 11, 2009

Callender GG, Rich TA, Perrier ND. Multiple endocrine neoplasia syndromes. *Surg Clin North Am.* 2008;88:863–895.Cohen MS, Moley JF. Surgical treatment of medullary thyroid carcinoma. *J Intern Med.* 2003;253:616–26

DeLellis RA, Lloyd RV, Heitz PU, Eng C (2004) Pathology and Genetics: Tumours of the Endocrine Organs. *World Health Organization Classification of Tumours* series, vol 8. IARC Press, Lyon, France.

Eng C, Clayton D, Schuffenecker I, Lenoir G, et. al. The relationship between specific RET proto-oncogene mutations and disease phenotype in multiple endocrine neoplasia type 2. International RET mutation consortium analysis. *JAMA.* 1996;276:1575–9.

Goldsmith S. To ablate or not to ablate: Issues and evidence involved in 131-I ablation of residual tissue in patients with differentiated thyroid carcinoma. *Semin Nucl Med* 41:96-104, 2011

Griffith O, Melk A, J, Wiseman S. Meta analysis and Meta review of thyroid cancer gene expression profiling studies identifies important diagnostic biomarkers. *Journal of Clinical Oncology* Vol. 24 No 31: 5043-5051, 2006

Handkiewicz D, Wloch J, Roskosz J et al. Total thyroidectomy and adjuvant radioiodine treatment independently decrease locoregional recurrence risk in childhood and adolescent differentiated thyroid cancer. *J Nuclear Medicine* 48: 879-888, 2007

Jarzab B, Handkiewicz D, Wloch J. Juvenile differentiated thyroid carcinoma and the role of radioiodine in its treatment: a quantitative review. *Endocrine related Cancer* 12: 773-803, 2005

Luster M, Lassmann M, Freudenberg L, Reiners C. Thyroid cancer in childhood: Management strategy, including dosimetry and long term results. *Hormones* 6(4): 269-278, 2007

Machens A, Gimm O, Hinze R, Hoppner W, Boehm BO, Dralle H. Genotype-phenotype correlations in hereditary medullary thyroid carcinoma: oncological features and biochemical properties. *J Clin Endocrinol Metab.* 2001;86:1104–9.

Machens A, Schneyer U, Holzhausen HJ, Raue F, Dralle H. Emergence of medullary thyroid carcinoma in a family with the Cys630Arg RET germline mutation. *Surgery.* 2004;136:1083–7.

Mitsutake N, Knauf J, Nisutake S. et al. Conditional BRAF expression induces DNA synthesis, apoptosis, dedifferentiation and chromosomal instability in thyroid PCCL3 cells. *Cancer Research* 65(6): 24652473, 2005

Niedziela M. Pathogenesis, diagnosis and management of thyroid nodules in children. *Endocrine-Related* Cancer 13: 427-453, 2006

Parisi M, Mankoff D. Differentiated Pediatric Thyroid Cancer: correlates with adult disease, controversies in treatment. *Seminars in Nuclear Medicine* 37:340-356, 2007

Shapiro N, Bhattacharyya N. Population Based Outcomes for Pediatric Thyroid Carcinoma. *Laryngospe* 115:337-340, 2005

Silva F, Laguna R, Nieves-Rivera F. Pediatric thyroid cancer with extensive disease in a Hispanic population: Outcome and long term survival. *Journal of Pediatric Endocrinology and Metabolism* 23: 59-64, 2010

Wada N, Sugino K, Mimura T et al. Pediatric differentiated thyroid carcinoma in stage 1: risk factor analysis for disease free survival. *BMC Cancer* 2009, 9:306

Xu X, Quiros R, Gatusso P, et al. High prevalence of BRAF gene mutation in papillary thyroid carcinoma and thyroid tumor cell lines. *Cancer Research* 63: 4561-4567, 2003

Zbuk KM, Eng C. Cancer phenomics: RET and PTEN as illustrative models. *Nat Rev Cancer.* 2007; 7:35–45.

9

Current Innovations and Opinions in the Surgical Management of Differentiated Thyroid Carcinoma

Brian Hung-Hin Lang
Department of Surgery, University of Hong Kong Medical Centre, Queen Mary Hospital, Hong Kong SAR, China

1. Introduction

Over the last decade, surgeons have witnessed dramatic changes in the surgical management of differentiated thyroid carcinoma (DTC). This is not only a result of the introduction of new technologies in surgery but also a result of better understanding of the disease and its behavior. DTC accounts for over 90% of all follicular-cell derived thyroid malignancies and is the commonest primary endocrine-related malignancy. In our locality, its age-adjusted incidence has doubled over the last 20-25 years with a similar trend being observed elsewhere.(Hong Kong Cancer Registry, 2011) Despite this, the cancer-specific mortality remains low with an overall 10-year survival above 90%.(Lang et al., 2007a) However, recurrent or persistent disease after seemingly curative surgery poses a problem for both clinicians and patients.(Mazzaferri et al.,2001) Since surgery remains to play a pivotal role in the overall management of DTC, the primary aim of any new changes would be to further reduce and if possible, to prevent these recurrences or persistent diseases from occurring. Examples of some of these new changes would include: 1. the adoption of new, innovative surgical approaches (i.e. endoscopic, robot-assisted and trans-oral thyroidectomy) in surgical management of DTC in order to reduce the surgical morbidity, shorten hospital stay and enhance patient satisfaction; 2 the use of several surgical adjuncts such as new alternate energy sources (Harmonic scalpel (Ethicon), Sonosurg® (Olympus) and LigaSure™ (Valleylab), intraoperative nerve monitoring (IONM) and quick intraoperative parathyroid hormone assay (IOPTH) 3. the routine adoption of prophylactic central neck dissection (pCND) in DTC during total thyroidectomy. The aims of this review were to examine and evaluate these 3 broad subjects in an evidence-based matter and see if these changes could lead to better patient outcomes when compared to the conventional open thyroidectomy with or without the help of the surgical adjunct(s).

2. Innovative surgical approaches

2.1 Endoscopic thyroidectomy

The application of endoscopic visualization to thyroid surgery has allowed surgeons to perform thyroidectomy through incisions far smaller and less visible than the conventional

Kocher's incision - the so-called "less is more". In general, these endoscopic techniques attempt to minimize the extent of dissection, improve cosmesis, reduce post-operative pain, shorten hospital stay and hasten postoperative recovery. Michel Gagner was the first surgeon to report the feasibility of endoscopic technique to neck surgery.(Gagner, 1996) He reported a totally endoscopic subtotal parathyroidectomy in a 37 year old man suffering from familial hyperparathyroidism. (Gagner, 1996) Although the endoscopic procedure took over 5 hours, it demonstrated the technical feasibility and safety. Over the turn of the last century, an increasing number of different endoscopic techniques have been described and may be categorized into namely cervical or direct and extracervical or indirect approaches.(Lang, 2010a) The former is considered as truly minimally invasive since the skin incisions are small in the neck with direct access to the thyroid gland. On the other hand, the extracervical approach is considered as an endoscopic instead of minimally invasive approach because incisions are made distant from the neck and so the approach requires more extensive tissue dissections.(Henry, 2008) However, despite its invasiveness, it offers superior early cosmetic outcome because potentially unsightly scars can be hidden and so patients remains "scarless in the neck". This approach has been adopted more often in Asian countries where remaining "scarless in the neck" after thyroidectomy is a priority for a select group of patients.(Lang & Lo, 2010b)

2.1.1 Cervical / direct approaches

These approaches include the endoscopic lateral cervical approach and the minimally invasive video-assisted thyroidectomy (MIVAT). In the endoscopic lateral cervical approach, two 2.5mm and one 10mm trocars are inserted under direct vision along the anterior border of the sternocleidomastoid muscle on the side of resection. Using endoscopic instruments, the dissection starts from the lateral aspect of the thyroid gland and moves medially with identification of the recurrent laryngeal nerve (RLN), parathyroid glands and skeletonisation of the superior and inferior thyroid vessels.(Palazzo et al., 2006) Excellent visualization of RLN and parathyroid glands is possible with magnification by the endoscope. However, this technique is limited to unilateral thyroid resection and its application in thyroid cancer surgery is restricted to sub-centimeter papillary thyroid carcinoma (PTC) detected by high-resolution ultrasound machines. In contrast, the MIVAT would be preferred if bilateral thyroid resection is necessary because the incision is made in the midline instead of the lateral aspect of the neck. A 2cm incision is made in the middle of the neck about 2cm above the sternal notch. Blunt dissection is then carried out to separate the strap muscle from underlying thyroid lobe. A 5mm 30 degree endoscope is placed inside the 1.5cm wound for lighting and visualization. The procedure is performed under endoscopic view with the operating space maintained by external retraction. This technique was first applied for selected benign thyroid conditions in 2000.(Miccoli et al., 2000) However, with improvement in techniques, MIVAT has become increasingly adopted for low- to intermediate risk DTC.(Miccoli et al., 2009) MIVAT was shown to achieve similar completeness of resection and 5-year survival outcomes as those with low- and intermediate risk PTC undergoing conventional thyroidectomy.(Miccoli et al., 2009; Miccoli et al., 2002; Lombardi et al.,2007a) In addition, it has been shown that a concomitant pCND is technically feasible in MIVAT during initial total thyroidectomy.(Bellantone et al., 2002) Also for patients with low risk PTC with concomitant lateral lymph node metastases, a minimally invasive video-assisted functional lateral neck dissection through a small neck incision is also technically possible.(Lombardi et al,, 2007b) A recent randomized trial comparing conventional thyroidectomy with MIVAT found that the latter was associated with a lower risk of wound infection.(5.3% vs 0.0%, $p<0.05$)(Dionigi et al.,2011)

2.1.2 Extra-cervical / indirect endoscopic approaches

Unlike the cervical approaches, these approaches involve making incisions either in the chest, breast and/or axilla to hide the scars with clothing.(Lang, 2010a) Ikede et al. first described these approaches by placing three ports in the axilla with low-pressure gas insufflation for maintaining the operating space. Although cosmetic results were excellent, the procedure was technically demanding and time consuming because of unintentional easy gas leakage and frequent interference of the 3 operating surgical instruments in the small available space in the axilla.(Ikeda et al., 2003) Chung et al. modified this technique by making this approach gasless with the space maintained by a specially designed skin-lifting external retractor.(Kang et al.,2009a) In this approach, the procedure began with a 4 to 5cm incision in the axilla and then a subcutaneous space was created from the axilla to the thyroid gland. To avoid the problem of interference of instruments, an additional 5mm port was inserted in the chest area for medial retraction of the thyroid gland. Chung et al. recently reported their experience with this approach after performing 581 cases.(Kang et al., 2009a) Among these patients, 410 patients had low-risk PTC. In their series, concomitant pCND was performed and the rate of lymph node metastasis was 27.3%.(Kang et al., 2009a)

To further increase the degree of angulations and freedom of interference between instruments, a combined axillo-breast approach was developed utilizing 2 circumareolar trocars in the breast and a single trocar in the ipsilateral axilla. This approach was later modified by using bilateral axillary ports to allow better exposure to both sides of the thyroid compartment. This approach is now known as the bilateral axillo-breast approach (BABA). Despite the extensive tissue dissection, when compared with the conventional open approach, BABA has been shown to have similar results in terms of transient hypocalcemia, bleeding, permanent RLN paralysis and length of hospital stay.(Chung et al., 2007) More recently, a Korean group tried to eliminate wounds around the chest or breast areas all together by making incisions in the axilla and post-auricular areas instead. They reported a small series of 10 patients using this approach and 7 underwent bilateral thyroid resection for low-risk PTC. They demonstrated the feasibility of this technique of scarless (in the neck) thyroid surgery.(Lee et al., 2009a)

2.2 Robotic-assisted thyroidectomy

The application and feasibility of the endoscopic approach was given a further boost with the availability of various robotic systems such as the da Vinci system (Intuitive Surgical, Sunnyvale, California). Unlike other cancers such as prostate cancer, the initial enthusiasm of using the robot in thyroid cancers was not great because of its relatively high cost, bulkiness of the robotic arm and long operating time. However, since the publication of two large surgical series demonstrating the feasibility and safety of robotic assisted thyroidectomy in DTC, an increasing number of specialized surgical centers worldwide are beginning to accept and perform this procedure. The theoretical advantages of using the robot over the endoscopic approach include the three-dimensional view offer to the operating surgeon, the flexible robotic instruments with seven degree of freedom and 90^0 articulation, the increased tactile sensation and the ability to filter any hand tremors.(Kang et al., 2009b) Kang et al. recently reported their experience of 200 robot-assisted total thyroidectomy using the gasless trans-axillary approach for low-risk PTC with concomitant pCND and found excellent short-term results in terms of postoperative pain and patients' satisfaction.(Kang et al., 2009c) This was followed briefly by another report of 338 benign and malignant cases using the same trans-axillary.(Kang et al., 2009d) To date, this group has performed over 1000 cases. A separate Korean group also reported similar results using the da Vinci robot via the BABA technique.(Lee et al., 2009b) Although both techniques have been demonstrated to be feasible and safe, they have been limited to a few high-volume specialized centers. The surgeons performing these operations have had years of operating experience with the endoscopic approach and so the learning curve for a novel, non-endoscopic thyroid surgeon or someone who predominantly perform open thyroid procedures, remains undefined but is likely to be longer than one might think. Furthermore, better comparative studies such as a randomized controlled trial between robotic-assisted and endoscopic thyroidectomy are needed in order to better assess the added patient outcome benefits over the latter approach.

2.3 Endoscopic vs robotic-assisted thyroidectomy via the transaxillary route

Since both approaches actually utilize the same surgical approach (i.e. the transaxillary route), an obvious question would be whether using the robot would have added benefits over the conventional endoscopic operation, perhaps in terms of operating time, complication rate or number of assistants required.(Lang et al., 2011a) Lang et al. first reported a small series of patients who underwent the endoscopic (i.e. without the robot) and the robot-assisted thyroidectomy for mostly benign cases and compared their outcomes. They found that the robotic group was associated with an increased total procedure time and resulted in higher pain score on day 0 than the endoscopic group but the robot was able to eliminate the need of an extra surgical assistant at the time of operation.(Lang & Chow, 2011b) Lee et al. reported a larger series of patients with mostly papillary thyroid microcarcinomas. In their series, the robotic group was associated with shorter operating time, more lymph nodes retrieval and shorter learning curve.(J.Lee, 2011) This was followed by another larger series reported by the same group comparing the two approaches. In this study, they confirmed that the robot assisted thyroidectomy was superior to endoscopic and postulated that the reason for this superiority was because of the limitations of the conventional endoscopic instruments. (S.Lee, 2011) These contradictory findings could be explained by the fact that the first series comprised mainly benign nodular cases and so no pCND was necessary whereas in the latter two series, pCND was performed at the time of the thyroidectomy. Therefore, perhaps more complex surgical procedures might benefit from the robot whereas a straightforward operation such as a hemithyroidectomy or total thyroidectomy, the robot might not be any extra benefits.(Lang et al., 2011a)

2.4 Transoral thyroidectomy

This remains one of the most contentious surgical approaches and one of the most extreme examples of preferring "scarless in the neck" in thyroidectomy. The concept began in 2008 when Witzel et al. presented an experimental "natural orifice surgery" or NOS approach for thyroidectomy.(Witzel et al.,2008) To minimize the surgical trauma, they presented a transoral access to the thyroid gland using a single port access via an axilloscope. Following this, Wilhelm et al. reported the first 8 cases of transoral thyroidectomy in humans. The incisions were made in the vestibule of the mouth and conventional endoscopic instruments were inserted in the subplatysmal layer, anterior to the thyroid cartilage. However, parathesia of the mental nerve was reported in the first six cases and two unilateral RLN palsies were also noted in two of eight cases. Also there was one patient who developed a minor infection at the vestibular incision 4 weeks after surgery.(Wilhelm & Metzig, 2011) Therefore, at this moment, one could say that this approach is technically feasible but remains experimental and is associated with a higher rate of complications than the conventional open approach.

3. Use of surgical adjuncts

3.1 IONM

RLN injury is a leading cause of litigation in thyroid surgery.(Ready & Barnes, 1994) To those with this injury, it not only affects the voice quality but also diminishes the overall quality of life because of communication, social and work-related problems.(Smith et al., 1998) Routine RLN identification is considered the standard of care in thyroid surgery. However, with the availability of IONM, the questions are whether this new piece of technology could further reduce the risk of iatrogenic RLN injury in thyroid surgery or thyroid cancer surgery in particular.

Although IONM has been around for over 3 decades, its widespread usage in the surgical practice only dates back 5-10 years. There has been an increased in interest on applying this technique for thyroid surgery because of the introduction of new and user-friendly devices from technological advance.(Chan & Lo, 2006a) Currently, there are two types of IONM systems, namely those with electromyographic (EMG) documentation and those without EMG documentation. The former involves RLN stimulation with registration of the elicited laryngeal muscle activity through endoscopic insertion of electrodes into the vocal fold or with the use of endotracheal surface electrodes. The latter utilizes RLN stimulation with observation of posterior cricoarythenoid muscle contraction or palpation or intraoperative inspection of vocal cord function.(Dralle et al., 2008; Dralle et al., 2004) To date, there is no consensus on which is the best system and the choice depends on the availability of which system in your institution and the operator familiarity or experience. Regardless of which systems, there are potential flaws and pitfalls. In general, the positive predictive value (PPV) is proportionally low with this technology. That means that when a nerve has no signal during stimulation, it does not mean that it is injured. In fact, in our experience, the PPV was only 15% in low-risk thyroid surgery i.e. approximately only 1 out of 9 RLNs with no signals had an actual injury. This might be due to some technical errors such as detachment or displacement of electrodes or poor contact of the probe with the nerve due to inadequate exposure.(Chan & Lo, 2006) Perhaps, direct vagal stimulation could possibly reduce some of these errors but need more unnecessary dissection. Even more intriguing is the fact that this technique is also associated with false negative results, albeit rarely. In our experience, among 271 nerves at risk, 15 (5.5%) ended with RLN palsy but of these, 7 still had a positive IONM signals. Therefore, it seems that IONM might not be able to detect "sub-lethal" injury to RLN. It is possible that the action potential could be propagated along the neural pathway, as detected by the IONM, but not to the extent of initiating laryngeal muscle contraction during the postoperative period.(Chan, 2006a,2006b) Fortunately, all these injuries would invariably recover.

On the other hand, although the objective of the use of this device is to avoid RLN injury during thyroid surgery, the evidence of supporting its routine use has been weak. The first multicenter study including 29,998 RLNs at risk confirmed that the incidence of RLN palsy was not significantly reduced by the additional use of IONM when routine RLN identification was performed.(Dralle et al., 2004) There were more than 20 publications addressing this issue but majority of these studies were heterogeneous in terms of patients' characteristics (such as primary operations vs reoperations or benign vs malignant goiters), IONM techniques and the extent of resection (i.e. total vs subtotal lobectomy). A recent literature review could not definitely draw confirm conclusions or evidence on the effectiveness of IONM in reducing RLN injury in thyroid surgery.(Dralle et al., 2008) Furthermore, most studies were either case-series with no control group or retrospective studies with inadequate statistical power to demonstrate a difference between those with or without using IONM. In fact, a randomized study utilizing approximately 7,000 patients in each arm of patients undergoing thyroidectomy with or without IONM will be required to have adequate statistical power to show a difference in outcome with reference to RLN paralysis.(Dralle et al., 2004; Dralle et al., 2008) Interestingly though, the first prospective randomized study comparing IONM with routine RLN visualization only was recently published.(Barczynski et al., 2009) In this study, approximately 500 patients were randomized into each arm. The number of patients recruited in each arm was based on the principle of detecting a 2% difference in the incidence of transient RLN injury with a 90% probability at $p<0.05$. This study did demonstrate a statistically significant difference in reducing transient RLN injury when IONM was adopted in comparison with RLN visualization only. However, as expected, the rate of permanent RLN injury was similar in the two study arms because of inadequate statistical power. Nevertheless, despite the inadequate power of most published IONM studies, there seemed to be a trend toward improved RLN protection with the use of this new technology.(Dralle et al. 2008) In addition, the IONM may be of potential benefit for "difficult" cases such as reoperative thyroidectomy, locally advanced thyroid cancers or central neck dissection for cancer recurrence. Perhaps, for the relatively inexperienced surgeons, the IONM might reduce the incidence of RLN injury in difficult cases.

3.2 IOPTH (intraoperative parathyroid hormone) for predicting post-thyroidectomy hypoparathyroidism

Hypoparathyroidism is a common complication after bilateral thyroid resections or total thyroidectomy. Up to 30% of patients after total thyroidectomy develop temporary hypoparathyroidism.(Pattou et al.,1998) There are many identifiable risk factors leading to postoperative hypoparathyroidism including thyroidectomy for thyrotoxicosis and thyroid cancer, thyroid reoperations, reduced stores of vitamin D, increased extent of thyroid resection and need of concomitant pCND.(McHenry et al., 1994;Abboud et al. 2002) Patients undergoing thyroidectomy for thyroid cancer are particularly prone to hypoparathyroidism because they often need a more complete thyroid resection together with neck dissection. In fact, total thyroidectomy and pCND is increasingly being performed for DTC to achieve lower recurrences, better disease-free survival and enhanced postoperative athyroglobulinemia.(Roh et al. 2007; Lang et al., 2011c) However, it has been shown that up to 60% of patients after pCND could develop transient hypocalcemia secondary to the frequent occurrence of unintentional or incidental parathyroidectomy.(Pereira et al.,2005) Therefore, in the presence of such a high incidence of postoperative hypoparathyroidism, the need of routine postoperative inpatient calcium monitoring remains questionable after thyroid cancer surgery while the early routine administration of oral calcium and/or vitamin D supplements seems to be relevant and can facilitate the early discharge from hospital shortly after surgery without developing unpleasant hypocalcemic symptoms.(Grodski & Serpell,2008) In fact, a recent randomized study supported this strategy because routine administration of oral calcium was shown to markedly reduce the severity and symptoms of hypocalcemia.(Roh et al.,2009) However, the adoption of this strategy could lead to over-treatment in patients who do not have hypocalcaemia leading to rebound hypercalcemia and increased medication costs. On the other hand, this strategy might lead to inadequate treatment in patients with severe symptomatic hypocalcaemia as oral calcium alone may not fully correct the hypocalcemia and so vitamin D supplements is indicated in such situation.(Lo,2003)

On the other hand, in-patient serial close monitoring of serum calcium is recommended after total thyroidectomy because most symptomatic hypocalcemia occurs around 24-28 hours after surgery.(Pfleiderer et al.,2009) A 24-hour or longer hospital stay is invariably required. Therefore, efforts are made to shorten hospital stays, decrease biochemical blood tests and reduce hospital costs by adopting other strategies to achieve early prediction of post-thyroidectomy hypocalcemia. With the availability of IOPTH and wide application in patients undergoing minimally invasive parathyroidectomy to predict postoperative cure, this new surgical adjunct has been applied to thyroid surgery to monitor parathyroid function and to predict the occurrence of postoperative normocalcaemia or hypocalcaemia. In our early prospective study of using IOPTH in predicting hypocalcemia in 100 consecutive patients (including 33 patients with DTC) who underwent either total or completion thyroidectomy, we found that a normal level of IOPTH at 10mins or a level less than 75% decline in IOPTH at 10 mins after excision of thyroid gland accurately identified normocalcemia.(Lo et al.,2002) It was suggested that intraoperative or early postoperative parathyroid hormone assay might be a sensitive tool to confirm postoperative normocalcaemia and identify patients at-risk of developing postoperative hypocalcaemia. Since then, up to 30 different investigators have published their results of using various different IOPTH assays in predicting hypocalcemia after total thyroidectomy. The IOPTH levels and their rate of decline at various time points after surgery could be utilized for prediction of postoperative hypocalcaemia with variable sensitivity, specificity and accuracy.(Lombardi et al.,2004,2006) However, based on two evidence-based reviews, it was recommended that the IOPTH level within a few hours after thyroid surgery could accurately predict postoperative normocalcaemia and identify patients at-risk of developing hypocalcemia, particularly severe, symptomatic hypocalcemia.(Grodski & Serpell, 2008; Noordzij et al.,2007) It was suggested that patients could be stratified into high or low risk groups and PTH should be measured at 1-6 hrs after operation in comparison to preoperative PTH. A < or > 65% decline at 6 hours after operation should allow early discharge or facilitate the decision of early calcium supplement. On the other hand, a strategy of 2 cut-off points should be considered with a high accuracy. A <50% decline within few hours after surgery allowed early discharge while a >90% decline necessitated early calcium supplement because of the accuracy in predicting normocalcaemia and hypocalcaemia respectively.(Noordzij et al.,2007) For those patients with 50-90% decline, either serial calcium monitoring or routine treatment should be considered. In the AES guideline, one single serum PTH measurement is recommended at 4 hrs after operation.(AES group, 2007) A normal PTH can predict normocalcaemia and patients can be discharged early with 7% subsequently developing mild hypocalcaemia. For patients with undetectable PTH level, oral calcium and vitamin D analogue should be administered early to avoid symptomatic hypocalcaemia. Intermediate or subnormal PTH level is a less accurate predictor of hypocalcaemia. In that case, oral calcium should commence or patients should be monitored with serial calcium levels for the need of calcium and/or vitamin D analogue.(AES group,2007) Therefore, PTH assay can now be considered as a perioperative adjunct to predict normocalcaemia or hypocalcaemia with reasonable accuracy. It can facilitate early discharge, avoid routine calcium replacement, facilitate early calcium replacement to avoid symptomatic hypocalcaemia and decrease overall cost as well as increase patients' satisfaction. However, probably in the community hospital setting where IOPTH may not be available, the least expensive alternative option for same day discharge is routine postoperative oral calcium +/- vitamin D supplementation.

3.3 Alternate energy source for intraoperative hemostasis in thyroidectomy

In addition to scalpels and ligatures, alternate energy such as electric (e.g. ligasure) and ultrasonic (e.g. harmonic scalpel (Ethicon) and Sonosurg®) have been used for cutting and hemostasis in surgery. An unique feature of thyroidectomy is that thyroid gland has one of the richest blood supplies among the organs, with numerous blood vessels and plexuses entering the parenchyma. These vessels are usually controlled with ligatures (or clamp and tie) but the ligation and division of these vessels is time consuming and so perhaps the use of these alternate energy sources may reduce the actual operating time and cost. Essentially both ligasure or harmonic scalpel were consistently shown to shorten the total operating time by approximately 15-30% but in terms of complication rates, there was no statistically difference when compared to the conventional clamp and tie technique. Similarly, a recent meta-analysis which included 7 randomized trials comparing harmonic scalpel with conventional clamp and tie technique found that there was a weighed mean reduction of operative time of 18.74 minutes (95% CI: 10.52 – 28.97 minutes, p<0.001) but there was no statistical difference in complication rates.(Cirocchi et al., 2010)

First author (year)	No. of patients	Design	Two arms	Type of surgery	Type of thyroid pathology	Conclusions
Voutilainen (2000)	36	RCT	CT vs HS	HT/TT	Benign and malignant	HS: ↓ operating time; short learning curve
Siperstein (2002)	171	RS	CT vs HS	HT/TT	Benign and malignant	HS: ↓ operative time by 30mins in HT and TT

First author (year)	No. of patients	Design	Two arms	Type of surgery	Type of thyroid pathology	Conclusions
Ortega (2004)	200	RCT	CT vs HS	HT/TT	Benign	HS: 15-20% reduction in operating time, less costs
Petrakis (2004)	517	RS	CT vs LS	TT	Benign	LS: ↓ operating time, less RLN injury, less blood loss, less hypocalcemia
Kiriakopoulos (2004)	80	PS	CT vs LS	TT	Benign and malignant	Similar operating time and blood loss
Kirdak (2005)	58	PS	CT vs HS	HT/TT	Benign and malignant	HS: ↓ operating time only
Cordon (2005)	60	RCT	CT vs HS	HT/TT	Benign and malignant	HS: ↓ operating time only
Franko (2006)	155	RS	CT vs LS	HT/TT	Benign and malignant	LS: ↓ operating time, less blood loss, less hypocalcemia
Lepner (2007)	403	RS	CT vs LS	HT/TT	Not specified	LS: ↓ operating time, less hypocalcemia
Sartori (2008)	150	RCT	CT vs LS/HS	HT/TT	Benign and malignant	HS: ↓ operating time, more hypocalcemia
Pons (2009)	60	RCT	CT vs LS/HS	TT	Not specified	HS: ↓ operating time, less pain and cost
Cirocchi (2010)	608	MA (7 RCTs)	CT vs HS	TT	Benign and malignant	HS: ↓ operating time, less cost but similar complication rates
Zarebczan (2011)	231	RS	HS vs LS	HT/TT	Benign and malignant	HS: ↓ operating time but complications were similar
Rahbari (2011)	90	RCT	HS vs LS	HT/TT	Benign and malignant	No difference in operating time, cost or complications

Abbreviations: RCT = randomized controlled trial; PS = prospective study; RS = retrospective study; MA = meta-analysis; CT = conventional technique; HS = harmonic scalpel; LS = ligasure; HT = hemithyroidectomy; TT = total thyroidectomy

Table 1. shows a summary of the trials and their conclusions comparing different hemostatic techniques in thyroidectomy.

4. The role of pCND in DTC

The role of pCND in DTC remains one of the most discussed surgical subjects in recent few years. To date, there is little good evidence to show that pCND improves cancer-specific survivals or reduces cancer-specific mortality in DTC.

First author /year of publication	Number of patients		Follow up duration (months)	Cancer-specific mortality		*p*-value
	CND+ group	CND- group		CND+ group	CND- group	
Tisell/ 1996	P/T - 195	199;167	156 months (median)	8.4% - 11.1%	1.6%	Not reported
Sywak/ 2006	P - 56, A	391	CND-: 70 months CND+: 25 months (median)	0%	0%	Not statistically significant
Roh/2007	P - 40, B T - 42 (26/42 with lateral neck dissection)	73	52 months (mean)	0%	0%	Not statistically significant

Abbreviations: CND-: thyroidectomy alone, CND+: thyroidectomy plus central neck dissection; P: prophylactic, T: therapeutic; A: unilateral, B: bilateral

Table 2. A literature summary of studies which specifically evaluated cancer-specific mortality between thyroidectomy alone or thyroidectomy with pCND.

To date, the strongest evidence supporting the role of pCND in DTC came from an earlier study carried out by a Swedish group. Tisell et al. evaluated 175 patients who underwent thyroidectomy with CND and compared with contemporaneous controls from other two studies of Scandinavian population conducted on patients in Norway and Finland.(Tisell et al. 1996;Kukkonen et al. 1990; Salvesen et al. 1992) They showed that patients who underwent thyroidectomy with pCND had a higher survival rate (1.6% vs. 8.4-11.1%). However, these studies were criticized for including patients with gross lymph node involvement requiring therapeutic neck dissections. (Tisell et al.,1996; Kukkonen et al.,1990; Salvesen et al.,1992)

Another important outcome parameter or survival surrogate is disease recurrence or disease-free survival.

However, it is difficult to interpret their results as there were great variations in terms of indication (therapeutic or prophylactic), extent (unilateral or bilateral) and duration of follow up among different studies. The majority of studies did not show any significant differences. Moo et al. reported a decrease in recurrence rate in patients who underwent bilateral pCND (4.4% vs 16.7% p=0.13).(Moo et al.,2010) Zungia et al. analyzed a cohort of 266 patients with 6.3 years mean follow up and reported the 5-year disease-free survival was comparable (88.2% vs. 85.6%; p= 0.72).(Zuniga et al.,2009) Interestingly, a recent meta-analysis comprising 5 retrospective comparative studies (n=1264) found that there was an insignificant trend toward lower overall recurrence rate in the group who underwent either unilateral or bilateral pCND when compared to those who had total thyroidectomy only (2.02% vs 3.92%,odds ratio (OR) = 1.05, 95% confidence interval (CI) = 0.48 - 2.31).(Zetoune et al.,2010) Their subgroup analysis revealed no decrease in central (1.86% vs. 1.68%, OR 1.31, 95% CI = 0.44-3.91) or lateral compartment recurrence (3.73% vs. 3.79%, OR 1.21, 95% CI = 0.52 -2.75).(Zetoune et al.,2010) Therefore, based on these findings, there might be a potential benefit of lower recurrence in those who underwent either unilateral or bilateral pCND, although larger-scale prospective studies are required to confirm this.

Study design	First author / year of publication	Number of patients		Follow up (mean)	Overall recurrence		*p*-value
		CND+ group	CND- group		CND+ group	CND- group	
Retro-spective	Gemsenjager / 2003	P - 29	88	8.1 years	3.4%	2.3%	Not mentioned
Retro-spective	Wada / 2003	P - 235	155	53 months	0.4%	0.6%	Not significant
Retro-spective	Sywak / 2006	P-56, A	391	CND-: 70 months CND+: 24.5 months (median)	3.6%	5.6%	Not mentioned
Retro-spective	Roh / 2007	P-40, B T - 42, B	73	52 months	P - 0% T - 1.2%	4.0%	Not mentioned
Retro-spective	Zungia / 2009	P-136,B	130	6.9 years	5yr DFS - 88.2%	5yr DFS - 85.6%	0.72
Retro-spective	Costa / 2009	P-126,B	118	CND-: 64 months CND+: 47 months	6.3%	7.7%	0.83
Retro-spective	Moo / 2010	P-45, B	36	3.1 years	4.4%	16.7%	0.13
Meta-analysis	Zetoune / 2010	P - 396, A/B	868		2.0%	3.9%	NS
Retro-spective	Lang / 2011c	P - 82, A	103	26 months	3.7%	2.9%	1.0

Table 3. A literature summary of studies which evaluated recurrence rates between thyroidectomy alone or thyroidectomy with pCND.

Serum Tg level is useful in detecting persistent or recurrent DTC after thyroidectomy and RAI ablation.(Hay et al.,2002) A detectable post-surgical Tg level is associated with risk of recurrence and so it may be applied as an surrogate marker of outcome in studying prognosis of DTC.(Cooper et al.,2009;Leboulleuz et al.,2005) Sywak et al. examined 447 patients with clinically node-negative papillary thyroid carcinoma, while 56 patients underwent thyroidectomy and pCND.(Sywak et al.,2006) Though there was no significant difference in recurrence or survival after a short median follow up (thyroidectomy plus pCND vs. thyroidectomy alone: 25 vs. 70 months), they showed that there was a significantly lower level of stimulated Tg at 6 months after RAI ablation (mean: 0.41 vs. 9.3, p=0.02), and higher proportion of athyroglobulinemia (72% vs. 43%; p< 0.001).(Sywak et al.,2006) In contrast, Hughes et al. found that there was no difference in post-ablation median stimulated Tg level or rate of athyroglobulinemia between patients undergoing thyroidectomy with or without bilateral pCND.(Hughes et al.,2010) However, in their subgroup analysis of patient undergoing pCND, they demonstrated that pre-ablation Tg level was significantly higher in node positive patient these patients achieved a comparable rate of post-ablation athyroglobulinemia after a higher dose of RAI.(Hughes et al.,2010) More recently, Lang et al. retrospectively analyzed 185 patients with PTC and of these, 82 (44.3%) patients had an unilateral pCND together with a total thyroidectomy (CND+ group).(Lang et al.,2011c) They found that the CND+ group had a significantly lower median pre-ablation stimulated Tg level (<0.5ug/L vs. 6.7ug/L,p<0.001) and achieved a higher rate of pre-ablation athyroglobulinemia (51.2% vs. 22.3%,p=0.024) than those who underwent a total thyroidectomy only but these differences were not observed 6 months after ablation. They also found that pCND was the only independent factor for pre-ablation athyroglobulinemia.(Lang et al.,2011c) In their experience, most of the residual microscopic disease, presumably not removed by the initial pCND, was still able to be ablated by RAI ablation and so the group without pCND achieved similar stimulated Tg levels and similar rate of athyroglobulinemia 6 months after ablation.(Lang et al.,2011c) The authors concluded that although performing pCND in total thyroidectomy may offer a more complete initial tumor resection than total thyroidectomy alone by minimizing any residual microscopic disease, such difference becomes less noticeable 6 months after RAI ablation.(Lang et al.,2011c) The other advantage of performing pCND is the fact that the status of central lymph nodes or pN1a is better known and so more accurate staging is possible.(Lang et al.,2007b)

Increased patient morbidity is one of the major concerns. Increased risk of transient hypoparathyroidism has been consistently shown in many studies.(Sywak et al., 2006;Hughes et al. 2010;Lang et al.,2011c;Palestini et al.,2008;Roh et al.,2007;Moo et al.,2010;Rosenbaum et al.,2009) The higher rate of temporary hypoparathyroidism could be explained by the higher rate of unintentional removal of parathyroid glands (i.e. unintentional parathyroidectomy) and subsequent auto-transplantation.(Sywak et al.,2006;Hughes et al.,2010;Lang et al.,2011c) Unintentional devascularization of parathyroid glands during dissection also contributes to the higher rate of temporary hypoparathyroidism. In terms of temporary recurrent laryngeal nerve injury, Palestini et al. reported a higher rate of transient recurrent laryngeal nerve injury in patients undergoing thyroidectomy plus unilateral pCND (5.4% vs. 1.4%, p< 0.05) (Palestini et al.,2008) while other studies failed to show any statistically significant differences.(Sywak et al., 2006;Hughes et al. 2010; Lang et al.,2011; Roh et al.,2007; Sadowski et al.2009;Rosenbaum et al.,2009) To date, no studies have shown an increase risk of permanent hypoparathyroidism or recurrent laryngeal nerve injury. A recent systematic review comprising 5 retrospective studies evaluated the morbidity of pCND and found that there was one extra case of transient hypocalcaemia for every eight pCND performed. (Chisholm et al.,2009) However, there was no increased risk of permanent hypocalcaemia, transient or permanent recurrent nerve injury.(Chisholm et al.,2009)

5. Conclusion

Despite numerous reports on the various cervical and extra-cervical endoscopic approaches, the only truly minimally invasive approach in DTC appears to be MIVAT because it is associated with a shorter skin incision, minimal tissue dissection, shortened hospital stay, less wound infection and less pain. Unlike the cervical approaches, the extra-cervical approaches appear to have similar but not better outcomes than the open or conventional thyroidectomy and randomized trials comparing these approaches with open thyroidectomy are currently lacking. However, the extra-cervical approaches remain a surgical option for patients who are motivated to remain "scarless in the neck". The addition of da Vinci robot in endoscopic thyroidectomy (i.e. robotic-assisted thyroidectomy) may shorten operating time and increase the number of lymph nodes retrieved during thyroidectomy for DTC. Trans-oral thyroidectomy is technically feasible but remains experimental and appears to be associated with a higher rate of morbidity than the open approach. Surgical adjuncts such as IONM, IOPTH and alternate energy sources appear to be useful for surgeons to have as part of their armamentarium. Whether they actually improve surgical outcomes of patients over a standard open thyroidectomy remains to be determined by future prospective randomized studies. The role of pCND remains controversial as there is no good evidence to show that it improves long-term outcomes such as cancer-specific or disease-free survivals when compared to thyroidectomy without pCND. However, analysis of short-term markers for recurrence suggests that pCND may be associated with better short-term outcomes.

6. References

Abboud, B. Sargi, Z. Akkam, M. Sleilaty, F.(2002) Risk factors for postthyroidectomy hypocalcemia. *Journal of the American College of Surgeons,* Vol .195, pp.456-61

AES Guidelines 06/01 Group. Australian Endocrine Surgeons Guidelines AES06/01. (2007) Postoperative parathyroid hormone measurement and early discharge after total thyroidectomy: analysis of Australian data and management recommendations. *ANZ Journal of Surgery,* Vol.77, pp.199-202

Barczynski, M. Konturek, A. Cichon, S. (2009) Randomized clinical trial of visualization versus neuromonitoring of recurrent laryngeal nerves during thyroidectomy. *British Journal of Surgery,* Vol.96, pp.240-6

Bellantone, R. Lombardi, CP. Raffaelli, M et al. (2002) Central neck lymph node removal during minimally invasive video-assisted thyroidectomy for thyroid carcinoma: a feasible and safe procedure. *Journal of Laparoendoscopic & Advanced Surgical Techniques,* Vol.12, pp.181-5

Chan, WF. Lo, CY.(2006a) Pitfalls of intraoperative neuromonitoring for predicting postoperative recurrent laryngeal nerve function during thyroidectomy. *World Journal of Surgery,* Vol.30, pp.806-12

Chan, WF. Lang, BH. Lo, CY. (2006b) The role of intraoperative neuromonitoring of recurrent laryngeal nerve during thyroidectomy: a comparative study of 1000 nerves at risk. *Surgery,* Vol.140, pp.866-72

Chung, YS. Choe, JH. Kang, KH. Kim, SW et al. (2007) Endoscopic thyroidectomy for thyroid malignancies: comparison with conventional open thyroidectomy. *World Journal of Surgery,* Vol.31, pp.2302-6

Cirocchi, R. D'Ajello, F. Trastulli, S. Santoro, A. Di Rocco, G. Ventdettuoli, F et al. (2010) Meta-analysis of thyroidectomy with ultrasonic dissector versus conventional clamp and tie. *World Journal of Surgical Oncology,* Vol.8, pp.112

Chisholm EJ, Kulinskaya E, Tolley NS. (2009) Systematic review and meta-analysis of the adverse effects of thyroidectomy combined with central neck dissection as compared with thyroidectomy alone. *Laryngoscope,* Vol.119,No.6,(June),pp.1135-9.

Cordon, C. Fajardo, R. Ramire, J. Herrera, MF. (2005) A randomized, prospective, parallel group study comparing the harmonic scalpel to electrocautery in thyroidectomy. *Surgery,* Vol.137, pp.337-41

Costa S, Giugliano G, Santoro L, Ywata De Carvalho A, Massaro MA, Gibelli B, et al. (2009) Role of prophylactic central neck dissection in cN0 papillary thyroid cancer. *Acta Otorhinolaryngologica Italica* , Vol 29, No.2,(April),pp.61-9

Dionigi, G. Boni, L. Rovera, F et al. (2011) Wound morbidity in mini-invasive thyroidectomy. *Surgical Endoscopy,* Vol.25, pp.62-67

Dralle, H. Sekulla, C. Lorenz, K. Brauckhoff, M. et al. (2008) Intraoperative monitoring of the recurrent laryngeal nerve in thyroid surgery. *World Journal of Surgery,* Vol.32, pp.1358-66

Dralle, H. Sekulla, C. Haerting, J. et al. (2004) Risk factors of paralysis and functional outcome after recurrent laryngeal nerve monitoring in thyroid surgery. *Surgery,* Vol.136, pp.1310-22

Franko, J. Kish, KJ. Pezzi, CM. Pak, H. Kukora, JS. (2006) Safely increasing the efficiency of thyroidectomy using a new bipolar electrosealing device (LigaSure) versus conventional clamp-and-tie technique. *The American Journal of Surgery,* Vol. 72, pp.132-6

Gagner, M. (1996) Endoscopic subtotal parathyroidectomy in patients with primary hyperparathyroidism. *British Journal of Surgery* Vol.83, pp.875

Gemsenjager E, Perren A, Seifert B, Schuler G, Schweizer I, Heitz PU. (2003) Lymph node surgery in papillary thyroid carcinoma. *Journal of the American College of Surgeons,* Vol.197, No.2,pp.182-90.

Grodski, S. Serpell, J. (2008) Evidence for the role of perioperative PTH measurement after total thyroidectomy as a predictor of hypocalcemia. *World Journal of Surgery,* Vol.32, pp.1367-73

Hay, ID. Thompson, GB. Grant, CS. Bergstralh, EJ. Dvorak, CE. Gorman, CA, et al. (2002) Papillary thyroid carcinoma managed at the Mayo Clinic during six decades (1940-1999): temporal trends in initial therapy and long-term outcome in 2444 consecutively treated patients. *World Journal of Surgery,* Vol.26, No.8, pp.879-85

Henry, JF. (2008) Minimally invasive thyroid and parathyroid surgery is not a question of the length of the incision. *Langenbeck's Archives of Surgery,* Vol.393, pp.621-6

Hong Kong Cancer Registry. Cancer incidence and mortality in Hong Kong 1983-2008. Hong Kong. Available: http://www3.ha.org.hk/cancereg/e_stat.asp [Accessed on 15th May 2011]

Hughes, DT. White, ML. Miller, BS. Gauger, PG. Burney, RE. Doherty, GM. (2010) Influence of prophylactic central lymph node dissection on postoperative thyroglobulin levels and radioiodine treatment in papillary thyroid cancer. *Surgery*, Vol.148, No.6, (December), pp.1100-6; discussion 1106-7

Ikeda, Y, Takami, H. Sasaki, Y. Takayama, J. et al. (2003) Clinical benefits in endoscopic thyroidectomy by the axillary approach. *Journal of the American College of Surgeons*, Vol.196, pp.189-195

Kang, SW. Jeong, JJ. Yun, JS. Sung, TY. et al. (2009a) Gasless endoscopic thyroidectomy using trans-axillary approach; surgical outcome of 581 patients.*Endocrine Journal*, Vol.56, pp.361-9

Kang, SW. Jeong, JJ. Yun, JS. et al. (2009b) Robot-assisted endoscopic surgery for thyroid cancer: experience with the first 100 patients. *Surgical Endoscopy*, Vol.23, pp.2399-406

Kang, SW. Jeong, JJ. Nam, KH. Chang, HS. et al. (2009c) Robot-assisted endoscopic thyroidectromy for thyroid malignancies using a gasless transaxillary approach. *Journal of the American College of Surgeons*, Vol.209, pp.e1-7

Kang, SW. Lee, SC. Lee, SH. Lee, KY. Jeong, JJ. et al. (2009d) Robotic thyroid surgery using a gasless, transaxillary approach and the da Vinci S system: the operative outcomes of 338 consecutive patients. *Surgery*, Vol.146, pp.1048-55

Kirdak, T. Korun, N. Ozguc, H. (2005) Use of ligasure in thyroidectomy procedures : results of a prospective comparative study. *World Journal of Surgery*, Vol.29, pp.771-4

Kiriakopoulos, A. Dimitrios, T. Dimitrios, L. (2004) Use of a diathermy system in thyroid surgery. *Archives of Surgery*, Vol. 139, pp.997-1000

Kukkonen, ST. Haapiainen, RK. Franssila, KO. Sivula, AH. (1990) Papillary thyroid carcinoma: the new, age-related TNM classification system in a retrospective analysis of 199 patients. *World Journal of Surgery*, Vol.14, No.6, (November-December), pp.837-41; discussion 41-2

Lang, BH. Lo, CY. Chan, WF. et al. (2007a) Prognostic factors in papillary and follicular thyroid carcinoma: their implications for cancer staging. *Annals of Surgical Oncology*, Vol.14, pp.730-8

Lang B, Lo CY, Chan WF, Lam KY, Wan KY. (2007b) Restaging of differentiated thyroid carcinoma by the sixth edition AJCC/UICC TNM staging system: stage migration and predictability. *Annals of Surgical Oncology*,vol.14,No.5,pp.1551-9

Lang, BH.(2010a) Minimally invasive thyroid and parathyroid operations: surgical techniques and pearls. *Advanced Surgery*, Vol.44, pp.185-98

Lang, BH. Lo, CY. (2010b) Technological innovations in surgical approach for thyroid cancer. *Journal of Oncology*, Vol.2010, pii:490719

Lang, BH. Chow, MP. Wong, KP. (2011a) Endoscopic vs robotic thyroidectomy: which is better? *Annals of Surgical Oncology*, [Epub] DOI:10.1245/s10434-011-1827-8

Lang, BH. Chow, MP.(2011b) A comparison of surgical outcomes between endoscopic and robotic assisted thyroidectomy: the authors' initial experience. *Surgical Endoscopy*, Vol.25, pp.1617-23

Lang, BH. Wong, KP. Wan, KY. Lo, CY.(2011c) Impact of routine unilateral central neck dissection on pre-ablative and post-ablative stimulated thyroglobulin levels after total thyroidectomy in papillary thyroid carcinoma. *Annals of Surgical Oncology*, [Epub] DOI: 10.1245/s10434-011-1833-x

Lee, J. Lee, JH. Nah, KY. Soh, EY. Chung, WY. (2011) Comparison of endoscopic and robotic thyroidectomy. *Annals of Surgical Oncology*, Vol.18, pp.1439-46

Lee, KE. Kim, HY. Park, WS. Choe, JH. Kwon, MR. et al. (2009a) Postauricular and axillary approach endoscopic neck surgery: a new technique. *World Journal of Surgery,* Vol.33,pp.767-72

Lee, KE. Rao, J. Youn, YK. (2009b) Endoscopic thyroidectomy with the da Vinci robot system using the bilateral axillary breast approach (BABA) technique: our initial experience. *Surgical Laparoscopy Endoscopy & Percutaneous Techniques,* Vol.19,pp.71-5

Lee, S. Ruy, HR. Park, JH. Kim, KH. Kang, SW. Jeong, JJ. Nam, KH. Chung, WY. Park. CS.(2011) Excellence in robotic thyroid surgery: a comparative study of robot-assisted versus conventional endoscopic thyroidectomy in papillary thyroid microcarcinoma patients. *Annals of Surgery,* Vol.253,pp.1060-6

Lepner, U. Vaasna, T.(2007) Ligasure vessel sealing system versus conventional vessel ligation in thyroidectomy. *Scandinavian Journal of Surgery,*Vol.96, pp.31-4

Lo, CY. Luk, JM. Tam, SC.(2002) Applicability of intraoperative parathyroid hormone assay during thyroidectomy. *Annals of Surgery,* Vol.236, pp.564-9

Lo, CY. (2003) Postthyroidectomy hypocalcemia. *Journal of the American College of Surgeons,* Vol.196, pp.497-8

Lombardi, CP. Raffaelli, M. Princi, P. et al.(2004) Early prediction of postthyroidectomy hypocalcemia by one single iPTH measurement. *Surgery,* Vol.136, pp.1236-41

Lombardi, CP. Raffaelli, M. Princi, P. De Crea, C. Bellantone, R. (2007a) Minimally invasive video-assisted functional lateral neck dissection for metastatic papillary thyroid carcinoma. *American Journal of Surgery,* Vol.193,pp.114-118

Lombardi, CP. Raffaelli, M. de Crea, C. Princi, P. et al.(2007b) Report on 8 years of experience with video-assisted thyroidectomy for papillary thyroid carcinoma. *Surgery,* Vol.142, pp.944-951

Lombardi, CP. Raffaelli, M. Princi, P. et al.(2006) Parathyroid hormone levels 4 hours after surgery do not accurately predict post-thyroidectomy hypocalcemia. *Surgery,* Vol.140, pp.1016-1023

Mazzaferri, EL. Kloos, RT. (2001) Clinical review 128: Current approaches to primary therapy for papillary and follicular thyroid cancer. *Journal of Clinical Endocrinology & Metabolism,* Vol.86, No.4, (April), pp.1447-63

McHenry, CR. Speroff, T. Wentworth, D. et al. (1994) Risk factors for postoperative hypocalcemia. *Surgery,* Vol.116, pp.641-8

Miccoli, P. Berti, P. Bendinelli, C. Conte, M. et al. (2000) Minimally invasive video-assisted surgery of the thyroid: a preliminary report. *Langenbeck's Archives of Surgery* Vol.385, pp.261-4

Miccoli, P. Elisei, R. Materazzi, G. Capezzone, M. et al. (2002) Minimally invasive video-assisted thyroidectomy for papillary thyroid carcinoma: a prospective study of its completeness. *Surgery,* Vol.132, pp.1070-73

Miccoli, P. Pinchera, A. Materazzi, G. et al. (2009) Surgical Treatment of low- and intermediate-risk papillary thyroid cancer with minimally invasive video-assisted thyroidectomy. *Journal of Clinical Endocrinology & Metabolism,* Vol.94, pp. 1618-22

Moo, TA. McGill, J. Allendorf, J. Lee, J. Fahey, T. 3rd, Zarnegar R. (2010) Impact of prophylactic central neck lymph node dissection on early recurrence in papillary thyroid carcinoma. *World Journal of Surgery,* Vol.34, No.6, pp.1187-91

Noordzij, JP. Lee, SL. Bernet, VJ. et al. (2007) Early prediction of hypocalcemia after thyroidectomy using parathyroid hormone: an analysis of pooled individual;

patient data from nine observational studies. *Journal of the American College of Surgeons*, Vol.205, pp.748-54

Oretga, J. Sala, C. Flor, B. Lledo, S. (2004) Efficacy and cost-effectiveness of the UltraCision Harmonic scalpel in thyroid surgery: an analysis of 200 cases in a randomized trial. *Journal of Laparoendoscopic & advanced surgical techniques*,Vol.14,No.1,pp.9-12

Palazzo, FF. Sebag, F. Henry, JF.(2006) Endocrine surgical technique: endoscopic thyroidectomy via the lateral approach. *Surgical Endoscopy*, Vol.20, pp.339-42

Palestini, N. Borasi, A. Cestino, L. Freddi M, Odasso C, Robecchi A.(2008) Is central neck dissection a safe procedure in the treatment of papillary thyroid cancer? Our experience. *Langenbeck's Archives of Surgery*. Vol.393, No.5, (September), pp.693-8.

Pattou, F. Combemale, Fabre S. et al. (1998) Hypocalcemia following thyroid surgery: incidence and prediction of outcome. *World Journal of Surgery*, Vol.22, pp.718-24

Pereira, JA. Jimeno, J. Miguel, J. Iglesias, M. et al. (2005) Nodal yield, morbidity, recurrence after central neck dissection for papillary thyroid carcinoma. *Surgery*, Vol.138, pp.1095-1100

Petrakis, IE. Kogerakis, NE. Lasithiotakis. et al. (2004) Ligasure versus clamp-and-tie thyroidectomy for benign nodular disease. *Head & Neck*, Vol.26, pp.903-9

Pons, Y. Gauthier, J. Ukkola-Pons, E. et al. (2009) Comparison of ligasure vessel sealing system, harmonic scalpel, and conventional hemostasis in total thyroidectomy. *Otolaryngology - Head & Neck Surgery*, Vol.141, pp.496-501

Pfleiderer, AG. Ahmad, N. Draper, MR. et al.(2009) The timing of calcium measurements in helping to predict temporary and permanent hypocalcemia in patients having completion and total thyroidectomies. *Annals of the Royal College of Surgeons of England*, Vol.91, pp.140-6

Rahbari R, Mathur A, Kitano M et al. (2011) Prospective randomized trial of Ligasure versus Harmonic hemostasis technique in thyroidectomy. *Annals of Surgical Oncology*,vol.18,pp.1023-27

Ready, AR. Barnes, AD.(1994) Complications of thyroidectomy. *British Journal of Surgery*, Vol.81, pp.1555-6

Roh, JL. Park, JY. Park, CI.(2007) Total thyroidectomy plus neck dissection in differentiated papillary thyroid carcinoma patients: pattern of nodal metastasis, morbidity, recurrence and postoperative levels of serum parathyroid hormone. *Annals of Surgery*, Vol.245, pp.604-10

Roh, JL. Park, JY. Park, CI.(2009) Prevention of postoperative hypocalcemia with routine oral calcium and vitamin D supplements in patients with differentiated papillary thyroid carcinoma undergoing total thyroidectomy plus central neck dissection. *Cancer*, Vol.115, pp.251-8

Rosenbaum MA, McHenry CR.(2009) Central neck dissection for papillary thyroid cancer. *Archives of Otolaryngology Head & Neck Surgery*, Vol.135,No.11,(November),pp.1092-7.

Salvesen, H. Njolstad, PR. Akslen, LA. Albrektsen, G. Soreide, O. Varhaug, JE. (1992) Papillary thyroid carcinoma: a multivariate analysis of prognostic factors including an evaluation of the p-TNM staging system. *European Journal of Surgery*, Vol.158, No.11-12, pp.583-9

Sartori, PV. Fina, SD. Colombo, G et. al.(2008) Ligasure versus Ultracision in thyroid surgery : a prospective randomized study. *Langenbeck's Archives of Surgery*, Vol.393, pp.655-58

Siperstein, AE. Berber, E. Morkoyun, E. (2002) The use of the harmonic scalpel vs conventional knot tying for vessel ligation in thyroid surgery. *Archives of Surgery*, Vol.137, pp.137-42

Smith, E. Taylor, M. Mendoza, M. (1998) Spasmodic dysphonia and vocal fold paralysis: outcomes of voice problems on wok related functioning. *Journal of Voice*, Vol.12, pp.223-32

Sywak M, Cornford L, Roach P, Stalberg P, Sidhu S, Delbridge L. (2006) Routine ipsilateral level VI lymphadenectomy reduces postoperative thyroglobulin levels in papillary thyroid cancer. *Surgery*, Vol.140,No.6,pp.1000-1005;discussion 1005-7

Tisell, LE. Nilsson, B. Molne, J. Hansson, G. Fjalling, M. Jansson, S. et al. (1996) Improved survival of patients with papillary thyroid cancer after surgical microdissection. *World Journal of Surgery*, Vol.20, No.7, pp.854-9

Voutilainen, PE. Haglund, CH. (2000) Ultrasonically activated shears in thyroidectomies: a randomized trial. *Annals of Surgery*, Vol.231, pp.322-8

Wada N, Duh QY, Sugino K, Iwasaki H, Kameyama K, Mimura T, et al. (2003) Lymph node metastasis from 259 papillary thyroid microcarcinomas: frequency, pattern of occurrence and recurrence, and optimal strategy for neck dissection. *Annals of Surgery*. Vol.237,No.3,pp.399-407

Wilhelm, T. Metzig, A. (2011) Endoscopic minimally invasive thyroidectomy (eMIT): A prospective proof-of-concept study in humans. *World Journal of Surgery*, Vol.35, pp.543-551

Witzel, K. von Rahden, BHA. Kaminski, C. et al. (2008) Transoral access for endoscopic thyroid resection. *Surgical Endoscopy*, Vol.22, pp.1871-7

Zarebczan B, Mohanty D, Chen H.(2011) A comparison of the Ligasure and harmonic scalpel in thyroid surgery: a single institution review. *Annals of Surgical Oncology*,Vol.18, pp.214-18

Zetoune T, Keutgen X, Buitrago D, Aldailami H, Shao H, Mazumdar M, et al. (2010) Prophylactic central neck dissection and local recurrence in papillary thyroid cancer: a meta-analysis. *Annals of Surgical Oncology*, Vol.17, No.12,pp.3287-93

Zuniga S, Sanabria A. (2009) Prophylactic central neck dissection in stage N0 papillary thyroid carcinoma. *Archives of Otolaryngology Head & Neck Surgery*, Vol 135, No.11,pp.1087-91

10

Sentinel Lymph Node Biopsy in Well Differentiated Thyroid Cancer

Tamara Mijovic, Keith Richardson, Richard J. Payne and Jacques How
McGill University, Montréal, Canada

1. Introduction

The management of occult cervical lymph node metastasis in well-differentiated thyroid cancer (WDTC) is controversial. Given the risks of hypocalcemia, recurrent laryngeal nerve injury, and increased operative time with a central compartment neck dissection (CCND), a routine adoption of prophylactic lymph node dissection has not been accepted by many as a standard management for occult metastasis (Henry et al., 1998; Pereira et al., 2005; Shen et al., 2010). Conversely, other thyroid surgeons feel that the complication rate is low and that the benefits of CCND outweigh the risks (Anand et al., 2009; Haigh et al., 2000; Keleman et al., 1998; Pelizzo et al., 2001; Pitman et al., 2003; Rettenbacher et al., 2000). As a result, sentinel lymph node biopsy (SLNB) has gained an increase in popularity in recent years.

The principle of SLNB and its historical rise in other fields will be the starting point of the chapter. The SLN is defined as the first lymph node in a regional lymphatic basin receiving lymph flow from a primary tumor. For the past nineteen years, SLNB has been an acceptable technique for identifying the presence of metastatic disease for cutaneous melanoma (Morton et al., 1992) and early breast cancer (Giuliano et al., 1994; Krag et al., 1993). Lymphatic mapping with SLN permits staging of malignant tumors in an effort to avoid complete nodal dissection and its associated morbidity. The ideology behind SLN surgery follows the concept that the sentinel node is predictive of a primary tumor that has the potential to metastasize. If the sentinel node is positive, the pathological status of additional lymph nodes may be positive as well. Recently, SLNB techniques have been proposed for other tumor types, including lung, gastrointestinal and gynecologic malignancies (Makar et al., 2001), squamous cell carcinoma of the head and neck (Pitman et al., 2003; Taylor et al., 2001), colorectal cancer (Saha et al., 2000) and thyroid cancer (Pelizzo et al., 2001; Dixon et al., 2000).

To understand the applicability of SLNB in thyroid cancer, the cervical lymphatic anatomy will be reviewed. The mechanism of lymphatic tumoral spread in thyroid cancer and the clinical significance of such lymph node metastases will then be discussed. The arguments in favor and against prophylactic CCND will follow thereby providing the context in which the idea of the SLNB shows its advantages in the management of WDTC. The benefits of SLNB over a formal CCND will be discussed in the chapter with emphasis on the major advantages such as a decreased risk of hypocalcemia, decreased risk to the recurrent laryngeal nerve (RLN) injury and decreased operative time. Different techniques of SLN biopsy will then be outlined and our detailed institutional protocol, the McGill Thyroid Injection Protocol, will be illustrated. A comprehensive review of the literature on the outcomes of SLNB in the approach to management of thyroid cancer will then follow. Our chapter will conclude by addressing the pitfalls of SLNB in WDTC including the potential causes of false-negative cases in addition to adverse events related to the procedure.

2. Sentinel lymph node biopsy, a tool for the surgeon

In the field of oncology, lymph node status is one of the most important prognostic factors and a key element of tumor staging. It is also a guide towards the appropriate therapy and overall a crucial component in the assessment of patients with cancer. The approach to management of metastatic lymph nodes goes from medical management to various degrees of surgical aggressiveness.

2.1 The principle

In 1960, Gould (Gould et al.,1960) was the first to introduce the concept of the sentinel lymph node. According to him, lymphatic flow is unidirectional, and there is orderly progression of cancer cells from the primary organ to the first lymph node in the chain before spreading to other regional lymph nodes. This first lymph node draining a regional lymphatic basin from a primary tumor is defined as the sentinel lymph node, and its histological status is thought to be representative of the status of the other nodes in the chain. The SLNB technique finds its place where formal lymph node dissection is associated with significant morbidity, such as the groin or axilla.

2.2 The history

In 1992, the technique for lymphatic mapping was first described by Morton (Morton et al., 1992) in patients with cutaneous malignancy, and was found to be not only simple and practical, but also reliable with a reported false-negative rate of less than 1%. This report introduced modern surgical oncologists to a new surgical technique with a wide range of applications. Subsequently, Giuliano (Giuliano et al., 1994) exported the technique to breast cancer and demonstrated a reliable identification of SLN using a vital blue dye. In the last two decades, SLNB has been validated as an accurate method for assessing lymph node status and has gained consensus as the standard of management for identifying regional lymphatic spread in melanoma and breast cancer. The use of this technique in the management algorithms is under investigations for other solid cancer including thyroid.

3. Cervical lymph nodes in thyroid cancer

3.1 The anatomy

There are 500 lymph nodes in the body and 200 of these are in the head and neck region (Grodski et al., 2007). Historically, the location of cervical lymphadenopathies has been described in terms of chains and triangles, but currently, the most used system of nodal mapping anatomically classifies lymph nodes into levels (Sakorafas et al., 2010).

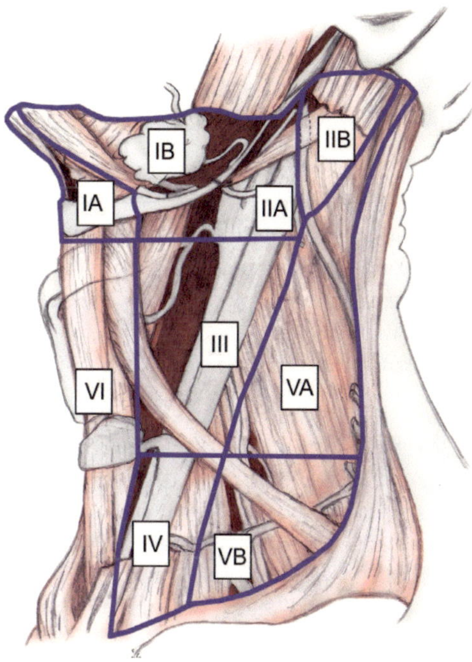

Fig. 1. Cervical lymph node levels (from Rugiero, 2008)

Level I is bound by the body of the mandible superiorly, stylohyoid muscle posteriorly, and the anterior belly of the digastric muscle on the contralateral side anteriorly. This level may be divided into level Ia, which refers to the nodes in the submental triangle (bound by the anterior bellies of the digastric muscles and the hyoid bone), and Ib, which refers to the submandibular triangle nodes.

Level II lymph nodes are related to the upper third of the jugular vein, extending from the skull base to the inferior border of the hyoid bone. The anterior border of level II is the stylohyoid muscle, and the posterior border is the posterior border of the sternocleidomastoid muscle. The spinal accessory nerve, which travels obliquely across this area, is used as a landmark to subdivide this group into IIb, the portion above and behind the nerve, and IIa, the part that lies anteroinferiorly and closer to the internal jugular vein.

Level III nodes are located between the hyoid superiorly and a horizontal plane defined by the inferior border of the cricoid cartilage. The sternohyoid muscle marks the anterior limit of level III, and the posterior border of the sternocleidomastoid muscle is the posterior border.

Level IV refers to the group of nodes related to the lower third of the jugular vein. These nodes are located between the inferior border of the cricoid cartilage and the clavicle, and, like level III, the anterior boundary is the sternohyoid muscle, and the posterior border is the posterior border of the sternocleidomastoid muscle.

Level V refers to the lymph nodes located in the posterior triangle of the neck. These include the spinal accessory, transverse cervical, and supraclavicular group of nodes. Level V is bound anteriorly by the posterior border of the sternocleidomastoid muscle and posteriorly by the anterior border of the trapezius muscle. Level V extends from the apex of the convergence of the sternocleidomastoid and trapezius muscle superiorly to the clavicle inferiorly as shown below. This level is subdivided by a plane defined by the inferior border of the cricoid cartilage into level Va superiorly and level Vb inferiorly.

Level VI refers to lymph nodes of the anterior, or central, compartment of the neck. Defined by the carotid arteries laterally, the hyoid bone superiorly, and the suprasternal notch inferiorly, it is rich in lymphatics that drain the thyroid gland, subglottic larynx, cervical trachea, hypopharynx, and cervical esophagus. Lymph nodes in this compartment are located in the tracheoesophageal groove (paratracheal nodes), in front of the trachea (pretracheal nodes), around the thyroid gland (parathyroidal nodes), and on the cricothyroid membrane (precricoid or Delphian node) (Rugiero, 2008).

The thyroid gland contains a dense network of intrathyroidal lymphatics with communication across the isthmus. Lymphatic flow tends to be to the ipsilateral level VI lymph nodes primarily since thyroid lymphatics usually accompany a venous drainage pattern into the central compartment of the neck (Roh & Kock, 2010). The upper poles, along with the pyramidal lobe and isthmus also drain superiorly toward lymph node levels II/III while the lateral aspect of each lobe drain towards lymph node levels III/IV. The lower pole of the gland drains initially into level VI then goes on to levels IV and VII (Roh & Koch, 2010; Sakorafas et al., 2010).

3.2 Lymph nodes metastases in well-differentiated thyroid cancer

Papillary thyroid cancer (PTC) is the most common thyroid malignancy. It represents 75% of thyroid malignancies and 90% of WDTC. It spreads predominantly via the lymphatics to the local draining lymph nodes (Balasubramanian & Harrison, 2011). It is generally believed that the central cervical compartment is the primary zone of lymphatic involvement for all thyroid cancers except those located in the upper pole of the glands from which lymphatic drainage may flow directly into the lateral neck nodes (Henry et al., 1998). In keeping with the theory, Nogychi in a study of 68 patients after elective neck dissection, found 78% of nodal metastases in the paratracheal region and 22% in the jugular chain (Nogychi et al., 1987, as cited in Kelemen et al., 1998). Many groups have, however, reported that the risk of lymphatic metastases was greatest for the lateral nodal groups (level II, III and IV) (Caron et al., 2006; Gimm et al., 1998; Lee et al., 2008; Roh et al., 2007, 2008; Shah et al., 1990) while others have shown comparable rates of involvements in both the central cervical and lateral neck compartments (Machens et al., 2002).

Irrespective of location, lymph node metastases are a common finding in PTC and tend to occur relatively early. The incidence of lymph node metastases has been reported to be as high as 90% and the incidence of palpable disease ranges between 30-50% (Dixon et al., 2000; Grodski et al., 2007). Histological evidence of nodal metastases in patients with clinically node negative PTC is approximately 50% (Balasubramanian & Harrison, 2011), but rates anywhere between 25 to 90% have been reported in studies where elective neck dissections were performed on patients without suspicious lymphadenopathies (Cunningham et al., 2010). Interestingly, in a similar group of patients who were observed and did not undergo a neck dissection, the rate of recurrence was only 1.4%, thus questioning the clinical significance of such lymph node metastases (Kelemen et al., 1998).

3.3 Clinical significance of lymph nodes metastases

Most clinical trials confirm that regional nodes are usually the first site of recurrence (Kelemen et al., 1998). In fact, metastases to lymph nodes account for 75% of locoregional recurrence (Grodski et al., 2007). It is estimated that the risk for nodal recurrence is 30% to 50% during 10 years. The overall recurrence rate has been documented at 20%, with most of them discovered within 24 months. Of these, 70% are detected through a radioactive iodine whole body scan with only 40% being clinically apparent (Kelemen et al., 1998).

In a series of patients with nodal metastases and a final histological diagnosis of papillary, follicular, or Hürthle cell carcinoma, a recurrence rate of 19% has been recorded vs 2% in patients free of nodal disease (Kelemen et al., 1998). In an age-matched study of patients with differentiated thyroid cancer, recurrences were also more common among patients with nodal involvement (32 vs. 14%) (Grodski et al., 2007). The presence of central node metastases in the lymphadenectomy specimen is therefore an independent predictor of disease free survival but its actual significance on the overall prognosis remains controversial.

Although PTC lymph node metastases are reported by some to have no clinically important effect on outcome in low risk patients, a study among 9904 patients with PTC has found that lymph node metastases, along with other factors, predicted poor outcome on multivariate analysis (Podnos et al., 2005). All-cause survival at 14 years was 82% for PTC without lymph node and 79% with lymph node metastases ($p < 0.05$). Another recent study showed that lymph node involvement is an independent risk factor for decreased survival, but only in patients with follicular carcinoma and patients with papillary carcinoma over age 45 years (Zaydfudim et al., 2008). Multiple metastases and extracapsular nodal extension are other factors increasing the risk of regional recurrence (Leboulleux et al., 2005). However, in an analysis of 5123 patients over a 30-year period, even when corrected for TNM staging, a significantly higher mortality rate for patients with lymph node involvement has been shown (Grodski et al., 2007).

Despite these data, PTC has an excellent prognosis, but there is no doubt that lymphatic spread is associated with increased risk of loco-regional recurrence which may require an additional and more complicated surgery, overall significantly affecting patients' quality of life not only through the major psychological impact of cancer recurrence, but also through increased rates of all complications of exploration of scarred necks (Kelemen et al., 1998). We are therefore assisting to a paradigm shift in the aims of treatment of PTC, from a focus on survival to a focus of disease-free status as a valid endpoint to evaluate the effectiveness of therapy.

3.4 Cervical neck dissection in well-differentiated thyroid cancer

While few would argue against a formal therapeutic neck dissection in cases of macroscopic clinically apparent lymph node metastases in patients with WDTC, there is great heterogeneity in the surgical approaches to a clinically negative neck. Recommendations in the management of adenopathy associated with PTC are quite varied and include blind nodal sampling, central compartment neck dissection, and modified radical neck dissection (Anand et al., 2009). To eliminate the probability of leaving behind residual disease, routine total thyroidectomy with cervical lymph node dissection (CLND) would be theoretically the ideal operation. However, such an aggressive surgical approach will represent over-treatment in a large percentage of patients, associated with longer surgical time and an unjustified increase of surgical morbidity (Sakorafas et al., 2010). Balancing the risk of increased morbidity from CLND with the benefit of removing a source of potential recurrence creates a controversial and difficult management decision. To help in the decision making process, guidelines for prophylactic CLND have been issued by different associations. Unfortunately, they remain vague and unclear with a certain degree of antagonistic recommendations.

3.4.1 In favor of prophylactic cervical lymph node dissection

Because of the high rate of occult lymph node metastases, their association with more frequent tumor recurrence and our inability to adequately indentify these cases pre-operatively, some experts argue in favor of routine prophylactic CLND in cases of WDTC. The British Thyroid Association (BTA) and the American Thyroid Association (ATA) are proponents of the prophylactic CLND (BTA, 2007; Cooper et al., 2009), especially in patients considered high risk. They maintain that the potential increased morbidity is small in experienced hands and hence a strong argument can be made for routine central CLND in all patients with WDTC and no known preoperative or intraoperative evidence of node involvement. More specifically, the ATA recommends prophylactic central neck dissection for patients with clinically uninvolved lymph nodes, especially for advanced tumors (T3 and T4 disease), and asserts that the central CLND may be appropriately omitted for T1 and T2 papillary and follicular thyroid cancers. They also acknowledge that omitting CLND for these smaller tumors, "may increase the chance of locoregional recurrence, but overall may be safer in less experienced surgical hands," to avoid the associated morbidity. This approach to microscopic nodal disease may result in fewer postoperative complications than routine dissection, but may fail to detect lymph node metastases in patients with smaller tumors, and may subject patients with larger tumors who do not have lymph node metastases to unnecessary lymph node resection. In addition, the guidelines allow for interpretation of these recommendations in the light of available surgical expertise at each institution, so that more invasive approaches are only recommended if experienced surgeons are available to carry them out, which is yet another factor contributing to the great variability in management.

Besides lower recurrence rates, prophylactic CLND has also the advantage of adequate staging, enhancing the effects of radioactive iodine by removing potentially positive lymph nodes while also lowering the postoperative thyroglobulin levels thereby facilitating follow-up (Grodski et al., 2007; Sakorafas et al., 2010).

In the discussion about the extent of prophylactic CLND in PTC, it should be remembered that the impact of the central compartment recurrence differs from that of a lateral compartment. It is generally accepted that lymph node metastases in the visceral compartment of the neck have greater clinical importance than metastases in the lateral neck areas (Henry et al., 1998). Reoperation for recurrence in the lateral compartment can be performed more easily than that for recurrence in the central compartment, where more critical structures (i.e., trachea, great vessels, etc) are located. Therefore, since metastases in the central compartment are very common, recurrences in the area are sometimes difficult to demonstrate, especially in males with a short and thick neck (Henry et al., 1998) and given that surgery for recurrence in the central compartment may be a complicated procedure, prophylactic central CLND during the initial thyroid surgery (usually through the same incision) seems for many to be a reasonable management option (Sakorafas et al., 2010).

3.4.2 Against prophylactic cervical lymph node dissection

The American Association of Clinical Endocrinology, the American Association of Endocrine Surgeons (Cobin et al., 2001) and the NCCN do not recommend routine central CLND, particularly in low-risk patients with PTC. The argument against prophylactic CLND resides in the added complications associated with the procedure. The possible complications of central compartment neck dissection include hypoparathyroidism, injury to the recurrent and superior laryngeal nerves, hemorrhage and seroma (Sakorafas et al., 2010). The morbidity of prophylactic central neck dissection was evaluated in a study of 100 patients who underwent total thyroidectomy of which 50 patients with papillary thyroid cancer and no evidence of macroscopic metastases also had a prophylactic central neck dissection (Henry et al., 1998). In the group that had no neck dissection, there was no permanent hypoparathyroidism, but there were four cases of transient hypoparathyroidism (8%). In the group that underwent the prophylactic procedure, seven patients presented transient hypoparathyroidism (14%) and two patients (4%) remained with permanent hypoparathyroidism. The authors were also able to conclude that after total thyroidectomy for PTC, prophylactic central neck dissection does not increase recurrent laryngeal nerve morbidity but is responsible for a higher rate of hypoparathyroidism, especially in the early postoperative course (Henry et al., 1998). They attributed the hypoparathyroidism associated with neck dissection to the insufficiency of blood supply generated by the dissection. Similar rates of permanent hypoparathyroidism were also reported by Pereira (Pereira et al., 2005) (4.6%) with the extent of hypocalcemia correlating with the extent of surgery. A recent study by Mitra convincingly showed that total thyroidectomy combined with CCND led to a marked increase in both transient as well as permanent hypocalcemia (Mitra et al., 2011). These authors therefore concluded that the morbidity of bilateral cervical neck dissections is significant, and cautioned against the systematic implementation of this technique in the absence of gross nodal involvement.

Another factor contributing to the opposition towards routine lymph node dissection is the questionable usefulness of the procedure in preventing recurrence. Recent data has not demonstrated any therapeutic gain in achieving a significant reduction in local recurrence by adding CCND to total thyroidectomy (Zetoune et al., 2010). Despite the high frequency of microscopic lymph node metastases, the recurrence rate in patients with occult nodal disease who have not undergone nodal excision procedures has been reported as only 1.4% to 15% (McHenry et al., 1991; Shen et al., 2010; Takami et al., 2002) and the 5-year mortality rate ranges from 0.9% to 17% (Takami et al., 2002). To some, it therefore appears that there might be no real benefit for the patient to undergo more extensive surgery in presence of a clinically negative neck.

4. Sentinel lymph nodes biopsy in thyroid cancer

4.1 The middle ground in the controversy

The lack of consensus on the matter of prophylactic CLND validates the need for a modality with which the surgeon can rely on to accurately predict the necessity for the procedure.

Accordingly, being able to identify those patients who would benefit from nodal dissection before a more extensive procedure is undertaken would improve PTC management (Anand et al., 2009).

Preoperative ultrasound is unable to detect all metastatic lymph nodes in the central compartment of the neck (Roh & Koch, 2010) while intraoperative palpation and lymph node size assessment are not accurate predictors of lymph node status (Fukui et al., 2001). In this perspective, the SLNB is theoretically appealing for PTC since it could detect subclinical lymph node metastases, thereby allowing the formal CLND to be performed only in patients with documented lymph node metastases, thus avoiding the morbidity of CLND in a significant percentage of patients with node-negative disease. In other words, SLNB may be helpful in selecting patients who would benefit from CLND, thus reducing unnecessary surgery and possible morbidity in other patients (Roh & Koch, 2010; Sakorafas et al., 2010).

The main advantage of an accurate SLNB technique would be the identification of node-negative patients with thyroid cancer in whom an unnecessary prophylactic central node dissection could be avoided (Roh & Koch, 2010). It allows the surgeon to alter the surgical procedure in real time. Completing a central neck dissection at the time of initial surgery can also potentially avoid the higher complication rates that have been reported with reoperation in the central compartment. Another advantage of SLNB biopsy is that it may help identify, at the time of initial operation, patients who are likely to develop a challenging central compartment recurrence. The SLNB technique may also permit early detection of patients who may benefit from adjuvant radioactive iodine ablation (Anand et al., 2009; Roh & Koch, 2010). Alternatively, biopsies of sentinel lymph nodes may avoid the use of ablative ^{131}I treatment in patients with low-risk thyroid cancers with SLNs that are negative for metastases. Furthermore, malignant Hürthle cell tumors and well-differentiated follicular carcinomas are difficult to identify histologically, and SLNB in such cases may aid in establishing the diagnoses if metastases can be identified in SLNs (Takami et al., 2002).

In summary, the SLNB is an alternative approach that may guide the decision to proceed with formal lymphadenectomy. For this tool to be truly useful, it needs to accurately identify lymph node metastases, have a low false-negative rate and be associated with less morbidity than the formal CCND. SLNB for PTC has therefore been studied in several settings using different techniques; the sections that follow will review that data.

4.2 The technique

Since the introduction of the SLNB in PTC by Keleman (Keleman et al., 1998) several variations of the technique have been described. The variability resides mainly in the type of dye or isotope injected, the volume that was injected, the timing of injection, the site of injection and the subsequent assessment of the sentinel lymph node. Table 1 modified from the largest meta-analysis of SLNB in PTC, summarizes the techniques used in all the studies performed up to now on the topic (Balasubramanian & Harrison, 2011).

Vital blue dyes are the most frequently injected medium with methylene blue, isosulphan blue and patent blue V being the most common types. In general, methylene blue is found to be the least expensive and to generate less hypersensitivity reactions than the others. All of them, however, have been shown to have minimal reactivity except isosulfan blue.

Indeed, since rosaniline dyes are used in many commercially available products, including cosmetics, paper, and textiles, patients may be sensitized to isosulfan blue by previous exposure to apparently unrelated compounds. Moderate and severe allergic reactions, including anaphylaxis, have been reported in up to 2% of patients receiving isosulfan blue (Kelley and Holmes, 2011). All blue dye disappears during histologic processing and does not affect histologic analysis (Roh and Koh, 2010).

In terms of radioisotopes, different forms of 99m-Technetium labeled colloids have been used. The sentinel lymph node in these cases is localized either by a marking on the skin overlying the lymph node; alternatively, it can be localized by radiotracer using a gamma-probe intraoperatively.

Reference	*n*	*Population*	*Dye/Isotope*	*Volume injected (mL)*	*Timing of injection*	*Injection site*	*Assessment of SLN*
Cunningham et al. 2010	211	PTC	1%isosulphan blue	0.5-2	After mobilization	IT	FS and H
Anand et al. 2009	97	Suspicious and PTC	1% methylene blue	0.2-0.3	Before mobilization	PT	H
Takeyama et al. 2009	37	Suspicious and diagnostic	1% sulphan blue	0.1	Before mobilization	PT	FS and H
Lee et al. 2009	54	DTC	2% methylene blue	0.1-0.5	Before mobilization	PT	FS and H
Bae et al. 2009	11	PTC	2% methylene blue	0.5	After strap muscle retraction	IT	FS and H
Roh and Park, 2008	50	PTC	2% methylene blue	0.2	After strap muscle retraction	PT	FS and H
Wang et al. 2008	25	PTC	2% methylene blue	1-2	NA	PT	H
Rubello et al. 2006	153	PTC	0.5% patent blue V	0.25ml/cm	After strap muscle retraction	IT	FS and H
Abdella 2006	30	Benign nodules	1% isosulphan blue	0.5-1	After strap muscle retraction	IT	H
Peparini et al. 2006	9	PTC	2.5% patent blue V	0.1-0.2	NA	PT or IT	NA
Falvo et al. 2006	18	PTC	Methylene blue	0.4	After mobilization	IT	H
Dzodic et al. 2006	40	DTC	1% methylene blue	0.2	After strap muscle retraction	PT	FS and H

Reference	*n*	*Population*	*Dye/Isotope*	*Volume injected (mL)*	*Timing of injection*	*Injection site*	*Assessment of SLN*
Chow et al. 2004	15	PTC	2.5% patent blue V	0.5-1	After strap muscle retraction	IT	H
Takami et al. 2003	68	PTC	1% isosulphan blue	0.3	After strap muscle retraction	PT	FS and H
Tsugawa et al. 2002	38	PTC	1% patent blue VF	0.2-0.5	NA	IT	H
Fukui et al. 2001	22	PTC	2% methylene blue	0.1	After mobilization	PT	FS and H (but not all cases)
Arch-Ferrer et al. 2001	22	PTC	1% isosulphan blue	0.5	After mobilization	IT	H
Catarci et al. 2001	8	Suspicious and PTC	2.5% patent blue V	0.2-0.4	Before mobilization	IT	H
Dixon et al. 2000	40	Suspicious and DTC	Isosulphan blue	0.1-0.7	After strap muscle retraction	IT	FS and H
Kelemen et al. 1998	17	Suspicious and DTC	1% isosulphan blue	0.1-0.8	After strap muscle retraction	IT	FS and H
Lee et al. 2009	43	DTC	99mTc-labelled tin colloid	0.1-0.2	Preop US	IT	FS and H
Boschin et al. 2008	65	PTC	99mTc-labelled nanocolloid	0.1-0.2	Preop US	IT	FS and H
Carcoforo et al. 2007	64	Suspicious and PTC	99mTc-labelled nanocolloid	0.3	Preop US	PT	H
Stoecki et al. 2003	10	Suspicious and DTC	99mTc-labelled sulphur colloid	0.2	Preop US	PT and later IT	H
Catarci et al. 2001	8	Suspicious and PTC	99mTc-labelled colloidal albumin	0.1	Preop US	IT	H
Rettenbacher et al. 2000	9	Suspicious and DTC	99mTc-labelled nanocolloid	0.5	NA	IT	H

(Adapted from Balasubramanian & Harrison, 2011)

Legend: SLN, sentinel lymph node; SLNB, sentinel lymph node biopsy; PTC, papillary thyroid cancer; IT, intratumoral; PT, peritumoral; FS, frozen section; H, histology; DTC, differentiated thyroid cancer; US, ultrasound; NA, data not available.

Table 1. Characteristics of studies evaluating sentinel lymph node biopsy in thyroid surgery

We have found that the protocol currently used at our institution was easy to apply and had good outcomes (Figure 1). We therefore describe our technique in details. Following splitting of the strap muscles to expose the thyroid nodule, four quadrants around the tumor are injected with a total of 0.2cc's of methylene blue with a tuberculin syringe. At this juncture, one minute without manipulation is set aside to allow for diffusion of the dye. The lymphatic channels which stain blue (tract of blue dye, Figure 2) are then followed into the central compartment and associated blue lymph nodes are harvested and sent for frozen section analysis (Figure 3). Thyroidectomy is then performed. If there are no blue lymph nodes identified, thyroidectomy is performed. In either case, re-examination of the central

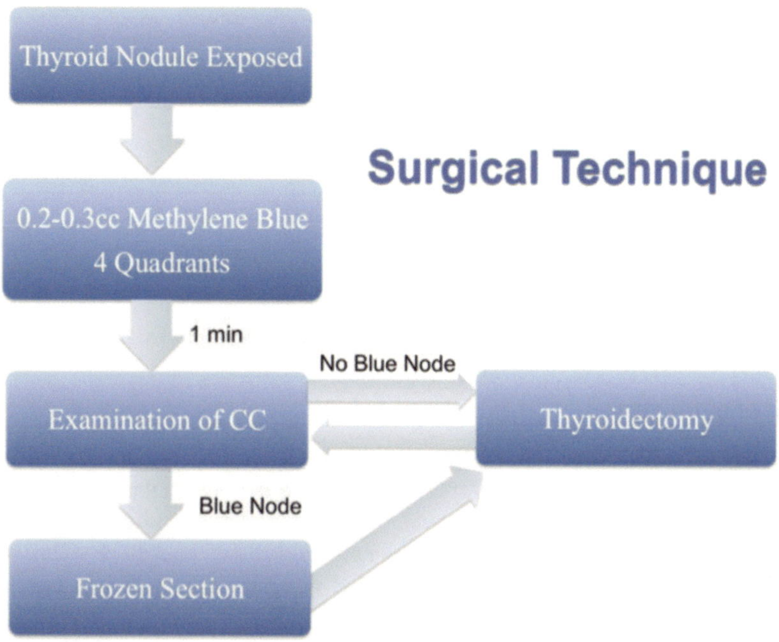

Fig. 1. Summary of the McGill Thyroid Injection Protocol

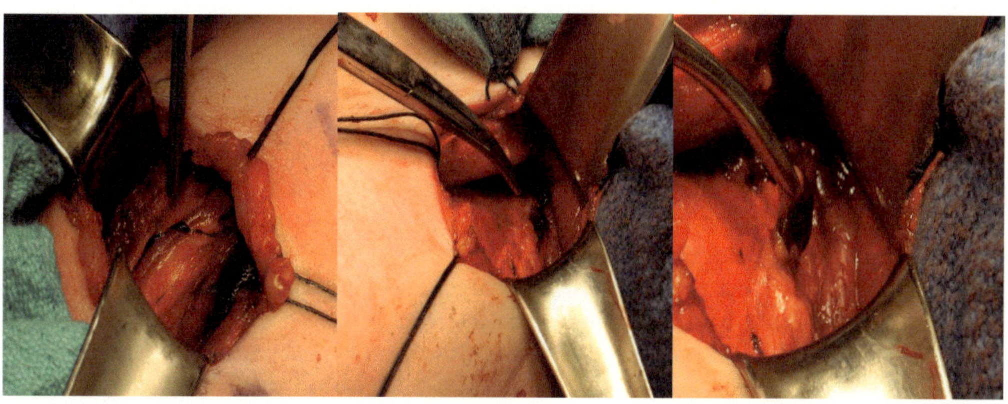

Fig. 2. Technique of SLN biopsy. Moments after injection of methylene blue, a tract of blue dye is seen heading towards the central compartment and pooling inside the SLN.

compartment is performed after thyroidectomy and all blue nodes are sent for frozen section analysis. All frozen section samples are submitted for permanent analysis following intra-operative assessment.

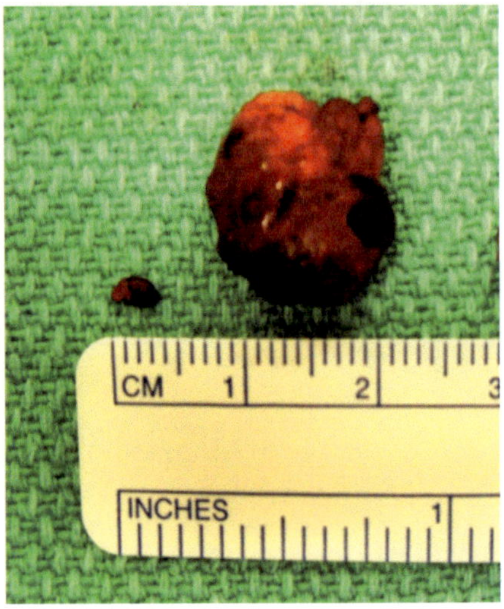

Fig. 3. The two lymph nodes above stained blue and were sent for frozen section analysis.

4.3 Review of outcomes

Keleman et al, in 1998, were the first to report the use of SLNB for thyroid carcinoma. Isosulfan blue dye was injected in 17 patients with thyroid neoplasms and the SLN was identified in 15 patients. SLN detection was missed in 11.8% of patients due to retrosternal localized SLN's and false-negative cases constituted 8%. Haigh & Giuliano in 2000 performed SLN biopsy in 17 cases and identified metastasis in 56% of cases. Notably, a control neck dissection was not carried out in all patients in both of these studies, and as such, positive and negative predictive values could not be determined. In a recent study, Cunningham et al (2010) performed a retrospective review of 211 patients and concluded that SLNB is feasible, safe and can identify patients who may benefit from CCND. As in the other previous studies, however, a CCND was not performed on all patients and thus a false negative rate could not be determined.

Given its aim of identifying the patients who do not require CCND, the single most critical qualitative descriptor for SLNB is the false-negative rate (FNR). This requires comparison of SLNB to a gold standard for the identification of occult metastases. The gold standard used varies from study to study. Most frequently, a control neck dissection is performed in all cases with its extent going from central compartment neck dissection only to a formal modified lateral neck dissection passing through a localized dissection of non-sentinel lymph nodes above and bellow the omohyoid (Dzodic, 2006). Another study used ^{131}I scan as the gold standard to help define the true-positive and true-negative SLN (Dixon et al., 2008).

Fukui et al conducted a study in 2001 on 22 patients with PTC who underwent a control lateral and central compartment neck dissection. SLN's were found in 21 of 22 patients and the prediction of disease status was accurate in 19 of 21 patients (90%). Two false negatives were reported in this study. Using peritumoral injection of blue dye, Takami et al (2002) reported a 12.5% SLN FNR in a prospective study of 68 patients. Similarly, Roh et al (2007) reported a 22% FNR using peritumoral blue dye in 50 patients. In 2009, Anand et al published the largest prospective series on SLN biopsy to date (N = 98) showing the reliability of SLN biopsy in the management of well differenciated thyroid cancer. The study showed with a sensitivity of 100% that a negative SLN on permanent pathological analysis represents a negative central compartment. The primary goal of this study was to determine if the SLN in WDTC was indeed a sensitive predictor of the status of the central compartment while avoiding the possible confounding affect of frozen section analysis. For this reason frozen section analysis was not performed. In a recent study encompassing the largest series to date on the technique, frozen section analysis was employed to clarify its role in surgical practice. They studied a total of 157 patients injected with methylene blue. The sensitivity, specificity, positive predictive value and negative predictive value of the SLN biopsy technique to remove all disease from the central compartment was 92.9%, 100%, 100% and 98.8% respectively ($p < 0.0001$). This protocol would have eliminated the need for a CCND in 92% (144/157) in press (Richardson et al., in preparation).

A systematic review and meta-analysis of SLNB in thyroid cancer was recently published and looked at all the possible outcomes with the use of this technique (Balasubramanian & Harrison, 2011). Twenty-four studies were included in the analysis and great heterogeneity in techniques, assessment methodology and extent of nodal surgery were noted. The overall detection rate of SLN was 86.3% (blue dye 83.7%, and radioisotope 98.4%). The combined use of blue dye and radioisotope reached a detection rate of 96%. Sentinel lymph nodes with evidence of metastasis were present in 42.9% of patients with PTC and an identified SLNB. Following this positive SLN biopsy, 60.5% of patients had additional lymph node metastases identified on the neck dissection. The FNR of the blue dye technique was 7.7% while the radioisotope technique had a FNR of 16%. The combined techniques FNR was 0%. This meta-analysis also evaluated the methods of assessment of SLNB. It demonstrated that in this context simple frozen section was unreliable since it had a FNR of 12% (i.e. the frozen section was negative but the final histopathology of the same lymph node was positive). However, with the use of intraoperative immunohistochemical staining such as anticytokeratin and antithyroglobulin antibody, additional cases could be adequately identified thereby decreasing the FNR. This analysis concluded that SNB in thyroid cancer is a promising technique that has the potential to avoid prophylactic lymph node surgery in up to 57% of patients with clinically node-negative thyroid cancer. However, at this stage the data is still inconsistent and there appears to be a need for a more rigorous assessment of the SLNB technique in thyroid cancer.

4.4 Pitfalls of sentinel lymph node biopsy in papillary thyroid cancer

4.4.1 The false-negative rate

As described above, despite the more promising recent studies, FNRs as high as 22% have been reported and remain a serious concern regarding the value of SLNB (Sakorafas et al., 2010). Others have demonstrated that falsely negative SLNB happen even in cases of grossly positive metastatic PTC in the neck and have hypothesized that this is possibly occurring because the normal path of lymphatic drainage was blocked by tumor-laden lymphatics (Dixon et al., 2000). In addition to blockage of lymphatics by tumor, lymphatic disruption during exposure of thyroid nodule or gland mobilization could also account for the lack of identification of the otherwise positive lymph node. We therefore recommend minimal dissection prior to injection of the dye.

It is also likely that the extensive lymphatic network in the neck complicates the practical application of the theoretical concept of SLNB in patients with thyroid cancer (Sakorafas et al., 2010). Noguchi et al., in 1987, demonstrated that up to 7% of thyroid metastases appear in the lateral compartment only, bypassing the central lymph nodes, which could explain the false-negative cases in studies limited to the central compartment.

Furthermore, the concept of "SLN blind spot" was introduced by some authors to account for some of the false-negative cases. They describe three such cases where a blue node adherent to the substance of the thyroid gland was found ex vivo by the pathologist, and might have not been found intraoperatively because the blue-stained thyroid gland masked the blue tract and blue node (Cunningham et al., 2010).

Given that lymph nodes harboring metastatic disease can be as small as 3 mm, the problem of a "crushed node" or a sample small enough that it may sacrifice permanent section has been reported. A pathologist with expertise in head and neck oncology, namely thyroid cancer, is therefore desirable for assessing the frozen section samples (Amir et al., 2011).

The lack of an approach toward multifocal disease is potentially another cause of false negatives. Indeed, while the dominant nodule may have been malignant, a non-dominant nodule also harboring disease that was not injected with methylene blue may be the source of the metastasis that is therefore missed because the nodule was not injected (Amir et al., 2011). Future studies designed to develop a novel approach to multifocal disease would therefore be very pertinent.

4.4.2 Adverse events related to sentinel node biopsy

In addition to the complications associated with a CCND that can follow a positive SLNB, the procedure of the SLNB has in itself been associated with some adverse events. From experience, we have noted that during injection, spillage of the dye may cause problems in identification of the sentinel lymph node, recurrent laryngeal nerve and parathyroid glands. This can, however, be easily overcome by slow intratumoral or peritumoral dye injection and immediate blotting of spillage at the injection site. One study has reported permanent hypoparathyroidism secondary to removal of a parathyroid gland that has stained blue (Cunningham et al., 2010). All degrees of skin responses to the blue dye have also been reported. For instance, methylene blue, despite its safety record, has been associated with intense erythema, superficial ulceration, and on one occasion a necrotic lesion (Kelley & Holmes 2011). Methylene blue-induced skin necrosis results from oxidation of surrounding tissues causing breakdown of cell membranes and inflammation, as well as a local vasoconstrictive effect due to methylene blue's inhibitory effect on nitric oxide. There is no increase in recurrent laryngeal injury rates associated with SLNB (Roh & Koch, 2010).

5. Conclusion

The management of occult cervical lymph node metastasis in WDTC is controversial. The SLNB is a safe and accurate method for assessing the possible involvement of the cervical lymph nodes by a primary thyroid tumour which allows for intraoperative decision making regarding the extent of neck dissection needed in each case. Despite the promising data, it might be too early to consider the SLNB technique as a standard of care in the management of patients with thyroid cancer. Several technicalities and pitfalls still need to be addressed. Most importantly, at this point, randomized controlled clinical trials are necessary to determine whether occult nodal metastases play a clinically significant role in longterm survival and disease-free survival, and whether SLNB and subsequent nodal management is associated with a survival benefit in patients with thyroid cancer.

6. References

Amir, A.; Payne RJ.; Richardson, K.; Hier, M.; Mlynarek, AM.; Caglar, D. (2011). Sentinel Lymph Node Biopsy in Thyroid Cancer: It Can Work But There Are Pitfalls. Otolaryngology Head and Neck Surgery, (in press).

Anand, SM.; Gologan, O.; Rochon L., Tamilia, M.; How, J.; Hier, MP.; Black, MJ.; Richardson, K.; Hakami, H.; Marzouki, HZ; Trifiro, M.; Tabah, R.; Payne, RJ. (2009) The Role of Sentinel Lymph Node Biopsy in Differentiated Thyroid Carcinoma. *Arch Otolaryngol Head Neck Surg,*Vol.135, pp. 1199-1204.

Balasubramanian, S. & Harrison, BJ. (2011) Systematic review and meta-analysis of sentinel node biopsy in thyroid cancer. *Br J Surg,* Vol.98, pp. 332-344.

British Thyroid Association, Royal College of Physicians. (2007) Guidelines for the management of thyroid cancer (Perros P, ed) 2nd edition. Report of the Thyroid Cancer Guidelines Update Group. London: Royal College of Physicians, 92p.

Caron, NR.; Tan, YY.; Ogivlie, JB.; Triponez, F.; Reiff, ES.; Kebebew, E. (2006) Selective modified radical neck dissection for papillary thyroid cancer, Is level I, II and V dissection always necessary? *World J Surg,* Vol.30, pp.833e40.

Cobin et al. (2001) AACE/AAES medical/surgical guidelines for clinical practice: management of thyroid carcinoma. *Endocr Pract,* Vol. 7, No.3, pp.(No. 3); 202-220.

Cooper, DS.; Doherty, GM.; Haugen, BR.; Kloos, RT.; Lee, SL.; Mandel, SJ.; Mazzaferri, EL.; McIver, B.; Pacini, F.; Schlumberger, M.; Sherman, SI.; Steward, DL.; Tuttle, RM. 2009 Revised management guidelines for patients with thyroid nodules and differentiated thyroid cancer. *Thyroid* Vol.19, pp.1167–1214.

Cunningham, DK.; Yao, KA.; Turner, RR.; Singer, FR.; VanHerle, AR.; Giuliano, AE. (2010). Sentinel Lymph Node Biopsy for Papillary Thyroid Cancer: 12 Years of Experience at a Single Institution. *Ann Surg Oncol.* Vol. 17, pp.2970-2975.

Dixon, E.; McKinnon, JG.; Pasieka, JL. (2000) Feasibility of Sentinel Lymph Node Biopsy and Lymphatic Mapping in Nodular Thyroid Neoplasms. *World J Surg,* Vol. 24, pp.1396-1401.

Dzodic, R. (2006). Sentinel Lymph Node Biopsy May Be Used to Support the Decision to Perform Modified Radical Neck Dissection in Differentiated Thyroid Carcinoma. *World J Surg,* Vol.30, pp.841-846.

Fukui, Y.; Yamakawa, T.; Taniki, T.; Numoto, S.; Miki, H.; Monden. Y. (2001). Sentinel Lymph Node Biopsy in Patients with Papillary Thyroid Carcinoma. *Cancer,* Vol. 92, pp. 2868-2874.

Gimm, O.; Rath, FW.; Dralle, H. (1998). Pattern of lymph node metastases in papillary thyroid carcinoma. *Br J Surg,* Vol. 85, pp.252e4.

Giuliano, AE. et al. (1994). Lymphatic mapping and sentinel lymphadenectomy for breast cancer. *Ann Surg,* Vol. 220, No. 3, pp. 391-398

Gould, E.; Winship, T.; Philbin, PH. (1960). Observations on a "sentinel node" in cancer of the parotid. *Cancer,* Vol.13, pp.77-78.

Grodski, S.; Cornford, L.; Sywak, M.; Sidhu, S.; Debridge L. (2007). Routine level VI lymph node dissection for papillary thyroid cancer: surgical technique. *ANZ J Surg.* Vol. 77, pp.203-208.

Henry, JF.; Gramatica, L.; Denizot, A.; Kvachenyuk, A.; Puccini, M.; Defechereux, T. (1998). Morbidity of prophylactic lymph node dissection in the central neck area in patients with papillary thyroid carcinoma. *Langenbeck's Arch Surg,* Vol.383, pp.167-169.

Kelemen, PR; VanHerle, AJ; Giuliano, AE. (1998). Sentinel Lymphadenectomy in Thyroid Malignant Neoplasms. *Arch Surg,* Vol. 133, pp.288-292.

Kelley, LM & Holmes, D.R. (2011). Tracer agents for the detection of sentinel lymph nodes in breast cancer: current concerns and directions for the future. *Surg Oncol,* Vol. 104, pp. 91-96.

Krag, DN, et al. (1993). Surgical resection and radiolocalization of the sentinel lymph node in breast cancer using a gamma probe. *Surg Oncol,*Vol. 2, No. 6, pp.335-339.

Leboulleux, S.; Rubino, C.; Baudin, E.; Caillou, B.; Hartl, DM.; Bidart, JM.; Travagli, JP.; Schlumberger, M. 2005 Prognostic factors for persistent or recurrent disease of papillary thyroid carcinoma with neck lymph node metastases and/or tumor extension beyond the thyroid capsule at initial diagnosis. J Clin Endocrinol Metab, Vol. 90, pp.5723–5729.

Lee, J.; Sung, TY.; Nam, KH.; Chung, WY.; Soh, EY.; Park, CS. (2008). Is level IIb lymph node dissection always necessary in N1b papillary thyroid carcinoma patients? *World J Surg,* Vol. 32, pp. 716e21.

Machens, A,; Hinze, R.; Thomusch, O.; Dralle H. Pattern of nodal metastasis for primary and reoperative thyroid cancer. *World J Surg,* Vol. 26, pp.22e8.

Makar, A.P.H., et al., (2001). Surgical management of stage I and II vulvar cancer: The role of the sentinel node biopsy. Review of literature. *Int J Gynecol Cancer,* Vol. 11, No. 4, pp. 255-262.

McHenry, C,; Rosenm IB.; Walfish PG. (1991). Prospective Management of Nodal Metastases in Differentiated Thyroid Cancer. *Am J Surg,* Vol. 162, pp. 353-356.

Mitra, I, et al. (2011). Effect of central compartment neck dissection on hypocalcemia incidence after total thyroidectomy for carcinoma. *J Laryngol Oto,* Vol.125, No.5, pp.497-501.

Moo, T & Fahey III, TJ. (2011). Lymph node dissection in papillary thyroid carcinoma. *Seminars in Nuclear Medicine March,* Vol. 41, pp. 84-88.

Morton, D.L., et al. (1992). Technical details of intraoperative lymphatic mapping for early stage melanoma. *Arch Surg,* Vol. 127, No.4, pp. 392-399.

Noguchi, S.; Murakami, N. (1987). The value of lymph-node dissection in patients with differentiated thyroid cancer. *Surg Clin North Am,* Vol. 67, pp. 251–261.

Pelizzo, MR.; Boschin, IM,; Toniato, A.; Bernante, P.; Piotto, A.; Rinaldo, A.; Ferlito A. (2001). The Sentinel Node Procedure with Patent Blue V Dye in the Surgical Treatment of Papillary Thyroid Carcinoma. *Acta Otolaryngol.* Vol. 121, pp. 421-424.

Pereira, JA.; Jimeno, J.; Miquel, J.; Iglesias, M.; Munne, A.; Sancho, JJ.; Sitges-Serra, A. (2005). Nodal yield, morbidity, and recurrence after central neck dissection for papillary thyroid carcinoma. *Surgery.* Vol. 138, pp.1095-1101.

Pitman, K.T., et al. (2003). Sentinel lymph node biopsy in head and neck cancer. *Oral Oncol,* Vol. 39, No, 4, pp. 343-349.

Podnos, YD.; Smith, D,; Wagman, LD.; Ellenhorn, JD. (2005). The implication of lymph node metastasis on survival in patients with well-differentiated thyroid cancer. *Am Surg,* Vol. 71, pp.731–734.

Rettenbacher, L.; Sungler, P.; Gmeiner, D.; Kässmann, H.; Galvan, G. (2000). Detecting the sentinel lymph node in patients with differentiated thyroid carcinoma. *Eur J Nucl Med,* Vol. 27, pp. 1399-1401.

Richardson, K, et al. (2011). Sentinel Lymph Node Biopsy in Well Differentiated Thyroid Cancer. *Head & Neck,* (in press).

Roh, JL.; Kim, JM.; Park, CI. (2008). Lateral cervical lymph node metastases from papillary thyroid carcinoma: pattern of nodal metastases and optimal strategy for neck dissection. *Ann Surg Oncol* Vol. 15, pp. 1177e82.

Roh, JL. and Koch, WM. (2010). Role of sentinel lymph node biopsy in thyroid cancer. *Expert Rev Anticancer Ther,* Vol. 10, No.9; 1429-37.

Roh, JL.; Park, JY.; Park. CI (2007). Total thyroidectomy plus neck dissection in differentiated papillary thyroid carcinoma patients: pattern of nodal metastasis, morbidity, recurrence, and postoperative levels of serum parathyroid hormone. *Ann Surg,* Vol. 245, pp. 604e10.

Rugiero, FP. (July 29, 2008) Classification of Neck Dissection, In: *E-Medicine,* July 11, 2011, Available from: http://emedicine.medscape.com/article/849834-overview.

Sakorafas, GH.; Sampanis, D.; Safioleas, M. (2010). Cervical lymph node dissection in papillary thyroid cancer: Current trends, persisting controversies, and unclarified uncertainties. *Surg Oncol,* Vol. 19, pp.e57-e70.

Saha, S., et al. (2000). Sentinel lymph node mapping in colorectal cancer--a review. *Surg Clin North Am,* Vol.80, No. 6, pp. 1811-9.

Shah JP. (1990). Cervical lymph node metastases diagnostic, therapeutic and prognostic implications. *Oncology,* Vol. 4, pp. 61e9.

Shen, WT et al. (2010). Central neck lymph node dissection for papillary thyroid cancer: The reliability of surgeon judgment in predicting which patients will benefit. *Surgery,* Vol.148, pp. 398-403.

Taylor, R.J., et al. (2001). Sentinel node localization in oral cavity and oropharynx squamous cell cancer. *Arch Otolaryngol Head Neck Surg,* Vol. 127, No.8, pp. 970-4.

Takami, H.; Sasaki, K.; Ikeda, Y.; Tajima, G.; Kameyama, K. (2002). Thyroid Sentinel lymph node biopsy in patients with thyroid carcinoma. *Biomed Pharmacother,* Vol. 56, pp.83s-87s.

Zaydfudim, V.; Feurer, ID.; Griffin, MR.; Phay, JE. (2008) The impact of lymph node involvement on survival in patients with papillary and follicular thyroid carcinoma. *Surgery,* Vol. 144, pp. 1070–1077.

Zetoune, T et al. (2010). Prophylactic Central Neck Dissection and Local Recurrence in Papillary Thyroid Cancer: A Meta-analysis. *Ann Surg Oncol*, pp 3287-3293.

11

Preparing Patients for Radioiodine Treatment: Increasing Thyroid Cell Uptake and Accelerating the Excretion of Unbound Radioiodine

Milovan Matović
University of Kragujevac, Medical Faculty; Clinical Centre Kragujevac, Department of Nuclear Medicine
Serbia

1. Introduction

The therapeutic application of radioiodine ^{131}I in postoperative ablation of the remaining thyroid tissue, as well as in the treatment of recidivism and/or local and remote metastases of differentiated thyroid carcinoma has been a part of the clinical practice for over 50 years. It is a regular segment of the standard therapeutic procedure in differentiated thyroid carcinoma treatment and it comes recommended by a number of authorities in the field (American Association of Clinical Endocrinologists/Associatione Medici Endocrinologi [AACE/AME], 2006; Cooper et al., 2006; Pacini et al., 2006; Society of Nuclear Medicine [SNM], 2006, British Thyroid Association [BTA], 2007; Dietlein et al., 2007; Luster et al., 2008; National Comprehensive Cancer Network [NCCN], 2010;). Certain differences in opinion on the subject are concerned only with the dose that is applied, as well as with whether radioactive iodine therapy should be utilized in lower risk patients (Иваницкая&Шантырь, 1981; Haq et al., 2004; Ringel&Ladenson, 2004; Cooper et al., 2006; Pacini et al., 2006; Gheriani, 2006). Several decades of experience have shown indisputable beneficial effects of the administration of ^{131}I as postoperative adjuvant therapy. However, there can be certain adverse effects, beside the beneficial ones, which are a consequence of radiation damage to other tissues and organs. The organs most exposed to the harmful radiation effect of ^{131}I in differentiated thyroid carcinoma treatment are salivary glands, nasolacrimal ducts, stomach epithelium, kidneys, bladder wall, colon, gonads, bone marrow, etc. But, most long-term follow-up studies report a very low risk of secondary malignancies in long-term survivors (Rubino et al., 2003; Brown et al., 2008). However, meta-analysis of two large multicenter studies showed that the risk of second malignancies was significantly increased relative to thyroid cancer survivors not treated with RAI (Sawka et al., 2009). The risk of secondary malignancies is dose related (Rubino et al., 2003), Cumulative ^{131}I activities above 500–600 mCi are associated with a significant increase in risk. There appears to be an increased risk of breast cancer in women with thyroid cancer (Brown et al., 2003; Sandeep et al., 2006; Chen et al., 2001). It is unclear whether this is due to RAI therapy, screening bias or other factors.

The question that arises regarding radioactive iodine administration is: how do we optimize the beneficial therapeutic effects of radioiodine on one hand and minimize the adverse effects on other tissues and organs on the other. The compromise can be achieved in two ways. The first is to increase radioiodine uptake in thyroid tissue/tumour tissue and increasing the therapeutic efficiency of ^{131}I. In other words, the aim is to achieve the best therapeutic effect in the target tissue with as low a dose of ^{131}I as possible. The second is to reduce the adverse effects, i.e. reduce the amount of radiation energy ^{131}I tissues by accelerating the elimination of radioiodine which hasn't been bound by thyroid/tumour tissue.

There is yet another reason why the accelerated elimination of radioiodine from the body of the patient should be striven for. The reason is legal and concerns regulations which exist in every country and which determine the amount of radioactive iodine that patients are allowed to have in their body without being required to receive their treatment in a 'restricted area'. With the doses of radioiodine normally applied in differentiated thyroid carcinoma treatment, hospitalisation of some duration is required in many countries. For this reason, it is in the best interest of the health system to shorten the hospitalisation, i.e. the isolation of the patient being treated with radioactive iodine, without reducing the therapeutic effect of ^{131}I.

There are significant variations in the regulations regarding ^{131}I administration from one country to another. These variations mostly have to do with the upper limit of the radionuclide that can be administered without the patient requiring isolation.

Legal regulations state that anything above that limit requires the therapy to be carried out on hospital premises, or more precisely, in special rooms designated as controlled radiation zones ('restricted areas'). This limit varies in different countries. For example, in Serbia, the upper limit is relatively low and special precautions have to be taken if the radioactivity of ^{131}I exceeds 400 MBq (10.81mCi). In other words, the patient can be released from hospital only when the radioactivity in his body decreases below the level of 400 MBq (the Republic of Serbia, Ministry of environmental protection, 2003). The limit is significantly higher in the EU and USA, where hospitalisation is obligatory only if the radioactivity of ^{131}I exceeds 1110 MBq (30mCi) (1110 MBq). In this case the patient is hospitalised and kept in isolation until their radioactivity level decreases to 30 mCi (1110 MBq) (Tuttle et al., 2000; Society of Nuclear Medicine [SNM], 2006).

In cases of differentiated thyroid carcinoma treatment the doses of ^{131}I vary from 30mCi for the remaining thyroid tissue ablation, to 200 mCi for the treatment of metastases, even though there are several records of the doses reaching as much as 333 mCi (9GBq) (Haq et al., 2004). With the application of these larger doses, the permitted radioactivity limit in the body is reached a few days following the application of the ablation/therapeutic dose of ^{131}I (Venencia et al., 2002). The time necessary to reach the limit depends primarily on the dose applied and the condition of kidney function, as well as on the size of the thyroid/tumour tissue being treated.

2. Methods for increasing radioiodine uptake

2.1 Thyrotropin stimulation (endogenous and exogenous TSH stimulation)

In order to optimize radioiodine uptake in the thyroid remnant or in thyroid tumour tissue, it is necessary either for the patient to have substantially elevated endogenous thyroid-stimulating hormone levels (serum TSH concentration above 30 mIU/mL), or to perform exogenous TSH stimulation by applying recombinant human TSH (rhTSH).

In the first case, sufficient levels of TSH are most commonly achieved if the patient is left without thyroid hormone replacement therapy for 4 to 6 weeks. The primary problem that frequently arises from thyroid hormone withdrawal as a way of increasing TSH levels is clinically evident hypothyroidism, which some patients find quite disagreeable. The condition is notable for hypometabolism, constipation, increased cholesterol levels in blood, the risk of cardiovascular disorders, and the most severe one - myxedema.

In the second case, exogenous TSH stimulation of the uptake is achieved by the application of rhTSH, available on the market as Thyrogen® (Genzyme). This medication is given to the patient intramuscularly for 2 days, in 0.9 mg doses.

Exogenous stimulation of thyroid minimises the chances of hypothyroidism, and at the same time enables better planning of radioiodine therapy. However, the application of rTSH increases the cost of the treatment significantly, as this medication is relatively expensive.

The results of a number of studies have shown that the final effects of uptake stimulation, both with endogenous TSH, and exogenous rhTSH are equally satisfactory and thus both come equally recommended (Haugen et al., 1999; Pacini et al., 2006).

2.2 Low iodine diet

In order to achieve a better uptake in thyroid/tumour tissue, a low iodine diet is recommended, i.e. the daily intake of not more than 25-75 μg of iodine. Patients should be put on the diet for 10 to 30 days prior to the diagnostic or therapeutic application of ^{131}I (Maxon et al., 1983; SNM, 2006; Thyroid Cancer Survivors' Association, 2007).

The consequence of the low intake of iodine is iodine depletion in the body, which should result in its increased uptake in thyroid remnants/tumour tissue. Since most countries have legal regulations by which producers are obliged to iodise table salt, this low iodine diet practically presupposes the limitation of table salt intake, which usually proves to be difficult for the patients to put into practice. One teaspoon of iodised table salt contains about 400 micrograms of iodine. Sea salt is also not recommended due to the fact that it contains a significant amount of iodine. The alternative is uniodised salt, which is often difficult to find. Apart from the limitation on table salt, it is essential that the patients avoid foods with high concentration of iodine (above 20 micrograms per meal), and these are the following:

- seafood (fish, shellfish, seaweed, seaweed tablets, kelp). These are all very high in iodine and should be avoided. Food containing sea-based additives, such as carrageenan, agar-agar, algin, alginate and nori should also be avoided.
- milk and dairy products such as cheese, cream, yogurt, butter, ice cream, milk chocolate, powdered dairy creamers, whey, casein and others which contain significant amounts of iodine (250 ml of milk- 1 cup or 16 tablespoons, contain from 88 to 168 micrograms of iodine, or an average of 115 micrograms).
- egg yolks or whole eggs
- bread and pastry
- salty processed foods such as potato chips and cured and corned foods such as hot dogs, ham, corned beef, sauerkraut, bacon, sausage, and salami.

- soybeans and most soy products (soy sauce, soy milk, tofu)
- red, orange, or brown processed food, pills and capsules, because the artificial colour (erythrosine) used for these foods contains significant amounts of iodine
- iodine-containing vitamins and food supplements

A limited daily intake of food which contains moderate amounts of iodine (5-20 micrograms per meal) is recommended. This includes the following:

- fresh meats (meat contains 56-290 micrograms of iodine per kilogram). Up to 140 grams a day of fresh meats such as chicken, beef, pork, lamb, and veal are fine on the low-iodine diet.
- grains, cereals. Up to 4 servings per day of grains, cereals, pasta, and breads without iodine-containing ingredients are fine for this diet. Homemade baked goods and cereals are best for this diet.
- rices. Similar to grains, rices vary in the amount of iodine depending on the region where they are grown, so rice should be eaten only in limited amounts. Some low-iodine diets recommend avoiding rice.

These instructions can often pose a problem because some guidelines only say that certain items or certain food categories should be avoided, and do not give details within categories, or else they just give lists of foods and ingredients that are allowed, without limits on quantities consumed.

Even though most recommendations and guides list iodine diet as an essential part of the preparation for radioiodine therapy application due to the fact that it increases the binding of iodine in thyroid/tumour tissue, there are also other, contrasting data. Some researches have shown that the effects of low iodine diet can include an increased iodine retention, instead of iodine depletion, especially if it is combined with the application of diuretics (Hamburger, 1969; Norfray & Quinn, 1974; Tepmongkol, 2002, Matovic et al. 2009a).

2.3 Lithium

The inhibiting effects of lithium carbonate on the release of iodine from the thyroid tissue are also useful in radioiodine treatment of differentiated thyroid carcinoma, for the purpose of achieving prolonged and increased radioiodine retention in the thyroid/tumour tissue (Briere et al., 1974; Gershengorn et al., 1976; Rasmusson et al., 1983; Pons et al., 1987). Researchers agree that the administration of 0.8-1.2 mmol/L of lithium carbonate results in an increased uptake and prolonged retention of radioiodine in thyroid/tumour tissue, which doubles the dose absorbed, without significant adverse whole-body irradiation. However, the majority of authors urge caution in using this medicine and suggest careful monitoring of its levels in plasma for the purpose of avoiding adverse effects, primarily intoxication, which affects the central nervous system and kidneys, and can potentially be fatal (Simard et al., 1989).

2.4 Retinoids and an increasing expression of NaI symporter system

Better accumulation of ^{131}I into the remnant thyroid/tumour tissue can be achieved through an increased expression of genes that enhance the synthesis of the NaI symporter. Retinoids or their metabolites, which bind with retinoic A and X receptors (RAR and RXR), are known to result in an increased expression of genes which lead to an increased synthesis of NaI symporters. This will theoretically lead to increased iodine uptake in thyroid/tumour tissue. However, there are contradictory data concerning the efficiency of this sort of adjuvant therapy in thyroid iodine uptake. While some researchers (Van Herle et al., 1990; Grunwald et al., 1998; Koerber et al., 1999) point out that the administration of 13-cis retinoic acid (in Accutan, Roche Laboratories, Nutley, NJ, USA) prior to radioiodine application increases its uptake in the tumour tissue, especially in follicular carcinomas, others (Gruning et al., 2003) do not find a significant efficiency in the increase of thyroid iodine uptake, based on studies of large groups of subjects.

However, the latest findings on NaI symporter system expression, as well as the identification of genes which encode its synthesis (Mandell et al., 1999; Spitzweg et al., 2001; Castro et al., 2001; Chung et al., 2002; Kogai et al., 2006) will probably allow for new approaches in radioiodine therapy of differentiated thyroid carcinomas, that focus on the optimisation of the dose administered to patients, by increasing the efficiency of this therapy.

3. Methods for increasing unbound iodine excretion

3.1 Hydration

The relevant literature suggests that the accelerated urinary excretion of ^{131}I can be achieved by extensive hydration. However, there are also data that do not support this. For example, Giebisch et al. (Giebisch et al., 1956) concluded in their research on dogs that water diuresis does not induce iodine diuresis, as 95% of the filtered iodine gets reabsorbed by the tubules in proximity to water absorption spots. Even so, extensive hydration is recommended in patients receiving radioiodine therapy, since it can lead to the dilution of radioiodine in the urine and a decrease in radioactive iodine retention in the urinary tract, which contributes to the decrease in the dose absorbed by the urinary bladder wall and surrounding organs.

3.2 Laxatives

In order to accelerate elimination of ^{131}I through stool, some experts prescribe laxatives to expedite bowel evacuation, especially in patients with constipation. Others, however, hold the opinion that only a small, insignificant amount of the applied radioiodine is eliminated in this way, and that therefore laxatives are not of great importance (Hays, 1993). For these reasons, it is considered that the administration of laxatives is not necessary in patients who have at least one stool a day.

3.3 rhTSH (Thyrogen®)

There are data that renal radioiodine excretion is ~50% faster during euthyroidism versus hypothyroidism due to reduced renal function in hypothyroidism. Administration of rhTSH minimises the chances of hypothyroidism and could be indirectly useful in accelerating of unbound radioiodine elimination. However, based on their meta anlaysis study, Freudenberg and co-workers (Freudenberg et al., 2010) suggests (but without statistically significant evidence), that rhTSH administration may results in a lower radiation dose to DTC metastases than does thyroid hormone withdrawal (THW). Furher studies should resolve this issue.

3.4 Diuretics

For the purpose of reducing the absorbed dose in critical organs and tissues of patients treated with radioiodine, a simple and efficient method is often recommended for the excretion of unbound ^{131}I - extensive hydration in combination with additional diuretic therapy.

In a study conducted on 49 adult subjects with and without thyroid and kidney function impairment, Bricker and Hlad (Bricker&Hlad, 1955) concluded that ^{131}I gets excreted from the body by means of passive filtration in glomeruli and gets partially reabsorbed by the tubuli by means of passive back-diffusion, without any active tubular transport mechanisms.

There are various, often contradictory data in the literature concerning the effects of diuretics on the biokinetics of radioiodine elimination. The majority of studies point to the fact that faster elimination of radioiodine can be achieved by the addition of diuretic therapy (Russell&Ingbar, 1965; Fregly&Gennaro, 1965; Fregly, 1966; McCarthy et al., 1967; Fregly& McCarthy, 1973; Seabold et al., 1993; Kapucu et al., 2003), but the results of other studies show that the administration of diuretics leads to increased radioiodine uptake in the thyroid tissue (Hamburger, 1969; Norfray&Quinn, 1974; Ding et al., 2004; Tepmongkol, 2002). The data concerning the studies of the urinary excretion of iodine and the effects of diuretics on its urinary excretion published so far are contradictory. They do not present a clear picture of what kind of benefits, if any, can be gained by adding diuretic therapy to radioactive iodine treatment protocols. This is probably at least in part due to the fact that the published data were obtained either from studies performed on animals (Fregly&Gennaro, 1965; Fregly, 1966; McCarthy et al., 1967), or from studies on patients who did not suffer from differentiated thyroid carcinoma and had not been operated on previously, and who received radioiodine doses far smaller than those given to patients suffering from differentiated thyroid carcinoma (Russell&Ingbar 1965; Fregly&McCarthy, 1973; Tepmongkol, 2002; Kapucu 2003).

There have been a small number of studies on the effects of diuretics on radioiodine clearance in patients who were treated with therapeutic doses of ^{131}I, but the conditions under which these studies were conducted were to a certain degree different to the ones typical for clinical practice and the way this therapy is normally carried out (Maruca et al., 1984; Seabold et al., 1993; Ding et al., 2004).

The effects of furosemide, hydrochlorotiazide, manitol, ethacrynic acid and acetozolamide on radioiodine urinary excretion have been studied so far. Out of all the diuretics, furosemide has been studied most.

3.4.1 Furosemide

Furosemide is effective, cheap and widely used. Abbott and associates (Abbott et al., 2008) have analysed the data concerning the effects of furosemide from both the medical and veterinary literature. Based on a considerable number of analysed papers, they concluded that one of the chief effects of furosemide includes iodine depletion in the body, which is achieved through a decrease in its reabsorption in the thick ascending limb of Henle's loop. Furosemide acts as the inhibitor of Na-K-Cl cotransporter 2 (NKCC 2), which is the mechanism present in the majority of other diuretics, excluding spironolactone. The inhibition of co-transporter NKCC 2 is dose-dependent with respect to the concentration of furosemide in the lumen, rather than in plasma. The administration of furosemide brings about an increase in sodium, chloride and water in distal collecting ducts, resulting in increased renal excretion of potassium and hydrogen. This can result in some patients developing hypokalemic and hypochloremic alkalosis, which is the most common adverse effects of this diuretic. For the purpose of hypokalemic and hypochloremic alcalosis prevention, it is advised that patients receive potassium chloride together with furosemide in cases of long term therapy.

When it comes to the influence of furosemide on radioiodine excretion, numerous and often contradictory data have been published. Some of them point to the fact that this diuretic influences the acceleration of iodine urinary excretion leading to iodine depletion. However, in one of our previous studies (Matovic et al., 2009a) it has been unmistakably shown that this diuretic, in combination with low iodine diet, slows down the elimination of radioiodine in patients treated with this radionuclide (figure 1. and figure 2.).

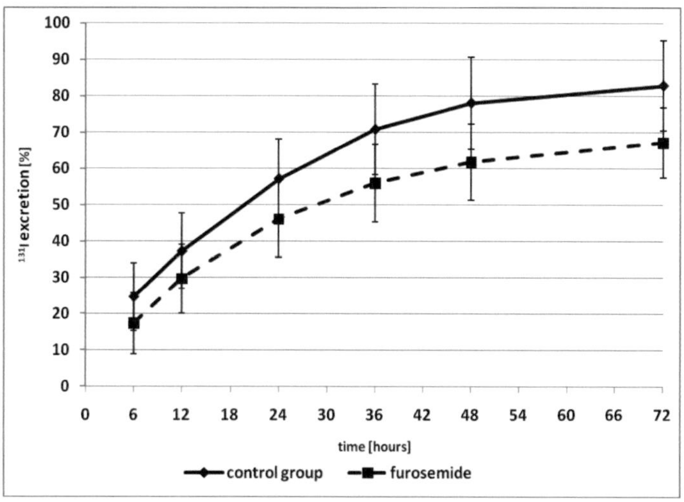

Fig. 1. Urinary excretion of radioiodine in patients treated with furosemide (■), and in the control group patients(•).

Our results were somewhat similar to the ones obtained by Maruca et al. (Maruca et al., 1984), who concluded that diuretic-mediated iodide depletion is not universally successful and that it is far less effective than it was considered before, therefore casting some doubt on its clinical benefits. Their aim was to achieve iodine depletion with low iodine diet and diuretics (Hydrochlorotiazide and Furosemide) in patients who had previously undergone thyroidectomy due to differentiated thyroid carcinoma. The results they obtained point to the fact that this low iodine diet and diuretics increase the uptake of iodine in the tumour tissue. According to their findings, the total iodine uptake and retention in the tumour tissue was mostly the consequence of total body retention, and not some specific mechanism at the cell level of thyroid/tumour tissue.

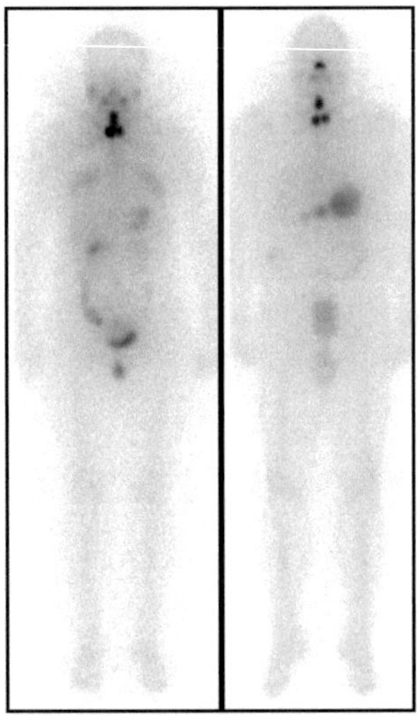

Fig. 2. Scintigrams obtained 72h post therapy with 3.70 GBq of ^{131}I in patients with (left) and without (right) furosemide aditional therapy. Increased amount of radioiodine in thyroid rest in case of previous furosemide therapy. Both patients had similar thyroid rest (uptake of radioidine was about 2% in both patients).

The presumption that low iodine diet plays an important role in how furosemide affects iodine biokinetics can be supported by the data obtained from a number of researchers, who found that furosemide and other diuretics cause an increase in iodine excretion in those patients who were not put on a prior low iodine diet. A comparison between a research by Seabold et al. (Seabold et al., 1993) and Norfray and Quin (Norfray&Quinn, 1974) provide possible further evidence for this. Specifically, Seabold et al. found that in patients who had not been on a low iodine diet and who had received radioiodine ablation therapy, furosemide as an adjuvant therapy accelerated the excretion of radioactive iodine, which enabled those patients to spend far less time on the hospital premises.

Based on experiments in animals, Norfray and Quinn found that intraperitoneal application of furosemide leads to an increased iodide excretion, which in turn results in a decrease in iodide pool in their bodies. The same authors found that supplemental iodide diet does not reduce this effect of furosemide, even though the thyroid radioiodine uptake increases in comparison to the control group under the influence of diuretic therapy, which reduces the iodide pool. This indirectly points to the fact that an uptake increase in thyroid/tumour tissue can be achieved by the administration of diuretics as well. However, they did not measure blood radioactivity, so the possibility that an increase in uptake under the influence of furosemide is at least in part a consequence of increased blood radioactivity, i.e. total body retention, instead of just an increase in the avidity of thyroid tissue for iodine cannot be excluded either.

Other researchers (Hamburger, 1969; Norfray&Quinn, 1974; Tepmongkol, 2002) also found that furosemide does not increase iodine excretion, but on the contrary, that it decreases it. According to the data provided by Kapucu and associates (Kapucu et al., 2003), the administration of Furosemide results in the loss of iodine from subjects' bodies (iodine depletion).

They noticed that after a 5-day furosemide therapy a better penetration of iodine into the thyroid gland was noted in patients who had not previously been on a low iodine diet, than in those who had been on the diet for 14 days, without receiving furosemide. The authors think the explanation for this lies in the loss of sodium from extracellular fluid which is greater when furosemide is administered than when preceded by a low iodine diet alone.

However, Russell and Ingbar (Russell&Ingbar, 1965) state that there is an intrathyroid, pituitary-independent mechanism of increasing thyroid function as an answer to the reduction in iodine concentration in plasma. As far back as 1965 they studied the effect of iodine depletion (with previous low iodine diet and the administration of manitol) on ^{131}I biokinetics and thyroid function, on a group of 8 patients.

According to their results, iodine depletion resulted in decreased iodine levels in blood, an increase in thyroid iodine transfer and the speed of thyroid clearance, as well as an increase in thyroid iodine uptake followed by a decrease in absolute iodine accumulation. These authors concluded within the same study that there is no increase in thyroid iodine clearance and ^{131}I uptake if NaI is applied together with manitol.

It should be stressed that in our research on mice (Matovic et al., 2009b) we did not note an increased radioiodine retention in thyroid tissue when we applied furosemide, even though they had undergone a low iodine diet. This can point to the fact that iodine biokinetics has certain species specific characteristics, either at the level of kidneys, or at the level of thyroid gland.

In our research, which included patients treated with radioiodine, we did not determine whether there is an increase in thyroid/tumour tissue uptake under the influence of furosemide therapy, but our results indirectly support the data provided by Maruca et al. that in cases of increase the most likely reason is, up to a certain point, an increase in ^{131}I levels in blood, i.e. an increase in total body retention of the radionuclide under the influence of additional furosemide therapy.

An important role in this mechanism is played by the preceding low iodine diet, which can be concluded based on the data provided by Hamburger et al. (Hamburger et al., 1969). They determined the uptake in thyroid/tumour tissue in a group of 25 patients with a confirmed diagnosis of inoperable thyroid carcinoma, who had previously been treated with diuretics and a low iodine diet. What was achieved by a combination of a low iodine diet and diuretics (manitol and ethacrynic acid) was doubled, or even tripled uptake in 16 patients, mild increase in 3, and no increase in 6 patients. According to their data, radioiodine levels in thyroid/tumour tissue remain high 96 hours following the diuretic preparation.

3.4.2 Other diuretics

Based on the results obtained from a controlled study, Tepmonkogol (Tepmongkol, 2002) concluded that the binding of radioiodine in the thyroid gland is as many as 7.18 times higher when hydrochlorothiazides were administered together with a low iodine diet. The control group comprised patients who were on a low iodine diet, but who received neither hydrochlorothiazide, nor other diuretics. The control group showed an increase in the uptake as well, even though a significantly smaller one, amounting to 1.33 times the original binding. The study was performed on patients suffering from hyperthyroidism who had been treated with radioiodine. Similar results were obtained by Ding and his associates (Ding et al., 2004), who showed that the administration of hydrochlorothiazide prior to the dosing of radioiodine can significantly increase the dose absorbed by the thyroid tissue. The study included patients suffering from differentiated thyroid carcinoma who had previously undergone thyroidectomy.

In a study performed on 18 young male subjects following an acute administration of hydrochlorothiazide and acetazolamide, Fregly and McCarthy (Fregly&McCarthy, 1973) analysed the fluctuations in urinary excretion of Na, K, Ca, Mg, Cl and I. Based on the results of this study, as well as on the previous studies done on animals (McCarthy et al., 1967, Fregly, 1966, Fregly&Gennaro, 1965), the authors concluded that hydrochlorothiazide has a significant effect on an increase in iodine excretion, which is closely tied to an increase in chloride excretion, while there was no increase in either iodine, or chloride excretion in those treated with acetazolamide.

Judging by all the aforementioned data, the most probable cause of the decrease in ^{131}I excretion under the influence of diuretics is the state of iodine depletion caused by the prior low iodine diet. For some reason this state is characterised by an absence of iodine reabsorption blockage in the tubuli under the influence of diuretic therapy, and paradoxically, results in increased iodine reabsorption.

Walser and Rahill (Walser&Rahill, 1965) concluded that the reabsorption of iodine and chlorine is done in the same part of the nephron by means of passive diffusion with a constant ratio of tubular permeability. Since the low iodine diet was at the same time low chloride, as well as a low sodium diet (due to the reduced table salt intake), it is possible that the explanation for this unexpected and paradoxical effect of diuretics on radioiodine excretion lies in that very fact.

Namely, it is possible that in cases where low iodine diet (i.e. low chloride/low sodium diet) was prescribed, the increase in the reabsorption of chlorine gets followed by an increase in iodine reabsorption at the level of the ascending segment of Henle's loop and the proximal tubules. As a consequence, iodine excretion decreases, instead of increasing, and the same goes for its blood levels, which directly influenc the prolongation of patient hospitalisation in the restricted area after the application of radioiodine therapy, due to the maintenance of high circulating levels. For this reason it is not advisable to use additional diuretic therapy for the purpose of speeding up the urinary excretion of radioiodine, at least not in patients who had previously been on a low iodine diet.

4. Methods for salivary glands and nasolacrimal ducts protection

Some authors recommend measures to prevent damage of the salivary glands and nasolacrimal ducts. Damage of those organs results with transient loss of taste and excessive tearing (epiphora), as clinical compliications. Methods for prevention of those complications have included usage of amifostine, hydration, sour candies, and cholinergic agents (Mandal&Mandal, 2003). However, in relevant literature there are not enough evidence to recommend for or against these methods. There are even authors (Nakada et al, 2005) who suggested sour candy may actually increase salivary gland damage.

5. Conclusion

With the aim of achieving a satisfactory compromise between high therapeutic efficiency of radioiodine therapy on thyroid/tumour tissue and the need to decrease its adverse effects on other tissues and organs, it is necessary for the patient to be carefully selected and adequately prepared.

The most basic part of the preparation is the achievement of high TSH stimulation in order to increase radioiodine uptake in the thyroid/tumour tissue. Both exogenous and endogenous methods of TSH stimulation are equally valid from the point of view of achieving the uptake, but keeping the patient without substitution for several weeks can be highly disagreeable, and in some patients even dangerous, due to the possible complications. On the other hand, the convenience that comes with the use of rhTSH comes at a higher cost. It is up to the patient and the physician to estimate which method of TSH stimulation to use by evaluating the cost/benefit of exogenous and endogenous TSH stimulation in each individual case.

The low iodine diet comes right after TSH stimulation as the second most important step in the preparation of patients for radioiodine therapy, its purpose being to increase the radioiodine uptake in thyroid/tumour tissue. However, it should be borne in mind that there can be a possible interference of this diet with the potential use of diuretics in patients treated with radioiodine. In any case, it is indisputable that a low iodine diet helps achieve a higher radioiodine uptake in the thyroid/tumour tissue, and it should therefore be prescribed to patients who are to receive the radioiodine therapy.

The administration of lithium is an efficient method of increasing the uptake of radioiodine in thyroid/tumour tissue, but it is not recommended in routine clinical practice, since its administration can have serious complications in case of an overdose. An increase in NaI symporter expression in thyroid/tumour tissue, achieved by the application of retinoids, results in a favorable increase in radioiodine uptake. Even though it does not belong to the clinical routine, this method can be useful in patients who have lost the ability to accumulate radioiodine in the tumour tissue. These patients are characterised by the secretion of thyroglobulin, a positive PET scan and a negative radioiodine scan. Further research on the identification of the gene responsible for the coding of NaI symporter system synthesis can provide a new approach to radioiodine treatment of thyroid carcinoma in the sense of dose optimisation, i.e. the prospects of increasing the efficiency of the therapy.

When it comes to methods aimed at accelerating the excretion of radioiodine that has not been bound to the thyroid/tumour tissue, extensive hydration of the patients is recommended, as it reduces the absorption in the critical organs by diluting the urine and increasing urinary volume, even though it does not result in increased iodine excretion.

Laxative administration in patients who have regular emptying of the bowel can cause certain discomfort to the patients, so this is not clinically justified nor necessary, having in mind the small quantity of radioiodine that gets eliminated in this way.

In patients who had been on a low iodine diet there is a decrease in excretion of ^{131}I under the influence of diuretics, which results in an increase in its levels in blood, which in turn indirectly prolongs the hospitalisation period. The patient has to be detained in the restricted area following the radioiodine therapy due to the high circulating levels that are maintained in their bodies. All this also results in a higher dose being absorbed by the patient's critical organs. For this reason, the administration of diuretics for the purpose of accelerating urinary excretion of radioiodine cannot be recommended, at least not in patients who had previously been on a low iodine diet.

6. Acknowledgment

This work was partially supported by Grants No 175007 and III41007, given by Ministry of Education and Science, Republic of Serbia and by Institute for Nuclear Sciences Vinča, Belgrade.

7. References

Abbott, L.A. & Kovacic J. (2008). The pharmacologic spectrum of furosemide. *J Vet Emerg Crit Care*,18(1):26-39

Bricker, N.S. & Hlad, C.J. Jr. (1955). Observations on the mechanism of the renal clearance of ^{131}I.*J Clin Invest*, 34(7, Part 1):1057-72

Briere, J.; Pousset, G.; Darsy, P.; Guinet, P. (1974). The advantage of lithium in association with iodine 131 in the treatment of functioning metastasis of thyroid cancer. *Ann Endocrinol*, 35:281–2

Brown, A.P.; Chen, J.; Hitchcock, Y.J.; Szabo, A.; Schrieve; D.C.&Tward, J.D. (2008). The risk of second primary malignancies up to three decades after the treatment of differentiated thyroid cancer. *J Clin Endocrinol Metab*, 93:504–515

Castro, M.R.; Bergert, E.R.; Goellner, J.R.; Hay, I.D. & Morris J.C. (2001). Immunohistochemical Analysis of Sodium Iodide Symporter Expression in Metastatic Differentiated Thyroid Cancer: Correlation with Radioiodine Uptake. *The Journal of Clinical Endocrinology & Metabolism*, 86(11): 5627-32

Chen, A.Y.; Levy, L.; Goepfert, H.; Brown, B.W.; Spitz, M.R.&Vassilopoulou-Sellin, R. (2001). The development of breast carcinoma in women with thyroid carcinoma. *Cancer*, 92:225–231

Chung, J.K. (2006). Sodium Iodide Symporter: Its Role in Nuclear Medicine. *Journal of Nuclear Medicine*, 43(9):1188-1200

Cooper, D.S.; Doherty, G.M., Haugen, B.R., Kloos, R.T., Lee, S.L., Mandel, S.J., Mazzaferri, E.L., McIver, B., Sherman, S.I. & Tuttle R.M. (2006). The American Thyroid Association Guidelines Taskforce. Management Guidelines for Patients with Thyroid Nodules and Differentiated Thyroid Cancer. *Thyroid*, 16(2):1-34

Dietlein, M.; Dressler, J.; Eschner, W.; Grünwald, F.; Lassmann, M.; Leisner, B.; Luster, M.; Moser, E.; Reiners, C.; Schicha, H.; Schober, O. (2007). Procedure guidelines for radioiodine therapy of differentiated thyroid cancer (version 3). *Nuklearmedizin*, 46: 213–19

Ding, H.; Kuang, A.R.; Guan, C.T. (2004). Randomized controlled trial of hydrochlorothiazide in augmenting the dose of 131I absorbed by thyroid remnant. *Sichuan Da Xue Xue Bao Yi Xue Ban*, 35(4):546-548

Fregly, M.J. & Gennaro J.F. Jr. (1965). Effect of thiazides on metacorticoid hypertension and on thyroid activity of rats. *Can J Physiol Pharmacol*, 43:521-30

Fregly, M.J. & McCarthy J.S. (1973). Effects of diuretics on renal iodide excretion by humans. *Toxicology and applied Pharmacology*, 25:289-298

Fregly, M,J. (1966). Effect of thiazides on the thyroid gland of rats. *Toxicol Appl Pharmacol*, 8(3):558-66

Freudenberg LS, Jentzen W, Petrich T, Frömke C, Marlowe RJ, Heusner T, Brandau W, Knapp WH, Bockisch A. (2010). Lesion dose in differentiated thyroid carcinoma metastases after rhTSH or thyroid hormone withdrawal: 124I PET/CT dosimetric comparisons. *Eur J Nucl Med Mol Imaging*, 37(12):2267-76

Gershengorn, M.C.; Izumi M.&Robbins J. (1976). Use of lithium as an adjunct to radioiodine therapy of thyroid carcinoma. *J Clin Endocrinol Metab*, 42:105–11

Gheriani H. (2006). Update on epidemiology classification, and management of thyroid cancer. *Libyan J Med*, AOP:060514

Giebisch, G. ; MacLeod, M.B.&Kavaler, F. (1956). Renal excretion of radioiodide in the dog. *Amer J Physiol*.187:529-535

Gruning, T.; Tiepolt, C.; Zophel, K.; Bredow, J.; Kropp, J.&Franke W.G. (2003). Retinoic acid for redifferentiation of thyroid cancer - does it hold its promise? *European Journal of Endocrinology*, 148:395–402

Grunwald, F.; Menzel, C.; Bender, H.; Palmedo, H.; Otte, R.; Fimmers, R.; Risse, J. & Biersack H.J. (1998). Redifferentiation therapyinduced radioiodine uptake in thyroid cancer. *Journal of Nuclear Medicine*, 39:1903–6

Guidelines for the management of thyroid cancer (2nd edition) (2007). British Thyroid Association. Royal College of Physicians; 106 pages

Hamburger, J.I. (1969). Diuretic augmentation of 131-I uptake in inoperable thyroid cancer. *N Engl J Med*, 280(20):1091–1094

Haq, M.S.; McCready, R.V.&Harmer, C.L. (2004). Treatment of advanced differentiated thyroid carcinoma with high activity radioiodine therapy. *Nuclear Medicine Communications*, 25(8):799-805

Haugen, B.R.; Pacini, F.; Reiners, C,; Schlumberger, M.; Ladenson, P.W.; Sherman, S.I.; Cooper, D.S.; Graham, K.E.; Braverman, L.E.; Skarulis, M.C.; Davies, T.F.; DeGroot, L.J.; Mazzaferri, E.L.; Daniels, G.H.; Ross, D.S.; Luster, M.; Samuels, M.H.; Becher, D.V.; Maxon, H.R.; Cavalieri, R.R.; Spencer, C.A.; McEllin, K.; Weintraub, B.D.&Ridgway, E.C. (1999). A comparison of recombinant human thyrotropin and thyroid hormone withdrawal for the detection of thyroid remnant or cancer. *J Clin Endocrinol and Metabolism*, 84: 3877–85

Hays, M.T. (1993). Colonic excretion of iodide in normal human subjects. *Thyroid*, 3(1):31-35

Kapucu, L.O.; Azizoglu, F.; Ayvaz, G.&Karakoc, A.(2003). Effects of diuretics on iodine uptake in non-toxic goiter: comparison with low-iodine diet. *Eur J Nucl Mol Imaging*, 30(9):1270–1272

Koerber, C.; Schmutzler, C.; Rendl, J.; Koehrle, J.; Griesser, H.; Simon, D.&Reiners, C. (1999). Increased I-131 uptake in local recurrence and distant metastases after second treatment with retinoic acid. *Clinical Nuclear Medicine*, 24:849–51

Kogai, T.; Taki, K.&Brent, G.A.(2006). Enhancement of sodium/iodide symporter expression in thyroid and breast cancer. *Endocrine-Related Cancer*, 13:797–826

Luster, M.; Clarke, S.E.; Dietlein, M.; Lassmann, M.; Lind, P.; Oyen, W.J.G.; Tennvall, J.&Bombardieri, E. (2008). Guidelines for radioiodine therapy of differentiated thyroid cancer. EANM guidelines, version of 23 April, 2008.pp 54

Mandel, S.J.&Mandel, L. (2003). Radioactive iodine and the salivary glands. *Thyroid*, 13:265–271

Mandell, R.B.; Leisa, Z.; Mandell, L.Z.& Link, C.J.Jr.(1999). Radioisotope Concentrator Gene Therapy Using the Sodium/Iodide Symporter Gene. *Cancer Research*, 59:661-8

Maruca, J.; Santner, S.; Miller. K.;&Santen, R.J.(1984). Prolonged iodine clearance with a depletion regimen for thyroid carcinoma: concise communication. *J Nucl Med*, 25:1089-1093

Matovic, D.M.; Jankovic, M.S.; Jeremic, M.; Tasic, Z.&Vlajkovic, M. (2009a). Unexpected effect of furosemide on radioiodine urinary excretion in patients with differentiated thyroid carcinomas treated with Iodine 131. *Thyroid*, 19(8):843-848

Matovic, D.M.; Jankovic, M.S.; Jeremic, M.; Novakovic, M.; Milosev, M.&Vlajkovic, M. (2009b). Effect of furosemide on radioiodine-131 retention in mice thyroid gland. *Hell J Nucl Med*, 12(2):129-131

Maxon, H.R.; Thomas, S.R.; Boehringer, A.; Drilling, J.; Sperling, M.I.; Sparks, J.C.&Chen, I.W. (1983). Low iodine diet in I-131 ablation of thyroid remnants. *Clin Nucl Med*, 8:123–126

McCarthy, J.S.; Fregly, M.J.&Nechay, B.R. (1967). Effects of diuretics on renal iodine excretion by rats and dogs. *The Journal of Pharmacology and Experimental Therapeutics*, 158(2):294-304

Medical guidelines for clinical practice for the diagnosis and management of thyroid nodules. Thyroid nodule guidelines. AACE/AME Task force on thyroid nodules. (2006). *Endocr Pract*, 12(1):63-102

Nakada, K.; Ishibashi, T.; Takei, T.; Hirata, K.; Shinohara, K.; Katoh, S.; Zhao, S.; Tamaki, N.; Noguchi, Y.&Noguchi, S. (2005). Does lemon candy decrease salivary gland damage after radioiodine therapy for thyroid cancer? *J Nucl Med*, 46: 261–266

Norfray, J.F.&Quinn, J.L.3rd. (1974). Furosemide mediated elevations of thyroid iodide uptake in the rat. *Proceedings of the society for experimenta biology and medicine*, 145: 286-288

Pacini, F.; Schlumberger, M.; Dralle, H.; Elisei, R.; Smit, J.; Wiersinga, W.&the European Thyroid Cancer Taskforce. Consensus statement. European consensus for the management of patients with differentiated thyroid carcinoma of the follicular epithelium. (2006). *Eur J Endocrinology*, 154: 787–803

Pons, F.; Carrio, I.; Estorch, M.; Ginjaume, M.; Pons, J.&Milian, R.(1987). Lithium as an adjuvant of iodine-131 uptake when treating patients with well-differentiated thyroid carcinoma.*Clin Nucl Med*, 12:644–647

Practice Guidelines in Oncology –Thyroid Carcinoma v.2., National Comprehensive Cancer Network, Inc. 2010

Rasmusson, B.; Olsen, K.&Rygard, J.(1983). Lithium as adjunct to I-131-therapy of thyroid carcinoma. *Acta Endocrinol (Copenh)*, 252(Suppl):74

Republic of Serbia, Ministry of eviromental protection. PRAVILNIK O NAČINU PRIMENE IZVORA JONIZUJUĆIH ZRAČENJA U MEDICINI. "Sl. list SRJ", br. 32/98 i 33/98 - ispr. i "Sl. list SCG", br. 1/2003. Pp 18 Avaliable from: http://www.ekologija.pf.ns.ac.yu/2%20jonizujuce%20zracenje.htm

Ringel, M.D.&Ladenson, P.W. (2004). Controversies in the follow-up and management of well-differentiated thyroid cancer. *Endocrine-Related Cancer,* 11:97-116

Rubino, C.; de Vathaire F. Dottorini, M.E.; Hall, P.; Schvartz, C.; Couette, J.E.; Dondon, M.G.; Abbas, M.T.; Langlois, C.&Schlumberger, M. (2003). Second primary malignancies in thyroid cancer patients. *Br J Cancer,* 89:1638–1644

Russell, M.B.&Ingbar, S.H.(1965). The Effect of Acute Iodide Depletion on Thyroid Function in Man. *J Clin Invest,* 44(7): 1117–24

Sandeep, T.C.; Strachan, M.W.; Reynolds, R.M.; Brewster, D.H.; Scelo, G.; Pukkala, E.; Hemminki, K.; Anderson, A.; Tracey, E.; Friis, S.; McBride, M.L.; Kee-Seng, C.; Pompe-Kirn, V.; Kliewer, E.V.; Tonita, J.M.; Jonasson, J.G.; Martos, C.; Boffetta, P.&Brennan, P. (2006). Second primary cancers in thyroid cancer patients: a multinational record linkage study. *J Clin Endocrinol Metab,* 91:1819–1825

Sawka, A.M.; Thabane, L.; Parlea, L.; Ibrahim-Zada, I.; Tsang, R.W.; Brierley, J.D.; Straus, S.; Ezzat, S.&Goldstein, D.P. (2009). Second primary malignancy risk after radioactive iodine treatment for thyroid cancer: a systematic review and metaanalysis. *Thyroid,* 19:451–457

Seabold, J.E.; Ben-Haim, S.; Pettit, W.A.; Gurli, N.J.; Rojeski, M.T.; Flanigan, M.J.; Ponto, J.A.&Bricker, J.A. (1993). Diuretic-enhanced I-131 clearance after ablation therapy for differentiated thyroid cancer. *Radiology,* 187:839-842

Simard, M.; Gumbiner, B.; Lee, A.; Lewis, H.&Norman, D. (1989). "Lithium carbonate intoxication. A case report and review of the literature". Archives of internal medicine 149 (1): 36–46. doi:10.1001/archinte.149.1.36 PMID 2492186. Available from: http://archinte.highwire.org/cgi/reprint/149/1/36.pdf

Society of Nuclear Medicine Procedure Guideline for Therapy of Thyroid Disease with Iodine-131(Sodium Iodide)Version 2.0, 2006. Accessible at: http://interactive.snm.org/docs/Therapy%20of%20Thyroid%20Disease%20with%20Iodine-131%20v2.0.pdf

Spitzweg, C.; Harrington, K.J.; Pinke, L.A.; Vile, R.G.&Morris, J.C. (2001). The Sodium Iodide Symporter and Its Potential Role in Cancer Therapy. *The Journal of Clinical Endocrinology & Metabolism,* 86(7): 3327-35

Tepmongkol, S. (2002). Enhancement of radioiodine uptake in hyperthyroidism with hydrochlorothiazide: a prospective randomised control study. *Eur J Nucl Med Mol Imaging,* 29:1307-10

ThyCa: Thyroid Cancer Survivors' Association, Inc. Low-Iodine Diet Guidelines – Summary. 6th Edition, 2007 Available from: http://www.thyca.org/rai.htm#diet

Tuttle, W.K. III&Brown, P.H.(2000). Applying Nuclear Regulatory Commission Guidelines to the Release of Patients Treated with Sodium Iodine-131. *J Nucl Med Technol,* 28:275–279

Van Herle, A.J.; Agatep, M.L.; Padua, D.N. 3rd; Totanes, T.L.; Canlapan, D.V.;, Van Herle, H.M.&Juillard G.J. (1990). Effects of 13 cis-retinoic acid on growth and differentiation of human follicular carcinoma cells (UCLA R0 82 W-1) in vitro. *Journal of Clinical Endocrinology and Metabolism*, 71:755–63

Venencia, C.D.; Germanier, A.G.; Bustos, S.R.; Giovannini, A.A.&Wyse, E,P. (2002). Hospital Discharge of Patients with Thyroid Carcinoma Treated with ^{131}I. *Journal of Nuclear Medicine*, 43 (1): 61-65

Walser, M.&Rahill, W.J. (1965). Renal tubular reabsorption of iodide as compared with chloride. *J Clin Invest*, 44:1371–1381

Иваницкая, В.И. & Шантырь, В.И. (1981). Лучевые методы диагностики и лечения рака щитоводной железы. Киев "Здоровя"; 160 pages

12

Differentiation Therapy in Thyroid Carcinoma

Eleonore Fröhlich[1,2] and Richard Wahl[1]
[1]Eberhard-Karls University Tübingen, Internal Medicine,
Department of Endocrinology, Metabolism, Nephrology and Clinical Chemistry,
[2]Medical University of Graz, Internal Medicine,
Dept. of Endocrinology and Nuclear Medicine,
[1]Germany
[2]Austria

1. Introduction

Thyroid cancer (TC) has a much lower incidence (0.74% in men, 2.3% in women worldwide) than cancers of breast, colon, prostate, lung and endometrium but is the seventh most frequent human malignancy and the most common neoplasm of the endocrine system. Thyroid cancer accounts for 1% of all newly diagnosed cancer cases. Over the past decades the incidence of thyroid cancer has increased significantly (50% in the last 25 years). It is suspected that the observed increase is mainly due to better detection methods because microcarcinoma are seen frequently (up to 35%) in autopsies (Harach et al., 1985). Most cancers of the thyroid originate from follicular thyrocytes, only a minority of cancers, namely medullary thyroid cancer, originate from calcitonin producing C-cells (C-cells). They belong to another entity of tumors and will not be addressed in this review.

Carcinomas of follicular cell origin include well-differentiated and poorly differentiated thyroid cancers (DTC) and anaplastic thyroid cancers. DTC comprises papillary thyroid carcinoma (PTC), which accounts for 80-90% of all thyroid cancer cases, follicular thyroid carcinoma (FTC) and Hürthle cell tumors. Undifferentiated/anaplastic thyroid cancer (ATC) is rare and accounts for only 1-2% of all TC.

The prognosis of DTC is good with a 10-year survival rate of 85% (Eustatia-Rutten et al., 2006). Recurrence, however, occurs in up to 30% of patients and only 30% of patients with distant metastases respond to radioiodine therapy with complete remission (Dohan et al., 2003). A total of 10-20% of patients develop distant metastases (Durante et al., 2006). In this group the 10-year survival rate drops to 40%. ATC usually has a fatal outcome.

2. Current treatment of thyroid carcinoma

The standard treatment of well-differentiated TC is surgery followed by radioiodine remnant ablation. As only thyrocytes are taking up iodide to a reasonable degree, radioiodine treatment is very specific and has a low rate of adverse effects. In case of insufficient iodine uptake options are few and survival is poor. External beam radiation is used as a palliative therapeutic option but these tumors usually are not responsive to this therapy. Adriamycin is the only cytostatic drug approved by the FDA for treatment of radioiodine refractory thyroid carcinoma. ATC do not express thyrotropin receptors; they neither take up iodide nor produce thyroglobulin. Surgical resection is only recommended for localized disease, which is rarely the case. In the advanced stage patients do not profit from removal of the tumor mass. Palliation to improve survival includes tracheotomy, radiation and chemotherapy or a combination of the three treatments.

Tyrosine kinase inhibitors, PPAR-y activators, retinoids, bortezomib, galdanomycin, VEGF receptor antagonists, stimulation of antigen presenting dendritic cells and p53 gene therapy are not yet approved for treatment of metastatic thyroid cancer and reserved for patients with life-threatening disease.

This review focuses on re-differentiation as mode of therapeutic action. Tyrosine kinase inhibitors, which target general tumor features like proliferation and apoptosis, currently represent the most promising group of compounds for the treatment of radioiodine-refractive TC. Their mode of action and the most promising candidates will be shortly addressed.

3. Targeted therapy

3.1 Definition and types of targeted therapies

Targeted therapies interfere with a specific molecular target, which has a critical role in tumor growth and progression. For targeted therapies antisense drugs, monoclonal antibodies and small molecules may be used. Targeted therapies, which intend to remove a block in normal cell differentiation, are termed 'differentiation therapy'.

The following molecules are involved in transformation and progression of TC and are, therefore, used in drug development for targeted therapies (Table 1).

3.2 Tyrosine Kinase Inhibitors (TKI)

Receptors over-expressed in cancer cells stimulate cell growth and proliferation through a cascade of tyrosine kinases (TKs) (Figure 2). TKIs may either compete with the ligand by binding to the extracellular domain or they may bind to the ATP-binding site of the kinase. Examples for ligand analogues are monoclonal antibodies like the anti-human epidermal growth factor receptor 2 antibody **Herceptin®** (trastuzumab), which is very successful in the treatment of breast cancer. By contrast, anti-EGFR antibodies show no significant anti-tumor action in PTC cell lines (Gabler et al., 1997).

Small molecule inhibitors, also called ATP mimetics, hinder the binding of ATP to the ATP binding pocket of protein kinases. Other compounds bind to the substrate-binding domain. By this binding autophosphorylation and signal transduction is inhibited. TKIs can inhibit proliferation and induce cell differentiation and apoptosis. As the catalytic domain of the TKs is very similar, most TKIs are not specific for one growth factor.

The most promising TKIs are briefly mentioned in the following section. For more information, the reader is referred to one of the more recent reviews (e.g. Coelho et al., 2007; Ho & Sherman, 2011; Kapiteijn et al., 2011).

Molecular target	Function	Role in TC
VEGF	Neo-angiogenesis	Increased expression in TC (Soh et al., 1997)
RET oncogene	Receptor for ligands of the glial-derived neurotropic factor family Trigger for autophosphorylation and intracellular signalling with stimulation of Ras/ERK/and PI3kinase/V-Akt cascade	In PTC chromosomal inversions and recombinations cause chimeric RET/PTC sequences, which are found in around 30% of thyroid carcinoma (Rabes et al., 2000). RET/PTC is frequently seen in microcarcinoma suggesting a role in the early phase of tumorigenesis.
c-Met	Proto-oncogene and receptor for hepatic growth factor, important for cell migration, proliferation, differentiation and angiogenesis.	It is over-expressed in 70% of PTC (Di Renzo et al., 1992). EGFR, RAS and RET regulate its expression.
BRAF	Member of the RAF familiy of serine/threonine kinases and are components of the RAF-MAPK kinase-ERK (RAF-MEK-ERK) intracellular signalling pathway	Point mutations seen in about 44% of PTCs and mutations are associated with a more and more aggressive phenotype. BRAF mutations are associated with impairment of NIS causing resistance to radioiodine uptake (Riesco-Eizaguirre et al., 2006; Romei et al., 2008).
Hsp90	Multichaperone heat shock protein, which mediates maturation and stability of several proteins involved in oncogenesis like EGF-R, Her-2, Akt, BRAF, CRAF, p53	mRNA expression of Hsp90 correlated to aggressive biological behaviour in TC (Boltze et al., 2003)
RAS	GTP-binding protein involved in proliferation, differentiation and cell survival. Ras acts via phosphatidyl inositol-3–phosphate kinase (PI3K) and through mitogen-activated protein kinase (MEK) and extracellular signal regulated kinases (ERKs).	Ras mutations in H-,N- and K-Ras oncogenes are common in TC and appear to be an early event in FTC tumorigenesis and are reported in about 50% of FTCs (Lemoine et al., 1989).
Farnesyltrans-ferase	Anchor of RAS in the plasma membrane. This anchorage is necessary for activation of RAS.	Involved in the activation of p21 (ras) in thyrocytes (Laezza et al., 1998)
MEK (MAPK/Erk kinase)	Key mediator in growth-promoting signals.	This kinase plays an important role in the pathogenesis of TC (Fagin, 2004)
EGFR (Her1, ErbB1)	Member of the Erb family of receptors and abnormally regulated in many cancer types. In addition	Overexpression is correlated to the presence of metastases in TC (Rodriguez-Antona et al., 2010).

Molecular target	Function	Role in TC
	to EGFR also ErbB2 (Her2/neu) is involved in the pathology of TC. EGFR tyrosine kinase activates Ras-Raf-MAPK cascade and the PI3K pathway.	
PI3K	Mediator of signals from many receptor tyrosine kinases.	Mutations and amplifications of PI3K have been described in differentiated and anaplastic primary tumors (Hou et al., 2007). Mutations in phosphoinositide-3-kinase alpha polypeptide and in Akt1 protein appear to be indicators for more aggressive, radioiodine refractory TC (Ricarte-Filho et al., 2009).
Mammalian target of rapamycin (**mTOR**)	Serine/threonine kinase, which serves as a downstream mediator of growth factors.	In thyrocytes, mTOR is also activated independent from Akt by direct stimulation through TSH (Brewer et al., 2007) and it may be suggested that mTOR is an especially useful target for the treatment of TC.
Akt/protein kinase B	Important mediator in apoptosis, proliferation and cell cycle progression.	Its expression is increased in sporadic FTC (Ringel et al., 2001).

Table 1. Overview on established targets for targeted therapies

3.2.1 Non thyroid specific targets: Neoangiogenesis

Strategies to reduce/inhibit angiogenesis include inhibition of VEGF signalling, where several TKIs showed efficacy in thyroid cancer. Although **Sutinimib®** (SU11248), Motesanib diphosphate (AMG-706) and Pazopanib (**Votrient®**, GW-786034) also inhibit other TKs, it is postulated that the therapeutic effect is caused mainly by inhibition of VEGF signalling. These compounds and the selective VEGF-R inhibitor **Axitinib®** (AG-013736) induced stable disease as best response in 42%-67% of the patients. Inhibition of angiogenesis is also the target for other compounds like thalidomide **(Thalidomid®)** and lenalidomide **(Revlimid®,** CC-5013**)**, which achieved stable disease in clinical trials. The prodrug Combre(ta)statin A4 phosphate binds to tubulin and destabilizes tumor blood vessels. In trials with ATC the compound induced stable disease in 30% of the patients.

3.2.2 Non thyroid specific targets: Proliferation and apoptosis

The BRAF inhibitor **Nexavar®** (Sorafenib) (BAY 43-9006) has been tested in patients with radioiodine refractory TC. Although no iodine uptake was seen, partial responses and stable disease have been reported. XL281, a pan RAF inhibitor, induced stable disease in PTC patients. AZD6244 (ARRY142886, Selumetinib), a MEK1 and MEK2 inhibitor, showed

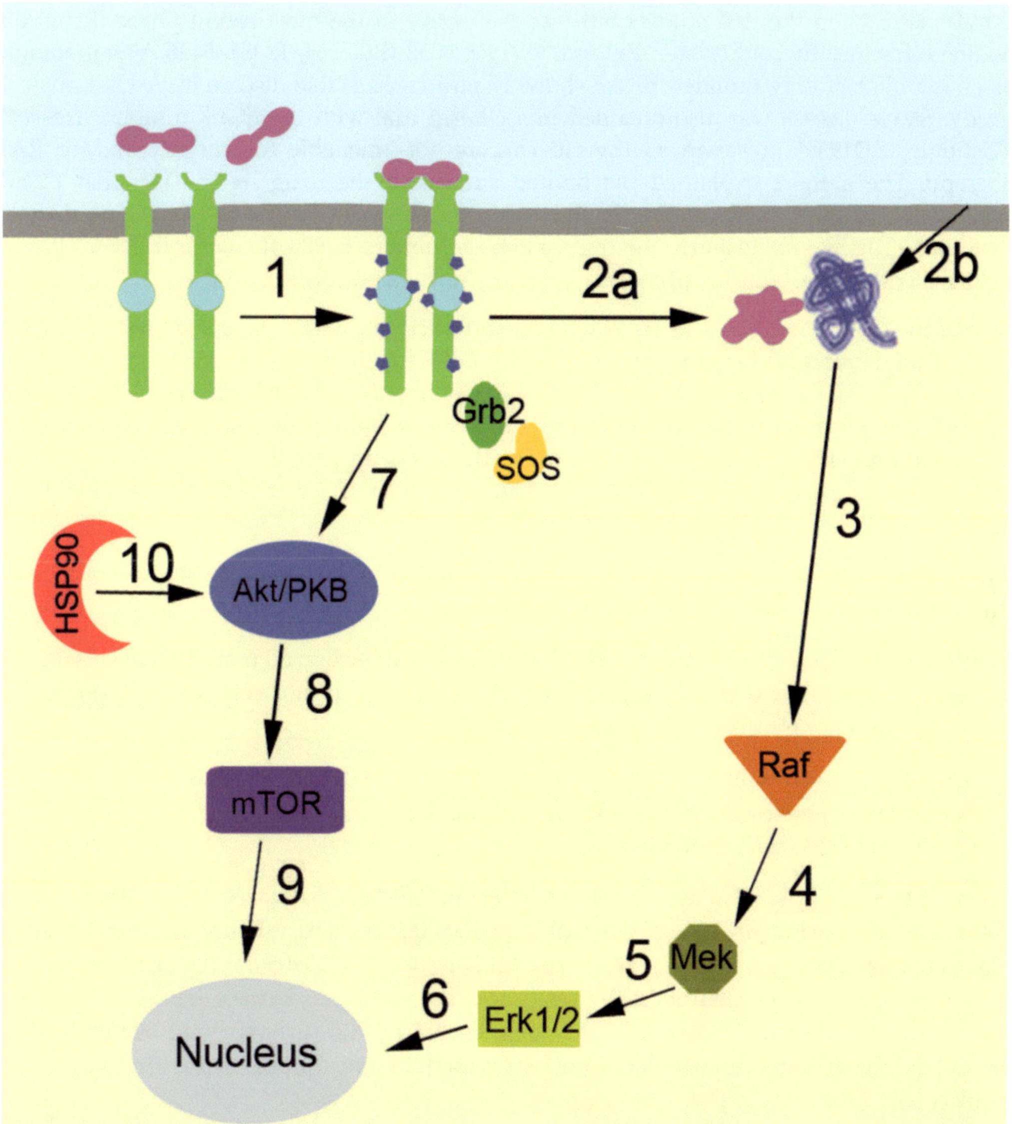

: growth factor like VEGF, EGF, HGF, : H-Ras; : GTP; : phosphate residue; : domain for kinase activity

Fig. 1. Activation of growth receptor TKs. 1: ligand binds to the receptor. Receptor dimerization and receptor binding to adapter protein, Grb2, coupled to the guanine nucleotide releasing factor, Son of Sevenless (SOS), occurs. Dimerization of the receptor leads to activation of Akt/PKB (7) and to activation of Ras (2a). Activation of Raf also needs anchorage of the Ras-GTP complex to the plasma membrane by farnesyltransferase (2b). Ras signalling acts through activation of Raf (3), MEK (4), ERK1/2 (5) that translocates into the nucleus (N) and acts (6) on transcription. Akt/PKB is activated by HSP90 (10) and stimulates through mTOR activation (8) transcription in the nucleus (9).

similar efficacy in the first studies but was ineffective in the most recent phase II trial on iodine refractory thyroid cancer. **Zelborat®** (PLX 4032 (RG7204, RO5185426, Vemurafenib) is an inhibitor of only mutated BRAF showing prolonged stable disease in a small phase I study. Stable disease was also obtained in a clinical trial with the EGFR inhibitor **Iressa®** (Gefitinib, ZD1939) in advanced thyroid cancers not amenable for surgery and/or RAI therapy. The authors explained the limited success of the drug by the fact that EGFR inhibitors, including Gefitinib, are ineffective in tumors with Raf mutations. Clinical trials on other TKIs like for instance the multi-kinase inhibitors **E7080 (Lenvatinib**[USAN]**)** and **AMG706 (Motesanib diphosphate)** are ongoing (www.clinicaltrials.gov).

Out of the several inhibitors of Hsp90, the ligand of c-Met, which have been tested in-vitro only 17-allylamino-17-demethoxygeldanamycin (17-AAG) appeared to be potent enough to justify phase I/II clinical trial in TC. The farnesyltransferase inhibitors BMS-214662 and L744832 have been evaluated in clinical phase I trials including thyroid carcinoma patients and no improvement in survival was reported. Results of a phase II trial with a combination of Everolimus **Zortress®, Afinitor®** (RAD001), an inhibitor of mTOR and sorafenib are pending.

The antiproliferative therapy with the COX-inhibitor **Celebrex®** (celecoxib) was not successful in TC.

Meta-analysis in a phase II trial on **Velcade®** (bortezomib) achieved mainly stable disease in metastased DTC, but due to increased Tg levels, efficacy is not certain. The compound displays antitumor effects also in cell lines from ATC.

JNJ-26854165, which inhibits the ubiquitin protein ligase HDM2, prevents the degradation of the tumor suppressor p53, and showed moderate success rates in patients with progressive Hurthle cell carcinoma.

Some of these TKIs act also as differentiating agents: 17-AAG increases the accumulation of iodide by decreasing its efflux, whereas NIS localization and amount are not changed (Marsee et al., 2004; Elisei et al., 2006). The MEK inhibitor PD98059, a flavonoid, increases NIS protein, but not iodide uptake (Vadysirisack et al., 2007). As surface expression was not decreased, it is suspected that a lower Vmax decreased the turnover rate of iodide. The mTOR inhibitor **Rapamune®** (sirolimus) increased iodide uptake in rat thyrocytes (de Souza et al., 2010).

4. Re-differentiation therapy: Thyroid-specific targets

Re-differentiation intends to reverse changes, which occurred during transformation of the cells. Proteins involved in thyroid hormone synthesis include sodium-iodide symporter (NIS), thyroperoxidase (TPO), pendrin (PDS) and thyroglobulin (Tg).

For the synthesis of the thyroid hormones triiodothyronine (T_3) and thyroxine (T_4), iodide is taken up from the blood stream by NIS localized at the basal side of the thyrocyte (Figure 2). Iodide is concentrated 20-40 fold with respect to the plasma concentration by NIS, the uptake is active and iodide is translocated towards the colloid by iodide efflux mediated mainly by PDS. Thyroglobulin is produced in the endoplasmic reticulum and Golgi apparatus and secreted in the follicular lumen. At the cell-colloid interface iodide is coupled to specific tyrosyl residues in thyroglobulin by the integral membrane protein TPO and monoiodotyrosine and diiodotyrosine is formed. Hydrogen peroxide for the oxidation of iodide by TPO is provided by the thyroid dual oxidase (DuOx). TPO also catalyzes the integration of hormone residues (coupling of iodotyrosines) in Tg. Excess hydrogen peroxide (H_2O_2) not involved in the oxidation of iodide may act mutagenic or carcinogenic. Selen-containing glutathione peroxidase is therefore typically upregulated to provide protection from oxidative damage. Some glutathione peroxidase gene polymorphisms are linked to an increased risk effect for TC presumably by lack of detoxification of hydrogen peroxide. Upon demand for thyroid hormones, endocytosis of iodinated Tg occurs. Iodinated Tg is hydrolysed in lysosomes and the hormones T_3 and T_4 secreted into the blood stream.

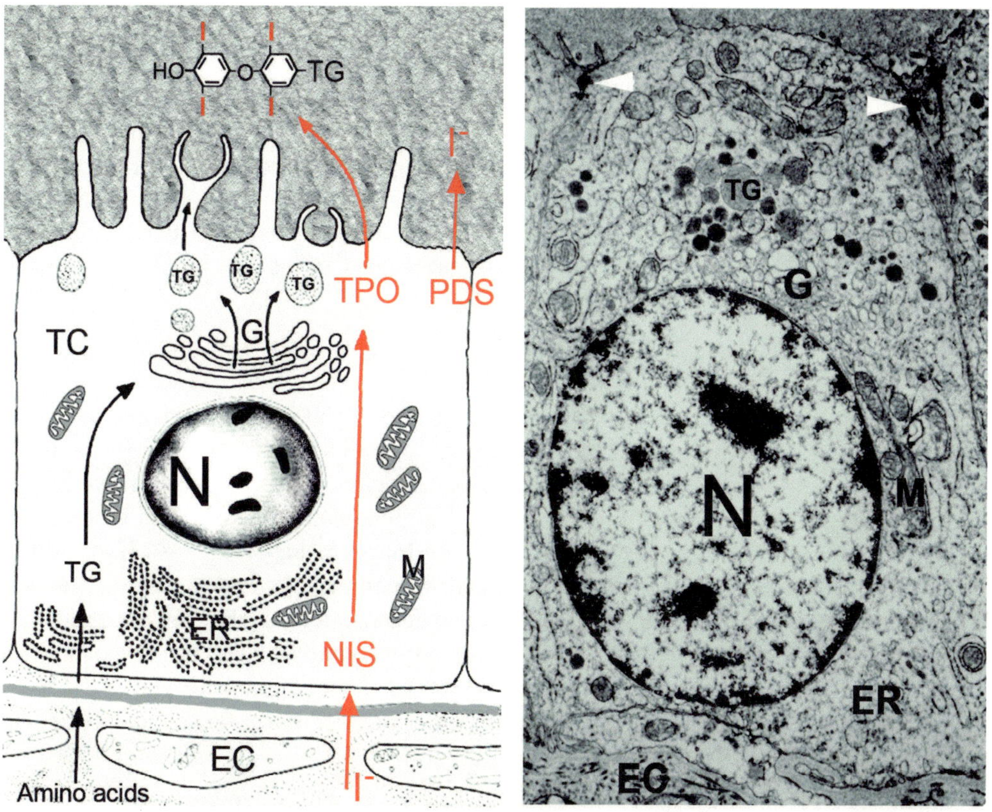

Fig. 2. Schematic drawing illustrating the synthesis of thyroid hormone in the thyroid gland and ultrastructure of a follicle cell. Iodide is taken up into the thyrocyte by NIS and Tg is synthetized from amino acids at the endoplasmic reticulum and the Golgi apparatus and transported in vesicles to the follicular lumen. PDS transports iodide into the lumen and TPO integrates iodide into Tg and couples iodotyrosines to hormone residues. The protein machinery for the synthesis of Tg, endoplasmic reticulum (ER), Golgi apparatus (G) as well as apical microvilli, tight junctions (arrowheads) and mitochondria (M) are clearly seen in the ultrastructure. N: nucleus, EC: endothelial cell.

In DTC NIS is expressed at different levels and pendrin expression is usually absent. TPO is expressed at low levels in FTC and follicular variants of PTC but below the detection limit in

PTC. The H_2O_2 generation system is present in DTC and levels increased in PTC. The TSH-R is present in most DTC. The capacity to synthesize iodinated and thyroxine rich Tg is lost in FTC due to defect in NIS and in PTC due to altered apical iodide transport and TPO activity (Gerard et al., 2003).

4.1 Sodium-iodide symporter (NIS)

NIS is an integral plasma membrane glycoprotein, which transports two sodium ions along with one iodide ion. The transmembrane gradient of sodium serves as the driving force for iodide uptake. The mature NIS protein has 13 transmembrane regions, the N-terminus is facing the extracellular milieu and the C-terminus is directed towards the intracellular milieu. Glycosylation occurs at three sites in the protein, but does influence neither stability nor membrane targeting. Phosphorylation occurs at the C-terminus. Affinity of NIS is higher for perchlorate and rhenium oxide than for iodide.

NIS is not only expressed in the thyroid but also in salivary gland, choroid plexus, gastric mucosa, lactating mammary gland and ciliary body of the eye. Potential expression of the protein has also been shown in colon, kidney, pancreas, rectum, thymus, placenta and non-lactating mammary gland (Wapnir et al., 2003). mRNA has been detected in almost all tissues but RT-PCR yields a large number of false positive results because of its high sensitivity (Dohan et al., 2003).

4.1.1 Regulation of NIS in the normal thyroid

TSH acts both on NIS transcription and on targeting of NIS to the plasma membrane through increase of c-AMP levels. The NIS promoter contains two important regions: (a) the proximal NIS promotor, where thyroid transcription factor-1, NIS-TSH-responsive factor-1 and Specificity protein 1 (Sp-1) bind and (b) the NIS upstream enhancer with binding sites for the paired domain factor Pax-1, thyroid transcription factor-1 and c-AMP-responsive element like sequences. The interaction of c-AMP-responsive element like sequences with Pax-1 is necessary for transcription of NIS. The localization to the plasma membrane appears to be mainly caused by binding of protein-recognition PDZ target motif at the carboxyl-terminus of the protein to PDZ-binding proteins, not by phosphorylation. TSH also regulates half-life of NIS: in the presence of TSH it is 5 days, in the absence 3 days (Riedel et al., 2001).

Cytokines like tumor necrosis factor α, interferon-γ, interleukin (IL)-1α, IL-1β and IL-6 inhibit NIS mRNA expression and iodide uptake. This inhibition may be the cause of hypothyroidism in autoimmune processes.

Tumor necrosis factor β in addition to decreasing TSH-induced NIS expression also changes the morphology of thyroid cells from cuboidal to flattened phenotype.

Estradiol down-regulates NIS expression and thereby may contribute to the higher incidence of goiter in women.

High intracellular iodide concentration down-regulates NIS. Similarly, follicular Tg acts as a potent suppressor of all thyroid-specific genes. This inhibition may represent a negative feedback autoregulatory mechanism and corresponds to the morphological heterogeneity of thyroid follicles: the active follicles display a cuboidal epithelium with high NIS expression and little Tg in the lumen, inactive follicles show a flattened epithelium, low or absent NIS expression and much Tg in the lumen.

High extracellular concentrations of iodide decrease the function of NIS, in addition to other effects. This phenomenon is called Wolff-Chaikoff effect (Wolff & Chaikoff, 1948). Although, the effect has been known for many years, its mechanism is still not well understood; transcriptional and post-transcriptional changes are involved.

4.1.2 NIS in thyroid cancer

NIS in thyroid cancer is not mutated (Russo et al., 2001), and various groups reported the amount of mRNA, compared to normal tissue, differently. As NIS protein is regulated at different levels (transcriptional, translational, posttranslational, targeting and intracellular distribution) the detection of mRNA is poorly predictive for normal function. NIS protein levels in thyroid cancer were reported to be higher than in normal tissue by some groups and lower than normal by others (Arturi et al., 1998; Saito et al., 1998; Lazar et al., 1999; Park et al., 2000). Impaired iodide uptake can be caused by absent or decreased NIS expression and by impaired targeting and insufficient retention at the plasma membrane. In the largest study on tissue, overexpression in combination with intracellular localization was seen in 70% of the TC samples (Dohan et al., 2001). Plasma membrane localization was rare and often not polarized but present at the apical and basal membrane. It is presumed that the altered trafficking of NIS causes NIS dysfunction. The pathological localization of NIS may also be induced by binding to the proto-oncogene pituitary tumor-transforming gene binding factor (PBF). Overexpression of this factor is associated with aggressive behaviour of TC. PBF binds to NIS, alters its subcellular localization and, thereby, inhibits its ability to take up iodide (Smith et al., 2009). Paired mRNA and protein analysis showed that decreased mRNA levels were associated with increased cytoplasmic staining of NIS (Wang et al., 2011). It was also suggested that NIS protein in cancer tissue is immature and has an abnormal turn-over rate (Saito et al., 1998, Dohan et al., 2001).

Intracellular NIS can cause negative feed-back on NIS mRNA synthesis. Reduced TSH-R may also cause low NIS mRNA levels and deficient NIS migration (Sodre et al., 2008). Activation of BRAF, Ras and RET decrease NIS mRNA. BRAF, in addition, also impairs targeting of NIS to the plasma membrane (Riesco-Eizaguirre et al., 2006).

4.2 Pendrin (PDS)

Pendrin is a transmembrane glycoprotein with three putative extracellular glycosylation sites on asparagine-residues. Both C- terminus and N-terminus are located inside the cytosol and contain a sulphate transporter/antisigma factor antagonist domain (Royaux et al., 2000). PDS was identified as the most important transporter for iodide export but its unique role is questioned because patients with biallelic mutation display only mild thyroid symptoms and PDS knock-out mice do not develop goiter (Wolff, 2005). On the other hand, TSH stimulates iodide transport across the apical membrane (Nilsson et al., 1990) and induces a rapid translocation of PDS from endosomes to the plasma membrane (Kopp et al., 2008) suggesting a causative link between translocation and iodide metabolism. Efflux by an additional transporter is hypothesized: the formerly named apical iodide transporter (AIT), which has been re-named to sodium/monocarboxylate transporter (SMCT), has been removed from the list of potential candidates (Paroder et al., 2006).

Extrathyroidal expression of PDS is more restricted than that of NIS. Expression has been detected in kidney, Sertoli cells, inner ear, mammary gland and placenta (Lacroix et al., 2001; Wangemann et al., 2004)

PTCs without iodide uptake have slightly reduced NIS and significantly reduced Tg, TPO and PDS levels (Mian et al., 2008). This shows that loss in iodide uptake depends not only on NIS function but also on other molecules in the intracellular thyroid metabolism. Together with NIS, PDS and Tg, TPO expression is decreased in PTC with BRAF mutation (Durante et al., 2007).

4.3 Thyroperoxidase (TPO)

TPO is a glycosylated transmembrane hemoprotein, which uses H_2O_2 as cofactor and catalyses the oxidation of iodide to iodines and the attachment of oxidized iodines to certain tyrosine residues on the protein Tg, producing 3-iodotyrosine (MIT) and 3,5'- diiodotyrosine (DIT). Thirdly, TPO and H_2O_2 are further used to couple two DIT residues, or one MIT with one DIT residue, to produce T4 or T3 and rT3, respectively (Dunn & Dunn, 2001). Expression of TPO is regulated by the transcription factors TTF-1, TTF-2 and Pax-8. Estrogen stimulates TPO in addition to NIS in rats (Lima et al., 2006). The action of estradiol is variable and depends on the gonadal status and the age of the animal.

Cancers with no iodide uptake contain approx. 30-fold less TPO and 20 fold less PDS (Mian et al., 2008). These TCs have a high frequency of BRAF mutation and 5-fold Glut-1 expression. TPO in TC is suppressed on the mRNA and on the protein level (Tanaka et al., 1996).

4.4 Thyroglobulin (Tg)

Tg is a large (660kD) dimeric protein, forming the main protein compound of the follicular colloid. Despite variable correlation of Tg levels and metastatic status, Tg mRNA in blood serves as a marker for TC and as follow-up of removed DTC. mRNA of Tg is significantly lower in TC and in adenoma and the decreases correlate to those in TSH-R mRNA. By contrast, mRNA of TPO showed no marked differences between normal and transformed thyroid tissues (Ohta et al., 1991). By other authors, levels of Tg mRNA varying from normal to complete loss in TC were reported (Brabant et al., 1991; Hoang-Vu et al., 1992)

4.5 TSH-receptor (TSH-R)

TSH and TSH-R are required for proliferation of thyrocytes and expression of differentiation markers like NIS (Garcia-Jimenez & Santisteban, 2007). The TSH-R is a 7-transmembrane spanning glycoprotein, also expressed in bone, brain, kidney, testes and cells of the immune system. In the extrathyroidal tissues its role is not clear (Matsumoto et al., 2008). TSH-R molecules are quite stable in the membrane and signalling occurs through TSH-binding. TSH activates the TSH-R and G-proteins such as G_S-alpha at the surface of thyrocytes. Intracellular production of cyclic AMP by adenylyl cyclase stimulates the cAMP-dependent protein kinase A, which in turn phosphorylates cytoplasmic and nuclear target proteins. One substrate is the nuclear transcription factor CREB, which activates the transcription of cAMP-responsive genes after being phosphorylated by PKA. TSH, at much higher levels, acts via phospholipase C and the phosphatidyl-inositol/Ca^{2+} signalling cascade with activation of protein kinase C (Hard, 1998). The cAMP pathway is functionally responsible for cell proliferation, iodide uptake, Tg and TPO expression, whereas the phosphatidyl-inositol/Ca^{2+} signalling pathway stimulates generation of hydrogen peroxide and iodide efflux. Insulin and IGF-1 control TSH-R and Tg gene expression in rats and are necessary co-factors for TSH in most species. Iodide, or the organic intermediate 2-iodohexadecanal, inhibits adenylate cyclase, TPO and NADPH oxidase. Another intermediate, the δ iodolactone 6-iodo-5-hydroxy-8,11,14- eicosatrienoic acid inhibits specifically IP3 formation induced by growth factors. The receptor is hyperactivated in adenoma, less expressed in DTC and silenced in ATC. Inactivating mutations of the TSH-R have been reported in TC but appear not to be related to tumor onset but to be a marker of the ongoing de-differentiation. Activating mutations have been reported in some TC (Cetani et al., 1999,Esapa et al., 1997). Expression of TSH-R is similar in cancer and in thyroid adenoma tissues and the mRNA levels are only slightly decreased compared to normal thyroid tissue (Lazar et al., 1999). Reduced expression of TSH-R protein was seen only in high risk PTC (Tanaka et al., 1997) and low protein levels of TSH-R correlate with high proliferation (high Mib-1 index) in poorly differentiated TC (Matsumoto et al., 2008). TSH-R expression decreases to a lesser extent in cancer tissues than other thyroid-specific proteins like NIS, TPO and Tg. Defective TSH-R cAMP signalling in FTC thyroid cancer cell lines (Demeure et al., 1997) and impairment in signal transduction have been demonstrated in TC (Kimura et al., 1992)

4.6 Molecular candidates for re-expression of thyroid-specific proteins

Re-expression of thyroid-specific proteins in thyroid cancer is expected to increase iodide uptake and thereby increase the efficacy of radioiodine treatment. For the re-induction of thyroid-specific genes, the following nuclear targets are the most promising candidates:

Retinoic acid receptors are crucial for the differentiation of tissues. Retinoids act as chemopreventive agents and increase differentiation in a variety of cancers.

Peroxisome proliferator-activated receptor gamma (PPAR-γ) activation leads to activation of PTEN, which inhibits PI3K. DTCs show a decreased expression of this receptor, therefore PPAR-γ agonists may have a beneficial effect.

Histone deacetylases and **DNA methylases** prevent transcription of genes linked to differentiation. Inhibitors of these enzymes may lead to re-differentiation.

5. Compounds for re-differentiation

5.1 Retinoids (RT)

Retinoids, retinol and its derivatives, act on the nuclear receptors retinoic acid receptor (RAR) and retinoid X receptor (RXR). Retinoids are related to vitamin A and three generations of retinoids have been developed so far. First generation retinoids include retinol, retinal, retinoic acid (all-trans RA, 9-cis RA and 13-cis RA) and isoretinon, second generation retinoids were etretinate and acitretin and third generation retinoids comprise tazarotene and bexarotene. The naturally occurring retinoids all-trans RA, 9-cis RA and 13-cis RA are interconverted in vivo. Thyrocytes mainly express receptors for RAR-α and RXR-γ. RXR-β expression was reduced in the majority of poorly differentiated and anaplastic cell lines and tumor samples (Schmutzler et al., 1998). Retinoids can act through homodimers of retinoid receptors or as heterodimers of the RXR receptor with the PPAR-γ receptor (Figure 3). It is hypothesized that retinoids upregulate NIS expression mainly by activation of RAR (Kogai et al., 2004).

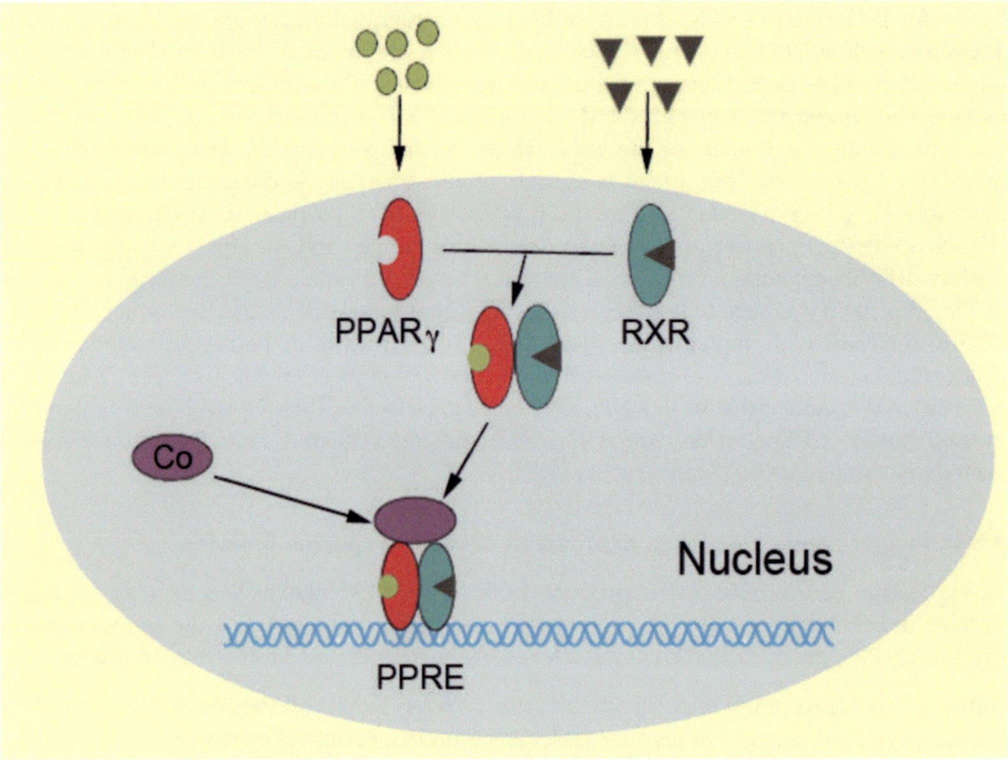

Fig. 3. Retinoids bind to the RXR/PPAR-γ receptor dimer and this heterodimer binds to peroxisome proliferator response elements (PPRE). Subsequently, a co-activator, possessing histone acetylase activity, attaches to the complex (Co) and induces gene transcription.

5.1.1 Compounds in clinical trials

Retinoids increased expression of thyroid-specific proteins (Schreck et al., 1994; Schmutzler et al., 1997; Kurebayashi et al., 2000; Jeong et al., 2006) and increased iodide uptake (van Herle et al., 1990). As retinoids were already approved for other indications, clinical trials were initiated. Varying results were obtained with isotretinoin **Accutane®, Roaccutane®** (13-cis-RA): iodide uptake was restored in 40% in the study by Simon et al. (Simon et al., 2002) but most other studies achieved much lower rates in the increase (Grunwald et al., 1998; Gruning et al., 2003; Kim et al., 2009). Similar inconsistent increases in iodide uptake were obtained by the use of tretinoin **Vesanoid®** (all-trans retinoic acid) and of **Targretine®** (bexarotene, Simon et al., 1996; Simon et al., 1998; Schmutzler & Kohrle, 2000; Simon et al., 2002; Coelho et al., 2004;

Short et al., 2004; Liu et al., 2006; Zhang et al., 2007). The expression of RAR-β and RXR-γ could serve as an indicator for the response to RA treatment but based on existing studies, retinoids alone appear not to be an effective therapy for radioiodine-refractory thyroid cancer.

5.1.2 Pre-clinical compounds

9-cis RA and retinol were both less well studied for application in TC. 9-cis RA was shown to induce cell cycle arrest and re-expression of RAR-β in TC cells (Fan et al., 2009) and retinol induced iodide uptake in differentiated cancer cell lines but had a low anti-proliferative effect (Fröhlich et al., 2009). Although retinol, compared to RA, shows a lower rate of adverse effects (e.g. Fluhr et al., 1999), the different intracellular concentrations of the active metabolite due to variations in serum retinol binding protein, in cellular transport proteins and in the activity of intracellular dehydrogenases diminishes its suitability as drug candidate in the treatment of TC.

5.2 Thiazolidinediones (TZDs)

Peroxisome proliferator-activated receptors (PPARs) are transcription factors belonging to the superfamily of nuclear receptors and related to the receptors for retinoic acid, estrogen, thyroid hormone, vitamin D and glucocorticoids. The three members of the PPAR family are PPAR-α, PPAR-β/δ and PPAR-γ. All members regulate energy metabolism. PPAR-γ promotes differentiation of mesenchymal stem cells into adipocytes and osteoclasts and plays a role in tumorigenesis (Wan, 2010). Rearrangements of PPAR-γ/PAX-8 occur in 36% to 45.5% of FTC and in 37.5% of follicular variants of PTC (Nikiforova et al., 2003; Castro et al., 2006). The rearrangement induces inactivation of PPAR-γ function. PPAR agonists bind to PPAR-γ and form a heterodimer with the RXR receptor at the response elements, activating the transcription of target genes (Figure 4). PPAR-γ is involved in the differentiation of pre-adipocytes. Ligands of PPAR-γ inhibit growth in PTC cell lines (Ohta et al., 2001). The growth inhibiting effect is not correlated to the degree of expression of PPAR-γ suggesting that mechanisms independent from signalling through this receptor are involved in the differentiating action of PPAR-γ agonists (Klopper et al., 2004).

5.2.1 Compounds in clinical trials

Clinical studies with **Avandia®** (rosiglitazone) showed increased radioiodide uptake in therapeutic ^{131}I scans (Kebebew et al., 2006; Tepmongkol et al., 2008). A current trial with rosiglitazone is ongoing and results are expected in the near future (www.clinicaltrial.gov). As PPAR-γ and RXRs form heterodimers there is the hope that, similar to results in other cancer types (Mehta et al., 2000), combinations of retinoids with TZDs may act synergistically. Based on data of an increased risk for cardiovascular events, however, the European Medicine Agency (EMA) has recommended in 9/2010 the withdrawl of all rosiglitazone-containing medications from the market.

5.2.2 Pre-clinical compounds

In vitro studies with troglitazone and rosiglitazone show that TZDs decrease proliferation and increase apoptosis and iodide uptake (Fröhlich et al., 2005). The anti-tumor effect of pioglitazone was much weaker than that of troglitazone and rosiglitazone. Also in primary cultured ATC cells **Actos®** (pioglitazone) reduced proliferation to a lesser extent than rosiglitazone (Antonelli et al., 2009). **Rezulin®** (troglitazone) was the most effective compound regarding re-differentiation (Fröhlich et al., 2005) but its use in the treatment of TC is prevented by the withdrawal of the drug from the market due to severe liver toxicity. Another new agent, Ciglitazone induced decreased proliferation and increased apoptosis in a panel of TC cell lines with PPAR-γ expression (Martelli et al., 2002).

5.3 Epigenetic alterations

Epigenetic alterations are changes around the gene that alter gene expression. These changes include histone modifications and DNA methylation (Figure 4). Transcriptionally active chromatin regions are hyperacetylated and hypomethylated. Epigenetic alterations in tumor cells often result in silencing of genes involved in cell differentiation. Transcription factors generally act on un-methylated promoters at local sites where histones are acetylated. The silencing of a gene may result from the binding of methyl-binding proteins (e.g. MeCP2) to methylated cytosines, which recruits histone deacetylases (HDAC). Hyperacetylated histones activate a pre-programmed set of genes that leads to cell cycle arrest, differentiation and apoptosis (inhibition of tumor growth). HDAC inhibitors may contribute to the removal of MeCP2 from methylated cytosines and allow histone acetylase to re-acetylate histones at gene promoter. Hyperacetylated histones may recruit DNA demethylase and further provide

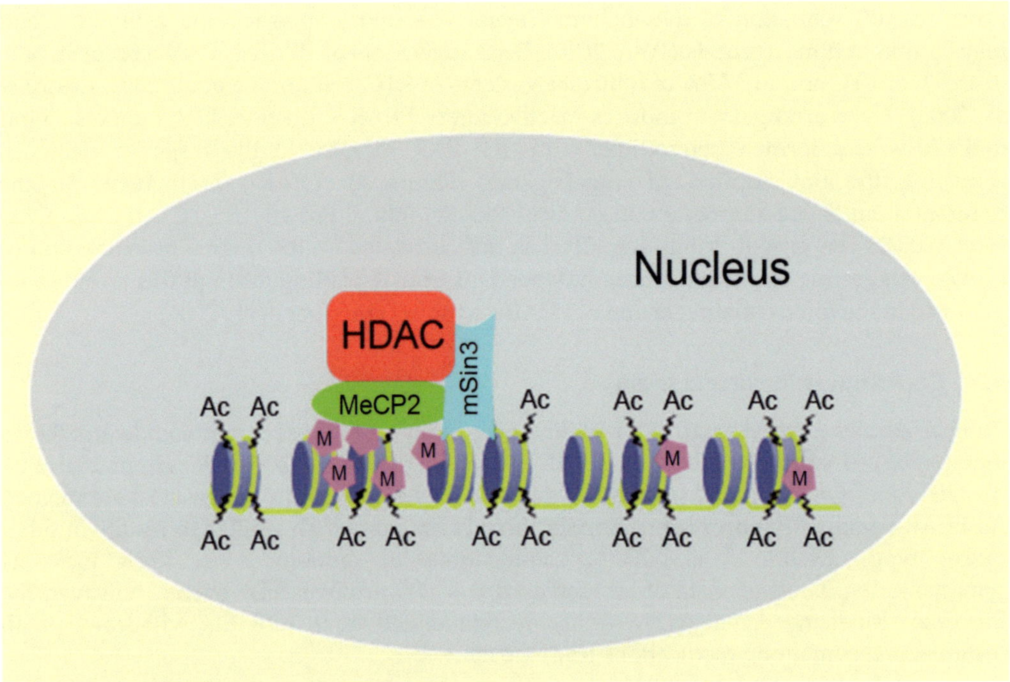

Fig. 4. Epigenetic changes include addition of acetyl-groups (Ac) by the action of histone acetylase and methylation of DNA (M) by DNA methyltransferase. The multiprotein repressor complex binds predominantly at cytosine- and guanine- rich DNA regions and consists of methyl-CpG-binding protein 2 and mammalian transcriptional repressor mSin3 and histone deacetylase (HDAC).

protection from DNA methylation. Inversely, demethylating agents can re-establish an active state by inducing the acetylation of histone. Via this mechanism inhibitiors of HDAC and of DNA methyltransferase could induce re-differentiation in thyroid cancer cells.

5.3.1 Histone deacetylase inhibitors (HDI)

In a nucleosome a DNA fragment is wrapped around a complex of histones (pair of H2A, H2B, H3 and H4). Acetylation occurs at lysine residues of the proteins. Deacetylation generates positively charged residues, which facilitate binding of histones to DNA leading to tightly packed chromatin. Thereby, binding to the promotor is prevented and gene transcription repressed (Xing, 2007). Genes silenced in TC include RAS, SF1A (signalling protein involved in RAS), tissue inhibitors of metalloproteinases, SLC5A8 (sodium coupled monocarboxylate transporter 1) as putative iodide transporter at the apical membrane), DARK (death associated protein kinase) and RAR-β2.

5.3.1.1 Compounds of HDI in clinical trials

Suberoyl anile hydroxamic acid (SAHA, vorinostat [rINN]) is the most advanced compound of this group for treatment of TC. In ATC and DTC cell lines significant increases in NIS expression and decreased growth rates were recorded (Fortunati et al., 2004). In one clinical study evaluating SAHA, patients with metastatic TC were included. One out of five patients showed an improved iodide uptake (Kelly et al., 2005). Based on these promising results a phase II trial with SAHA, approved by the FDA as **Zolinza®**, was initiated. Medication resulted in slightly more patients with stable disease than with progressive disease (Woyach et al., 2008). In a phase II study romidepsin, a depsipeptide with the trade name **Istodax®** (FK 228, FR 901228), restored radioiodine avidity in 2 of the 20 patients treated, but there were no objective responses even after ^{131}I treatment (Sherman et al., 2009). A phase II study on the new hydroxamic acid derived histone deacetylase inhibitor **panobinostat/panbinostat®** (LBH589) is currently recruiting participants. The recruitment status of a phase II study on **Depakene®** (valproic acid) initiated in 2007, is unknown (http://www.clinicaltrials.gov).

5.3.1.2 Pre-clinical compounds

Encouraging results on differentiated and poorly differentiated thyroid carcinoma cell lines were also obtained with other HDIs.

Trichostatin A® acted pro-apoptotic and increased NIS mRNA expression in TC cell lines (Puppin et al., 2005; Shen & Chung, 2005; Kondo et al., 2009). mRNA expression of PDS was reduced by trichostatin A treatment (Zarnegar et al., 2002).

Entinostat® (SNDX275, MS 275) restored functional NIS activity in FTC and ATO cell lines 20- 45 fold (Altmann et al., 2010).

Phenylacetate (Ammonul®) increased iodide uptake and decreased secretion of Tg in two of the five evaluated TC cell lines (Kebebew et al., 1999). The inhibition of Tg secretion was interpreted as increase in intracellular accumulation of this protein.

Apicidine and APHA compound 8 demonstrated a similar mode of action as valproic acid: all compounds strongly increased iodide-uptake with only a weak effect on proliferation (Fröhlich et al., 2009).

5.3.1.3 Combinations of HDIs with other compounds

SAHA in combination with the mTOR inhibitor temsirolimus and the Akt and PI3K inhibitor perifosine showed a strong synergistic effect on NIS expression and on TSH receptor expression (Hou et al., 2010). The expression of the latter raised hope that the tumors would become responsive to TSH, which together with a functional NIS could enhance iodide uptake markedly. Other studies also suggested strong synergistic effects between HDIs and other compounds: ATRA in combination with tributyrin strongly enhanced NIS mRNA and protein expression and radioiodine uptake in FTC133 cells (Zhang et al., 2011). Although no increases were obtained in TSH-R and TPO mRNA expression upon combined treatment of vitamin D3 and SAHA, growth arrest was achieved in several poorly differentiated cells (Clinckspoor et al., 2011).

5.3.2 Inhibitors of DNA methyltransferase (DMI)

Upon DNA methylation CH_3 groups are added to the fifth carbon position of the pyrimidine ring of cytosine residue in a CpG dinucleotide. CpG islands (regions rich in CpG dinucleotides) are usually located in the 5′ flanking promotor areas of genes. Gene promotor methylation near the transcription start site is usually associated with gene silencing (Xing, 2007). Methylated cytosine residues are bound by methyl-binding proteins that subsequently recruit HDACs and histone methytransferases, forming a complex with mSin3, a mammalian transcriptional co-repressor. In thyroid carcinoma cells TTF-1, the key transcription factor for thyroid-specific genes (Tg, TPO, TSH-R, PDS and NIS), is silenced by hypermethylation.

5.3.2.1 Compounds in clinical trials

A phase II trial on **Vidaza®** (5-azacytidine) in metastatic TC has been completed and results will be published soon. A phase II study on **Decitabine®** (5-Aza-2′-deoxycytidine) is listed as ongoing clinical trial evaluating re-differentiation for TC (http://www.clinicaltrials.gov).

5-Azacytidine was able to restore Tg expression in Ras-transfected TC lines (Avvedimento et al., 1989). In a study on mRNA expression of NIS, Tg, TPO and TSH-R and on iodide uptake in the PTC cell line B-CPAP, 5-Azacytidine compared to ATRA and trichostatin was very effective: it was the only compound, which increased iodide uptake (Tuncel et al., 2007). Also 5-Aza-2′-deoxycytidine increased differentiation and restored NIS expression in FTC, PTC and ATC cell lines (Kondo et al., 2009). 5-Aza-2′-deoxycytidine also induced mRNA expression of type I iodothyronine-5′-deiodinase, another thyroid-specific protein (Mentrup et al., 2002).

5.3.2.2 Combinations with other agents

Combination with retinoids may increase the efficacy of the treatment because 5-Aza-2′-deoxycytidine induced re-expression of the RAR-β receptor (Miasaki et al., 2008). 5-Azacytidine and RA together induced re-expression of differentiation-related proteins. In the human TC cell line FRO, TTF-1 and thyroglobulin were increased; in TT and WRO cell lines Pax-8 was increased; and in FRO and TT cell lines RAR-β and NIS mRNA were increased. Iodide uptake, however, was not increased and NIS localized in the cytoplasm

(Vivaldi et al., 2009). 5-Azacytidine and sodium butyrate increase NIS mRNA and iodide uptake in DRO cells. The NIS promotor region is often methylated and iodide-uptake apparently can be restored by the reversal of epigenetic changes (Venkataraman et al., 1999).

5.4 Other strategies for re-differentiation

Several compounds have been investigated in a less systematic way for their action in TC. In this section, compounds, belonging to other classes but displaying positive effects on TC cell lines and in patients, are discussed. Since mRNA expression of NIS alone may not reflect protein levels and, even if the protein is expressed, it may not be correctly localized and not be functional, it is difficult to predict whether these compounds will have beneficial effects in clinical trials.

5.4.1 Pre-clinical compounds

5.4.1.1 Lovastatin '(e.g. Mevacor®)

This inhibitor of 3-hydroxy-3-methyl-glutaryl-CoA reductase is used for lowering cholesterol in hypercholesterolemia to prevent cardiovascular disease. Inhibition of protein prenylation by lovastatin has anti-proliferative effects in normal and transformed thyrocytes (Bifulco et al., 1999) and reduced growth and invasion and caused re-differentiation in ATC cell lines by increasing Tg expression (Wang et al., 2003; Zhong et al., 2005). Lovastatin reduced proliferation but did not increase iodide uptake in cell lines derived from DTC (Fröhlich et al., 2009) and reduced the growth of ATCs in mouse xenografts (Wang et al., 2010).

5.4.1.2 1,25-dihydroxyvitamin D(3) (VitD3) '(e.g. Rocaltrol®)

VitD3 acts through nuclear receptors expressed in most cell types. In addition to its main function on calcium and bone metabolism, the hormone also acts on proliferation, apoptosis and differentiation of cells. VitD3 appears to be a good target for cancer therapy because decreased levels have been demonstrated in breast, prostate and colon cancer. The situation in TC is not clear: whereas one study reported normal VitD3 levels in TC patients, another study reported decreased VitD3 levels in TC, though not in goiter patients (Laney et al., 2010; Stepien et al., 2010). In cancers with proven deficiency VitD3 shows cytostatic effects and was tested successfully in a phase II clinical trial on prostate cancer (Srinivas & Feldman, 2009). VitD3 reduced tumor growth and increased differentiation (NIS and Tg mRNA) in vitro and in tumor xenografts (Drackiw et al. 2004; Okano et al. 1994; Akagi et al., 2008). In combination with SAHA, VitD3 showed growth arrest but no effects on mRNA expression of TSH-R and of TPO in ATC cell lines (Clinckspoor et al., 2007).

5.4.1.3 Arsenic trioxide (ATO)

Clinical-grade ATO, **Trisenox®**, is used as second-line therapy in retinoic acid refractive acute promyelocytic leukemia (Shen et al., 1997). In the treatment of solid cancers, however ATO is not routinely used and only few clinical trials, like a phase II trial on hormone-refractory prostate cancer, have been successfully performed (Gallagher et al., 2004). ATO acts by multiple mechanisms: depletion of glutathione, increase of reactive oxygen species, loss of mitochondrial potential and activation of caspase (Miller, 2002). Akt/protein kinase B pathway is also involved in the action. In several cell lines of differentiated TC the compounds reduced proliferation and increased apoptosis and iodide uptake (Fröhlich et al., 2008). Protein levels of NIS and PDS were not changed but in ATO-treated cells PDS displayed a polarized expression pattern. Depletion of glutathione increased the differentiating effect of ATO while Akt-inhibitors did not. Independent of the proliferation rate, ATO significantly decreased glucose uptake in TC cells as one additional mechanism of its multi-modal action.

5.4.1.4 Gene therapy

Transfection of TTF-1 and NIS together by an adenoviral vector into ATC cells achieved significant retention of iodide, whereas transfection with TTF-1 alone induced re-expression of TPO and Tg but not of NIS (Furuya et al., 2004). In extrathyroidal tissues, where no organification of iodide can occur, promising results were obtained. Re-circulation of iodide in the blood circulation of the liver results in high iodide-uptake rates and retention despite high efflux of iodide from the cells (Faivre et al., 2004). The successful introduction of functional and localized NIS was also demonstrated in dog prostate glands (Dwyer et al., 2005). Stable transfection of thyroid cancer cells with Pax8 leads to recovery of iodide uptake (Presta et al., 2005) but transfection with TPO is not sufficient to restore iodide trapping in ATC cell lines (Haberkorn et al., 2001).

5.4.1.5 Phosphatidylinositol-3-kinase inhibitors (PI3K inhibitors)/Akt-inhibitors

These agents are used in the treatment of several solid cancers but efficacy has not been shown in in-vivo studies for TC. PI3K-inhibition increased functional expression of NIS in FRTL-5 and PTC cell lines (de Souza et al., 2010) and the PI3K inhibitor LY294002 increased iodide accumulation in TC lines (Furuya et al., 2007). In parallel to increased iodide uptake, this inhibitor increased the expression of PAX-8, suggesting a posttranslational stimulation effect on NIS (Kogai et al., 2008). In the same study the Akt1/Akt2 selective inhibitor Akti-1/2 increased the expression of NIS-transfected TC cells not significantly. In non-transfected TC cell lines the re-differentiating effects of Akt inhibitor I (hydroxymethyl-chiro-inositol 2-(R)-2-O- methyl-3-O-octadecylcarbonate) and Akt inhibitor V (triciribine) were small (Fröhlich et al., 2008): the inhibitors showed an anti-proliferative effect but no increase in iodide uptake was seen. It appears that other Akt-inhibitors (e.g. KP372-1 and MK2206) also markedly reduce cell growth in various TC cell lines but have little effect on the expression of thyroid specific proteins (Mandal et al., 2005; Liu et al., 2011). Only in combination with MAPK inhibition Akt-inhibitors significantly induced NIS mRNA expression in several TC cell lines (Hou et al., 2007).

5.4.2 Compounds in clinical trials

5.4.2.1 Lithium

Eskalith®, Lithobid (lithium carbonate) is used in the treatment of manic depression and depressive disorders. It also causes an increased retention of iodide due to inhibition of the efflux of iodide leaving uptake of iodide unaffected (Temple et al., 1972). Despite causing an increase in radioiodine uptake, no beneficial effect was recorded in several studies on patients with metastatic DTC (Gershengorn et al., 1976; Pons et al., 1987; Koong et al., 1999; Liu et al., 2006).

5.4.2.2 Reverse transcriptase inhibitors

Reverse transcriptase inhibitors like **Sustiva®** (efavirenz) and **Viramune®** (nevirapine) are part of the antiretroviral therapy for the treatment of human immunodeficiency virus type 1 infection and AIDS. In addition, these compounds increase gene expression of TSH-R, thyroglobulin, TPO and NIS in the ATC lines (Landriscina et al., 2005). In a case report, up-regulation of Tg and NIS was shown in a patient treated with nevirapine resulting in improved survival of the patient with PTC. (Modoni et al., 2007).

6. Conclusion

Although DTC is generally regarded as a less problematic tumor, metastatic DTC has a poor prognosis and is unresponsive to conventional treatments. Novel therapies include inhibitors of various growth factor tyrosine kinases and of kinases involved in dys-regulated intracellular signalling. In addition, re-expression of thyroid specific proteins, mainly NIS, by retinoids, PPAR-γ agonists as well as DNA methyltransferase and histone deacetylase inhibitors have potential as novel therapies.

The TKIs sorafenib and sunitinib have entered clinical trials and appear to induce disease stabilization in treated patients. Differentiation therapy with retinoids did not live up to expected outcomes. The results of clinical trials with TZDs and HDIs are not yet known, though combination therapy with HDIs and conventional chemotherapy has shown promising early results. The final evaluation of these compounds is complicated by the fact that the achievement of stable disease cannot be regarded as a great success as many DTC do not progress rapidly any way. The inclusion of patients who only have progressive disease into clinical trials could enhance the clinical value of the induction of stable disease.

7. References

Akagi, T., Luong, Q. T., Gui, D., Said, J., Selektar, J., Yung, A., Bunce, C. M., Braunstein, G. D. & Koeffler, H. P. (2008). Induction of sodium iodide symporter gene and molecular characterisation of HNF3 beta/FoxA2, TTF-1 and C/EBP beta in thyroid carcinoma cells. *British Journal of Cancer*, Vol. 99, No 5, (Sepember 2008), pp. 781-788, ISSN 1532-1827

Altmann, A., Eisenhut, M., Bauder-Wust, U., Markert, A., Askoxylakis, V., Hess-Stumpp, H. & Haberkorn, U. (2010). Therapy of thyroid carcinoma with the histone deacetylase inhibitor MS-275. *European Journal of Nuclear Medicine and Molecular Imaging*, Vol. 37, No 12, (December 2010), pp. 2286-2297, ISSN 1619-7089

Antonelli, A., Ferrari, S. M., Fallahi, P., Berti, P., Materazzi, G., Minuto, M., Giannini, R., Marchetti, I., Barani, L., Basolo, F., Ferrannini, E. & Miccoli, P. (2009). Thiazolidinediones and antiblastics in primary human anaplastic thyroid cancer cells. *Clinical Endocrinology*, Vol. 70, No 6, (June 2009), pp. 946-953, ISSN 1365-2265

Arturi, F., Russo, D., Schlumberger, M., du Villard, J. A., Caillou, B., Vigneri, P., Wicker, R., Chiefari, E., Suarez, H. G. & Filetti, S. (1998). Iodide symporter gene expression in human thyroid tumors. *Journal of Clinical Endocrinology and Metabolism*, Vol. 83, No 7, (July 1998), pp. 2493-2496, ISSN 0021-972X

Avvedimento, E. V., Obici, S., Sanchez, M., Gallo, A., Musti, A. & Gottesman, M. E. (1989). Reactivation of thyroglobulin gene expression in transformed thyroid cells by 5-azacytidine. *Cell*, Vol. 58, No 6, (September 1989), pp. 1135-1142, ISSN 0092-8674

Bifulco, M., Laezza, C. & Aloj, S. M. (1999). Inhibition of farnesylation blocks growth but not differentiation in FRTL-5 thyroid cells. *Biochimie*, Vol. 81, No 4, (April 1999), pp. 287-290, ISSN 0300-9084

Boltze, C., Schneider-Stock, R., Roessner, A., Quednow, C. & Hoang-Vu, C. (2003). Function of HSP90 and p23 in the telomerase complex of thyroid tumors. *Pathology, Research and Practice*, Vol. 199, No 9, 2003), pp. 573-579, ISSN 0344-0338

Brabant, G., Maenhaut, C., Kohrle, J., Scheumann, G., Dralle, H., Hoang-Vu, C., Hesch, R. D., von zur Muhlen, A., Vassart, G. & Dumont, J. E. (1991). Human thyrotropin receptor gene: expression in thyroid tumors and correlation to markers of thyroid differentiation and dedifferentiation. *Molecular and Cellular Endocrinology*, Vol. 82, No 1, (November 1991), pp. R7-12, ISSN 7500844

Brewer, C., Yeager, N. & Di Cristofano, A. (2007). Thyroid-stimulating hormone initiated proliferative signals converge in vivo on the mTOR kinase without activating AKT. *Cancer Research*, Vol. 67, No 17, (Sepember 2007), pp. 8002-8006, ISSN 0008-5472

Castro, P., Rebocho, A. P., Soares, R. J., Magalhaes, J., Roque, L., Trovisco, V., Vieira de Castro, I., Cardoso-de-Oliveira, M., Fonseca, E., Soares, P. & Sobrinho-Simoes, M. (2006). PAX8-PPARgamma rearrangement is frequently detected in the follicular variant of papillary thyroid carcinoma. *Journal of Clinical Endocrinology and Metabolism*, Vol. 91, No 1, (January 2006), pp. 213-220, ISSN 0021-972X

Cetani, F., Tonacchera, M., Pinchera, A., Barsacchi, R., Basolo, F., Miccoli, P. & Pacini, F. (1999). Genetic analysis of the TSH receptor gene in differentiated human thyroid carcinomas. *Journal of Endocrinological Investigation*, Vol. 22, No 4, (April 1999), pp. 273-278, ISSN 0391-4097

Clinckspoor, I., Verlinden, L., Overbergh, L., Korch, C., Bouillon, R., Mathieu, C., Verstuyf, A. & Decallonne, B. (2011). 1,25-dihydroxyvitamin D3 and a superagonistic analog in combination with paclitaxel or suberoylanilide hydroxamic acid have potent antiproliferative effects on anaplastic thyroid cancer. *Journal of Steroid Biochemistry and Molecular Biology*, Vol. 124, No 1-2, (March 2011), pp. 1-9, ISSN 1879-1220

Clinckspoor, I., Verlinden, L., Verstuyf, M., Bouillon, R. & Decallonne, B. (2007). Effects of 1,25(OH)2D3 and analog WY1112 on proliferation and differentiation of FRO cells. Annual Meeting of the European Thyroid Association Leipzig, Hormone Research.

Coelho, S., Corbo, R., Buescu, A., Carvalho, D. & Vaisman, M. (2004). Retinoic acid in patients with radioiodine non-responsive thyroid carcinoma. *Journal of Endocrinological Investigation*, Vol. 27, No 4, (April 2004), pp. 334-339, ISSN 0391-4097

Coelho, S. M., Carvalho, D. P. & Vaisman, M. (2007). New perspectives on the treatment of differentiated thyroid cancer. *Arquivos brasileiros de endocrinologia e metabologia*, Vol. 51, No 4, (June 2007), pp. 612-624, ISSN 0004-2730

Dackiw, A. P., Ezzat, S., Huang, P., Liu, W. & Asa, S. L. (2004). Vitamin D3 administration induces nuclear p27 accumulation, restores differentiation, and reduces tumor burden in a mouse model of metastatic follicular thyroid cancer. *Endocrinology*, Vol. 145, No 12, (December 2004), pp. 5840-5846, ISSN 0013-7227 de Souza, E. C., Padron, A. S., Braga, W. M., de Andrade, B. M., Vaisman, M., Nasciutti, L. E., Ferreira, A. C. & de Carvalho, D. P. (2010). MTOR downregulates iodide uptake in thyrocytes. *Journal of Endocrinology*, Vol. 206, No 1, (July 2010), pp. 113-120, ISSN 1479-6805

Demeure, M. J., Doffek, K. M. & Wilson, S. D. (1997). Defective thyrotropin receptor G-protein cyclic adenosine monophosphate signaling mechanism in the FTC human follicular thyroid cancer cell line. *Surgery*, Vol. 122, No 6, (December 1997), pp. 1195-1201, ISSN 1365-2168

Di Renzo, M. F., Olivero, M., Ferro, S., Prat, M., Bongarzone, I., Pilotti, S., Belfiore, A., Costantino, A., Vigneri, R., Pierotti, M. A. & et al. (1992). Overexpression of the c-MET/HGF receptor gene in human thyroid carcinomas. *Oncogene*, Vol. 7, No 12, (Dec 1992), pp. 2549-2553, ISSN 0950-9232

Dohan, O., Baloch, Z., Banrevi, Z., Livolsi, V. & Carrasco, N. (2001). Rapid communication: predominant intracellular overexpression of the Na(+)/I(-) symporter (NIS) in a large sampling of thyroid cancer cases. *Journal of Clinical Endocrinology and Metabolism*, Vol. 86, No 6, (Jun 2001), pp. 2697-2700, ISSN 0021-972X

Dohan, O., De la Vieja, A., Paroder, V., Riedel, C., Artani, M., Reed, M., Ginter, C. S. & Carrasco, N. (2003). The sodium/iodide Symporter (NIS): characterization, regulation, and medical significance. *Endocrine Reviews*, Vol. 24, No 1, (February 2003), pp. 48-77, ISSN 0163-769X

Dunn, J. T. & Dunn, A. D. (2001). Update on intrathyroidal iodine metabolism. *Thyroid : official journal of the American Thyroid Association*, Vol. 11, No 5, (May 2001), pp. 407-414, ISSN 1050-7256

Durante, C., Haddy, N., Baudin, E., Leboulleux, S., Hartl, D., Travagli, J. P., Caillou, B., Ricard, M., Lumbroso, J. D., De Vathaire, F. & Schlumberger, M. (2006). Long-term outcome of 444 patients with distant metastases from papillary and follicular thyroid carcinoma: benefits and limits of radioiodine therapy. *Journal of Clinical Endocrinology and Metabolism*, Vol. 91, No 8, (August 2006), pp. 2892-2899, ISSN 0021-972X

Durante, C., Puxeddu, E., Ferretti, E., Morisi, R., Moretti, S., Bruno, R., Barbi, F., Avenia, N., Scipioni, A., Verrienti, A., Tosi, E., Cavaliere, A., Gulino, A., Filetti, S. & Russo, D. (2007). BRAF mutations in papillary thyroid carcinomas inhibit genes involved in iodine metabolism. *Journal of Clinical Endocrinology and Metabolism*, Vol. 92, No 7, (July 2007), pp. 2840-2843, ISSN 0021-972X

Dwyer, R. M., Schatz, S. M., Bergert, E. R., Myers, R. M., Harvey, M. E., Classic, K. L., Blanco, M. C., Frisk, C. S., Marler, R. J., Davis, B. J., O'Connor, M. K., Russell, S. J. & Morris, J. C. (2005). A preclinical large animal model of adenovirus-mediated expression of the sodium-iodide symporter for radioiodide imaging and therapy of locally recurrent prostate cancer. *Molecular Therapy*, Vol. 12, No 5, (November 2005), pp. 835-841, ISSN 1525-0016

Elisei, R., Vivaldi, A., Ciampi, R., Faviana, P., Basolo, F., Santini, F., Traino, C., Pacini, F. & Pinchera, A. (2006). Treatment with drugs able to reduce iodine efflux significantly increases the intracellular retention time in thyroid cancer cells stably transfected with sodium iodide symporter complementary deoxyribonucleic acid. *Journal of Clinical Endocrinology and Metabolism*, Vol. 91, No 6, (June 2006), pp. 2389-2395, ISSN 0021-972X

Esapa, C., Foster, S., Johnson, S., Jameson, J. L., Kendall-Taylor, P. & Harris, P. E. (1997). G protein and thyrotropin receptor mutations in thyroid neoplasia. *Journal of Clinical Endocrinology and Metabolism*, Vol. 82, No 2, (February 1997), pp. 493-496, ISSN 0021-972X

Eustatia-Rutten, C. F., Corssmit, E. P., Biermasz, N. R., Pereira, A. M., Romijn, J. A. & Smit, J. W. (2006). Survival and death causes in differentiated thyroid carcinoma. *Journal of Clinical Endocrinology and Metabolism*, Vol. 91, No 1, (January 2006), pp. 313-319, ISSN 0021-972X

Fagin, J. A. (2004). Challenging dogma in thyroid cancer molecular genetics--role of RET/PTC and BRAF in tumor initiation. *Journal of Endocrinology and Metabolism*, Vol. 89, No 9, (Sep 2004), pp. 4264-4266, ISsN 0021-972X

Faivre, J., Clerc, J., Gerolami, R., Herve, J., Longuet, M., Liu, B., Roux, J., Moal, F., Perricaudet, M. & Brechot, C. (2004). Long-term radioiodine retention and regression of liver cancer after sodium iodide symporter gene transfer in wistar rats. *Cancer Research*, Vol. 64, No 21, (November 2004), pp. 8045-8051, ISSN 0008-5472

Fan, H., Xiao, J. & Li, N. (2009). Effects of 9-cis-retinoic acid on proliferation of thyroid squamous cell carcinoma cell line SW579. *Chinese Journal of Control of Endemic Disease*, Vol. 2, No 1, (February 2009), pp. 4-10, ISSN 1001-1889

Fluhr, J. W., Vienne, M. P., Lauze, C., Dupuy, P., Gehring, W. & Gloor, M. (1999). Tolerance profile of retinol, retinaldehyde and retinoic acid under maximized and long-term clinical conditions. *Dermatology*, Vol. 199 Suppl 1, 1999), pp. 57-60, ISSN 1018-8665

Fortunati, N., Catalano, M., Arena, K., Brignardello, E., Piovesan, A. & Boccuzzi, G. (2004). Valproic acid induces the expression of the Na+/I- symporter and iodine uptake in poorly differentiated thyroid cancer cells. *Journal of Clinical Endocrinology and Metabolism*, Vol. 89, No 2, (February 2004), pp. 1006-1009, ISSN 0021-972X

Fröhlich, E., Brossart, P. & Wahl, R. (2009). Induction of iodide uptake in transformed thyrocytes: a compound screening in cell lines. *European Journal of Nuclear Medicine and Molecular Imaging*, Vol. 36, No 5, (May 2009), pp. 780-790, ISSN 1619-7089

Fröhlich, E., Czarnocka, B., Brossart, P. & Wahl, R. (2008). Antitumor Effects of Arsenic Trioxide in Transformed Human Thyroid Cells. *Thyroid*, Vol. 18, No 11, (November 2008), pp. 1183-1193, ISSN 1557-9077

Fröhlich, E., Macchicao, F. & Wahl, R. (2005). Action of thiazolidinediones on differentiation, proliferation and apoptosis of normal and transformed thyrocytes in culture. *Endocrine Related Cancer*, Vol. 12, No 2, (June 2005), pp. 1-13, ISSN 1351-0088

Furuya, F., Lu, C., Willingham, M. C. & Cheng, S. Y. (2007). Inhibition of phosphatidylinositol 3-kinase delays tumor progression and blocks metastatic spread in a mouse model of thyroid cancer. *Carcinogenesis*, Vol. 28, No 12, (December 2007), pp. 2451-2458, ISsN 1460-2180

Furuya, F., Shimura, H., Miyazaki, A., Taki, K., Ohta, K., Haraguchi, K., Onaya, T., Endo, T. & Kobayashi, T. (2004). Adenovirus-mediated transfer of thyroid transcription factor-1 induces radioiodide organification and retention in thyroid cancer cells. *Endocrinology*, Vol. 145, No 11, (November 2004), pp. 5397-5405, ISSN 0013-7227

Gabler, B., Aicher, T., Heiss, P. & Senekowitsch-Schmidtke, R. (1997). Growth inhibition of human papillary thyroid carcinoma cells and multicellular spheroids by anti-EGF-receptor antibody. *Anticancer Research*, Vol. 17, No 4B, (July-August 1997), pp. 3157-3159, ISSN 0250-7005

Gallagher, R., Ferrari, A., Kaubisch, A., Makower, D., Stein, C., Rajdev, L., Gucalp, R., Wadler, S., Mandeli, J. & Sarta, C. (2004). Arsenic trioxide (ATO) in metastatic hormone-refractory prostate cancer (HRPC): Results of phase II trial T99-0077. *Journal of Clinical Oncology, 2004 ASCO Annual Meeting Proceedings*, Vol. 22,14S, No, 2004), pp. 4638, ISSN 0732-183X

Garcia-Jimenez, C. & Santisteban, P. (2007). TSH signalling and cancer. *Arquivos brasileiros de endocrinologia e metabologia*, Vol. 51, No 5, (July 2007), pp. 654-671, ISSN 0004-2730

Gerard, A., Daumerie, C., Mestdagh, C., S, G., De Burbure, C., Costagliola, S., Miot, F., Nollevaux, M., Denef, J., Rahier, J., Franc, B., De Vijlder, J., Colin, I. & Many, M. (2003). Correlation between the loss of thyroglobulin iodination and the expression of thyroid-specific proteins involved in iodine metabolism in thyroid carcinomas. *Journal of Clinical Endocrinology and Metabolism*, Vol. 88, No 10, (October 2003), pp. 4977-4983, ISSN 0021-972X

Gershengorn, M. C., Izumi, M. & Robbins, J. (1976). Use of lithium as an adjunct to radioiodine therapy of thyroid carcinoma. *Journal of Clinical Endocrinology and Metabolism*, Vol. 42, No 1, (January 1976), pp. 105-111, ISSN 0021-972X

Gruning, T., Tiepolt, C., Zophel, K., Bredow, J., Kropp, J. & Franke, W. (2003). Retinoic acid for redifferentiation of thyroid cancer--does it hold its promise? *European Journal of Endocrinology*, Vol. 148, No 4, (April 2003), pp. 395-402, ISSN 0804-4643

Grunwald, F., Pakos, E., Bender, H., Menzel, C., Otte, R., Palmedo, H., Pfeifer, U. & Biersack, H. J. (1998). Redifferentiation therapy with retinoic acid in follicular thyroid cancer. *Journal of Nuclear Medicine*, Vol. 39, No 9, (November 1998), pp. 1555-1558., ISSN 0161-5505

Haberkorn, U., Altmann, A., Jiang, S., Morr, I., Mahmut, M. & Eisenhut, M. (2001). Iodide uptake in human anaplastic thyroid carcinoma cells after transfer of the human thyroid peroxidase gene. *European Journal of Nuclear Medicine* Vol. 28, No 5, (May 2001), pp. 633-638, ISsN 0340-6997

Harach, H. R., Franssila, K. O. & Wasenius, V. M. (1985). Occult papillary carcinoma of the thyroid. A "normal" finding in Finland. A systematic autopsy study. *Cancer*, Vol. 56, No 3, (August 1985), pp. 531-538, ISSN 0008-543X

Hard, G. C. (1998). Recent developments in the investigation of thyroid regulation and thyroid carcinogenesis. *Environmental health perspectives*, Vol. 106, No 8, (August 1998), pp. 427-436, ISSN 0091-6765

Ho, A. L. & Sherman, E. (2011). Clinical development of kinase inhibitors for the treatment of differentiated thyroid cancer. *Clinical Advances in Hematology & Oncology*, Vol. 9, No 1, (January 2011), pp. 32-41, ISSN 1543-0790

Hoang-Vu, C., Dralle, H., Scheumann, G., Maenhaut, C., Horn, R., von zur Muhlen, A. & Brabant, G. (1992). Gene expression of differentiation- and dedifferentiation markers in normal and malignant human thyroid tissues. *Experimental and Clinical Endocrinology*, Vol. 100, No 1-2, (January 1992), pp. 51-56, ISSN 0232-7384

Hou, P., Bojdani, E. & Xing, M. (2010). Induction of thyroid gene expression and radioiodine uptake in thyroid cancer cells by targeting major signaling pathways. *Journal of Clinical Endocrinology and Metabolism*, Vol. 95, No 2, (February 2010), pp. 820-828, ISSN 1945-7197

Hou, P., Liu, D., Ji, M. & Xing, M. (2007). Potent inhibition of thyroid cancer cells and reexpression of thyroid genes by dual knockdown of the PI3K/Akt and MAP kinase pathways. American Thyroid Association, New York.

Hou, P., Liu, D., Shan, Y., Hu, S., Studeman, K., Condouris, S., Wang, Y., Trink, A., El-Naggar, A. K., Tallini, G., Vasko, V. & Xing, M. (2007). Genetic alterations and their relationship in the phosphatidylinositol 3-kinase/Akt pathway in thyroid cancer. *Clinical Cancer Research*, Vol. 13, No 4, (February 2007), pp. 1161-1170, ISSN 1078-0432

Jeong, H., Kim, Y. R., Kim, K. N., Choe, J. G., Chung, J. K. & Kim, M. K. (2006). Effect of all-trans retinoic acid on sodium/iodide symporter expression, radioiodine uptake and gene expression profiles in a human anaplastic thyroid carcinoma cell line. *Nuclear Medicine and Biology*, Vol. 33, No 7, (October 2006), pp. 875-882, ISSN 0969-8051

Kapiteijn, E., Schneider, T. C., Morreau, H., Gelderblom, H., Nortier, J. W. & Smit, J. W. (2011). New treatment modalities in advanced thyroid cancer. *Annals of Oncology*, Vol., No, (April 2011), pp., ISSN 1569-8041

Kebebew, E., Peng, M., Reiff, E., Treseler, P., Woeber, K. A., Clark, O. H., Greenspan, F. S., Lindsay, S., Duh, Q. Y. & Morita, E. (2006). A phase II trial of rosiglitazone in patients with thyroglobulin-positive and radioiodine-negative differentiated thyroid cancer. *Surgery*, Vol. 140, No 6, (December 2006), pp. 960-966, ISSN 0039-6060

Kebebew, E., Wong, M. G., Siperstein, A. E., Duh, Q. Y. & Clark, O. H. (1999). Phenylacetate inhibits growth and vascular endothelial growth factor secretion in human thyroid carcinoma cells and modulates their differentiated function. *Journal of Clinical Endocrinology and Metabolism*, Vol. 84, No 8, (Aug 1999), pp. 2840-2847, ISSN 0021-972X

Kelly, W. K., O'Connor, O. A., Krug, L. M., Chiao, J. H., Heaney, M., Curley, T., MacGregore-Cortelli, B., Tong, W., Secrist, J. P., Schwartz, L., Richardson, S., Chu, E., Olgac, S., Marks, P. A., Scher, H. & Richon, V. M. (2005). Phase I study of an oral histone deacetylase inhibitor, suberoylanilide hydroxamic acid, in patients with advanced cancer. *Journal of Clinical Oncology*, Vol. 23, No 17, (June 2005), pp. 3923-3931, ISSN 0732-183X

Kim, W. G., Kim, E. Y., Kim, T. Y., Ryu, J. S., Hong, S. J., Kim, W. B. & Shong, Y. K. (2009). Redifferentiation therapy with 13-cis retinoic acids in radioiodine-resistant thyroid cancer. *Endocrine Journal*, Vol. 56, No 1, (March 2009), pp. 105-112, ISSN 1348-4540

Kimura, H., Yamashita, S., Namba, H., Usa, T., Fujiyama, K., Tsuruta, M., Yokoyama, N., Izumi, M. & Nagataki, S. (1992). Impairment of the TSH signal transduction system in human thyroid carcinoma cells. *Experimental Cell Research*, Vol. 203, No 2, (December 1992), pp. 402-406, ISSN 0014-4827

Klopper, J., Hays, W., Sharma, V., Baumbusch, M., Hershman, J. & Haugen, B. (2004). Retinoid X receptor-gamma and peroxisome proliferator-activated receptor-gamma expression predicts thyroid carcinoma cell response to retinoid and thiazolidinedione treatment. *Molecular Cancer Therapeutics* Vol. 3, No 8, (August 2004), pp. 1011-1020, ISSN 1535-7163

Kogai, T., Kanamoto, Y., Che, L. H., Taki, K., Moatamed, F., Schultz, J. J. & Brent, G. A. (2004). Systemic retinoic acid treatment induces sodium/iodide symporter expression and radioiodide uptake in mouse breast cancer models. *Cancer Research*, Vol. 64, No 1, (January 2004), pp. 415-422, ISSN 0008-5472

Kogai, T., Sajid-Crockett, S., Newmarch, L. S., Liu, Y. Y. & Brent, G. A. (2008). Phosphoinositide-3-kinase inhibition induces sodium/iodide symporter expression in rat thyroid cells and human papillary thyroid cancer cells. *Journal of Endocrinology*, Vol. 199, No 2, (November 2008), pp. 243-252, ISSN 1479-6805

Kondo, T., Nakazawa, T., Ma, D., Niu, D., Mochizuki, K., Kawasaki, T., Nakamura, N., Yamane, T., Kobayashi, M. & Katoh, R. (2009). Epigenetic silencing of TTF-1/NKX2-1 through DNA hypermethylation and histone H3 modulation in thyroid carcinomas. *Laboratory Investigation;*, Vol. 89, No 7, (July 2009), pp. 791-799, ISSN 1530-0307

Koong, S. S., Reynolds, J. C., Movius, E. G., Keenan, A. M., Ain, K. B., Lakshmanan, M. C. & Robbins, J. (1999). Lithium as a potential adjuvant to 131I therapy of metastatic, well differentiated thyroid carcinoma. *Journal of Clinical Endocrinology and Metabolism*, Vol. 84, No 3, (March 1999), pp. 912-916, ISSN 0021-972X

Kopp, P., Pesce, L. & Solis, S. J. (2008). Pendred syndrome and iodide transport in the thyroid. *Trends in Endocrinology and Metabolism*, Vol. 19, No 7, (September 2008), pp. 260-268, ISSN 1043-2760

Kurebayashi, J., Tanaka, K., Otsuki, T., Moriya, T., Kunisue, H., Uno, M. & Sonoo, H. (2000). All-trans-retinoic acid modulates expression levels of thyroglobulin and cytokines in a new human poorly differentiated papillary thyroid carcinoma cell line, KTC-1. *Journal of Clinical Endocrinology and Metabolism*, Vol. 85, No 8, (August 2000), pp. 2889-2896, ISSN 0021-972X

Lacroix, L., Mian, C., Caillou, B., Talbot, M., Filetti, S., Schlumberger, M. & Bidart, J. M. (2001). Na(+)/I(-) symporter and Pendred syndrome gene and protein expressions in human extra-thyroidal tissues. *European Journal of Endocrinology*, Vol. 144, No 3, (March 2001), pp. 297-302, ISSN 0804-4643

Laezza, C., Di Marzo, V. & Bifulco, M. (1998). v-K-ras leads to preferential farnesylation of p21(ras) in FRTL-5 cells: multiple interference with the isoprenoid pathway. *Proceedings of the National Academy of Sciences of the United States of America*, Vol. 95, No 23, (November 1998), pp. 13646-13651, ISSN 0027-8424

Landriscina, M., Fabiano, A., Altamura, S., Bagala, C., Piscazzi, A., Cassano, A., Spadafora, C., Giorgino, F., Barone, C. & Cignarelli, M. (2005). Reverse transcriptase inhibitors down-regulate cell proliferation in vitro and in vivo and restore thyrotropin signaling and iodine uptake in human thyroid anaplastic carcinoma. *Journal of Clinical Endocrinology and Metabolism*, Vol. 90, No 10, (October 2005), pp. 5663-5671, ISSN 0021-972X

Laney, N., Meza, J., Lyden, E., Erickson, J., Treude, K. & Goldner, W. (2010). The Prevalence of Vitamin D Deficiency Is Similar between Thyroid Nodule and Thyroid Cancer Patients. *International Journal of Endocrinology*, Vol. 2010, No Article ID 805716, 2010), pp. 805716-805723, ISSN 1687-8345

Lazar, V., Bidart, J. M., Caillou, B., Mahe, C., Lacroix, L., Filetti, S. & Schlumberger, M. (1999). Expression of the Na+/I- symporter gene in human thyroid tumors: a comparison study with other thyroid-specific genes. *Journal of Clinical Endocrinology and Metabolism*, Vol. 84, No 9, (September 1999), pp. 3228-3234, ISSN 0021-972X

Lemoine, N. R., Mayall, E. S., Wyllie, F. S., Williams, E. D., Goyns, M., Stringer, B. & Wynford-Thomas, D. (1989). High frequency of ras oncogene activation in all stages of human thyroid tumorigenesis. *Oncogene*, Vol. 4, No 2, (February 1989), pp. 159-164, ISSN 0950-9232

Lima, L. P., Barros, I. A., Lisboa, P. C., Araujo, R. L., Silva, A. C., Rosenthal, D., Ferreira, A. C. & Carvalho, D. P. (2006). Estrogen effects on thyroid iodide uptake and thyroperoxidase activity in normal and ovariectomized rats. *Steroids*, Vol. 71, No 8, (August 2006), pp. 653-659, ISSN 0039-128X

Liu, R., Liu, D., Trink, E., Bojdani, E., Ning, G. & Xing, M. (2011). The Akt-specific inhibitor MK2206 selectively inhibits thyroid cancer cells harboring mutations that can activate the PI3K/Akt pathway. *Journal of Clinical Endocrinology and Metabolism*, Vol. 96, No 4, (April 2011), pp. E577-585, ISSN 1945-7197

Liu, Y. Y., Stokkel, M. P., Pereira, A. M., Corssmit, E. P., Morreau, H. A., Romijn, J. A. & Smit, J. W. (2006). Bexarotene increases uptake of radioiodide in metastases of differentiated thyroid carcinoma. *European Journal of Endocrinology*, Vol. 154, No 4, (April 2006), pp. 525-531, ISSN 0804-4643

Liu, Y. Y., van der Pluijm, G., Karperien, M., Stokkel, M. P., Pereira, A. M., Morreau, J., Kievit, J., Romijn, J. A. & Smit, J. W. (2006). Lithium as adjuvant to radioiodine therapy in differentiated thyroid carcinoma: clinical and in vitro studies. *Clinical Endocrinology*, Vol. 64, No 6, (June 2006), pp. 617-624, ISSN 0300-0664

Mandal, M., Kim, S., Younes, M. N., Jasser, S. A., El-Naggar, A. K., Mills, G. B. & Myers, J. N. (2005). The Akt inhibitor KP372-1 suppresses Akt activity and cell proliferation and induces apoptosis in thyroid cancer cells. *British Journal of Cancer*, Vol. 92, No 10, (May 2005), pp. 1899-1905, ISSN 0007-0920

Marsee, D. K., Venkateswaran, A., Tao, H., Vadysirisack, D., Zhang, Z., Vandre, D. D. & Jhiang, S. M. (2004). Inhibition of heat shock protein 90, a novel RET/PTC1-associated protein, increases radioiodide accumulation in thyroid cells. *Journal of Biological Chemistry*, Vol. 279, No 42, (October 2004), pp. 43990-43997, ISSN 0021-9258

Martelli, M., Iuliano, R., Le Pera, I., Sama, I., Monaco, C., Cammarota, S., Kroll, T., Chiariotti, L., Santoro, M. & Fusco, A. (2002). Inhibitory effects of peroxisome poliferator-activated receptor gamma on thyroid carcinoma cell growth. *Journal of Clinical Endocrinology and Metabolism*, Vol. 87, No 10, (October 2002), pp. 4728-4735, ISSN 0021-972X

Matsumoto, H., Sakamoto, A., Fujiwara, M., Yano, Y., Shishido-Hara, Y., Fujioka, Y. & Kamma, H. (2008). Decreased expression of the thyroid-stimulating hormone receptor in poorly-differentiated carcinoma of the thyroid. *Oncology Reports*, Vol. 19, No 6, (June 2008), pp. 1405-1411, ISSN 1021-335X

Mehta, R. G., Williamson, E., Patel, M. K. & Koeffler, H. P. (2000). A ligand of peroxisome proliferator-activated receptor gamma, retinoids, and prevention of preneoplastic mammary lesions. *Journal of the National Cancer Institute*, Vol. 92, No 5, (March 2000), pp. 418-423, ISSN 0027-8874

Mentrup, B., Herbert, S., Schmutzler, C. & Koehrle, J. (2002). The expression of the human type I 5′ Iodothyronine deiodinase depends on the methylation status of the cell. *Journal of Endocrinological Investigation*, Vol. 25, No Suppl 7, 2002), pp. 29, ISSN 0391-4097

Mian, C., Barollo, S., Pennelli, G., Pavan, N., Rugge, M., Pelizzo, M. R., Mazzarotto, R., Casara, D., Nacamulli, D., Mantero, F., Opocher, G., Busnardo, B. & Girelli, M. E. (2008). Molecular characteristics in papillary thyroid cancers (PTCs) with no 131I uptake. *Clinical Endocrinology*, Vol. 68, No 1, (January 2008), pp. 108-116, ISSN 1365-2265

Miasaki, F. Y., Vivaldi, A., Ciampi, R., Agate, L., Collecchi, P., Capodanno, A., Pinchera, A. & Elisei, R. (2008). Retinoic acid receptor beta2 re-expression and growth inhibition in thyroid carcinoma cell lines after 5-aza-2'-deoxycytidine treatment. *Journal of Endocrinological Investigation*, Vol. 31, No 8, (August 2008), pp. 724-730, ISSN 1720-8386

Miller, W. H., Jr. (2002). Molecular targets of arsenic trioxide in malignant cells. *Oncologist*, Vol. 7, No Suppl 1, 2002), pp. 14-19, ISSN 1083-7159

Modoni, S., Landriscina, M., Fabiano, A., Fersini, A., Urbano, N., Ambrosi, A. & Cignarelli, M. (2007). Reinduction of cell differentiation and 131I uptake in a poorly differentiated thyroid tumor in response to the reverse transcriptase (RT) inhibitor nevirapine. *Cancer Biotherapy & Radiopharmaceuticals*, Vol. 22, No 2, (April 2007), pp. 289-295, ISSN 1084-9785

Nikiforova, M. N., Lynch, R. A., Biddinger, P. W., Alexander, E. K., Dorn, G. W., 2nd, Tallini, G., Kroll, T. G. & Nikiforov, Y. E. (2003). RAS point mutations and PAX8-PPAR gamma rearrangement in thyroid tumors: evidence for distinct molecular pathways in thyroid follicular carcinoma. *Journal of Clinical Endocrinology and Metabolism*, Vol. 88, No 5, (May 2003), pp. 2318-2326, ISSN 0021-972X

Nilsson, M., Bjorkman, U., Ekholm, R. & Ericson, L. E. (1990). Iodide transport in primary cultured thyroid follicle cells: evidence of a TSH-regulated channel mediating iodide efflux selectively across the apical domain of the plasma membrane. *European Journal of Cell Biology*, Vol. 52, No 2, (August 1990), pp. 270-281, ISSN 0171-9335

Ohta, K., Endo, T., Haraguchi, K., Hershman, J. & Onaya, T. (2001). Ligands for peroxisome proliferator-activated receptor gamma inhibit growth and induce apoptosis of human papillary thyroid carcinoma cells. *Journal of Clinical Endocrinology and Metabolism*, Vol. 86, No 5, (May 2001), pp. 2170-2177, ISSN 0021-972X

Ohta, K., Endo, T. & Onaya, T. (1991). The mRNA levels of thyrotropin receptor, thyroglobulin and thyroid peroxidase in neoplastic human thyroid tissues. *Biochemical and Biophysical Research Communications*, Vol. 174, No 3, (February 1991), pp. 1148-1153, ISSN 0006-291X

Okano, K., Usa, T., Ohtsuru, A., Tsukazaki, T., Miyazaki, Y., Yonekura, A., Namba, H., Shindoh, H. & Yamashita, S. (1999). Effect of 22-oxa-1,25-dihydroxyvitamin D3 on human thyroid cancer cell growth. *Endocrine Journal*, Vol. 46, No 2, (April 1999), pp. 243-252, ISSN 0918-8959

Park, H. J., Kim, J. Y., Park, K. Y., Gong, G., Hong, S. J. & Ahn, I. M. (2000). Expressions of human sodium iodide symporter mRNA in primary and metastatic papillary thyroid carcinomas. *Thyroid*, Vol. 10, No 3, (March 2000), pp. 211-217, ISSN 1050-7256

Paroder, V., Spencer, S. R., Paroder, M., Arango, D., Schwartz, S., Jr., Mariadason, J. M., Augenlicht, L. H., Eskandari, S. & Carrasco, N. (2006). Na(+)/monocarboxylate transport (SMCT) protein expression correlates with survival in colon cancer:

molecular characterization of SMCT. *Proceedings of the National Academy of Sciences of the United States of America,* Vol. 103, No 19, (May 2006), pp. 7270-7275, ISSN 0027-8424

Pons, F., Carrio, I., Estorch, M., Ginjaume, M., Pons, J. & Milian, R. (1987). Lithium as an adjuvant of iodine-131 uptake when treating patients with well-differentiated thyroid carcinoma. *Clinical Nuclear Medicine,* Vol. 12, No 8, (August 1987), pp. 644-647, ISSN 0363-9762

Presta, I., Arturi, F., Ferretti, E., Mattei, T., Scarpelli, D., Tosi, E., Scipioni, A., Celano, M., Gulino, A., Filetti, S. & Russo, D. (2005). Recovery of NIS expression in thyroid cancer cells by overexpression of Pax8 gene. *BMC Cancer,* Vol. 5, No 80, (July 2005), pp. 80, ISSN 1471-2407

Puppin, C., D'Aurizio, F., D'Elia, A. V., Cesaratto, L., Tell, G., Russo, D., Filetti, S., Ferretti, E., Tosi, E., Mattei, T., Pianta, A., Pellizzari, L. & Damante, G. (2005). Effects of histone acetylation on sodium iodide symporter promoter and expression of thyroid-specific transcription factors. *Endocrinology,* Vol. 146, No 9, (September 2005), pp. 3967-3974, ISSN 0013-7227

Rabes, H. M., Demidchik, E. P., Sidorow, J. D., Lengfelder, E., Beimfohr, C., Hoelzel, D. & Klugbauer, S. (2000). Pattern of radiation-induced RET and NTRK1 rearrangements in 191 post-chernobyl papillary thyroid carcinomas: biological, phenotypic, and clinical implications. *Clinical Cancer Research,* Vol. 6, No 3, (March 2000), pp. 1093-1103, ISSN 1078-0432

Ricarte-Filho, J. C., Ryder, M., Chitale, D. A., Rivera, M., Heguy, A., Ladanyi, M., Janakiraman, M., Solit, D., Knauf, J. A., Tuttle, R. M., Ghossein, R. A. & Fagin, J. A. (2009). Mutational profile of advanced primary and metastatic radioactive iodine-refractory thyroid cancers reveals distinct pathogenetic roles for BRAF, PIK3CA, and AKT1. *Cancer Research,* Vol. 69, No 11, (June 2009), pp. 4885-4893, ISSN 1538-7445

Riedel, C., Levy, O. & Carrasco, N. (2001). Post-transcriptional regulation of the sodium/iodide symporter by thyrotropin. *Journal of Biological Chemistry,* Vol. 276, No 24, (June 2001), pp. 21458-21463, ISSN 0021-9258

Riesco-Eizaguirre, G., Gutierrez-Martinez, P., Garcia-Cabezas, M. A., Nistal, M. & Santisteban, P. (2006). The oncogene BRAF V600E is associated with a high risk of recurrence and less differentiated papillary thyroid carcinoma due to the impairment of Na+/I- targeting to the membrane. *Endocrine-related Cancer,* Vol. 13, No 1, (March 2006), pp. 257-269, ISSN 1351-0088

Ringel, M. D., Hayre, N., Saito, J., Saunier, B., Schuppert, F., Burch, H., Bernet, V., Burman, K. D., Kohn, L. D. & Saji, M. (2001). Overexpression and overactivation of Akt in thyroid carcinoma. *Cancer Research,* Vol. 61, No 16, (August 2001), pp. 6105-6111, ISSN 0008-5472

Rodriguez-Antona, C., Pallares, J., Montero-Conde, C., Inglada-Perez, L., Castelblanco, E., Landa, I., Leskela, S., Leandro-Garcia, L. J., Lopez-Jimenez, E., Leton, R., Cascon, A., Lerma, E., Martin, M. C., Carralero, M. C., Mauricio, D., Cigudosa, J. C., Matias-Guiu, X. & Robledo, M. (2010). Overexpression and activation of EGFR and VEGFR2 in medullary thyroid carcinomas is related to metastasis. *Endocrine-related Cancer,* Vol. 17, No 1, (March 2010), pp. 7-16, ISSN 1479-6821

Romei, C., Ciampi, R., Faviana, P., Agate, L., Molinaro, E., Bottici, V., Basolo, F., Miccoli, P., Pacini, F., Pinchera, A. & Elisei, R. (2008). BRAFV600E mutation, but not RET/PTC rearrangements, is correlated with a lower expression of both thyroperoxidase and sodium iodide symporter genes in papillary thyroid cancer. *Endocrine-related cancer,* Vol. 15, No 2, (June 2008), pp. 511-520, ISSN 1351-0088

Royaux, I. E., Suzuki, K., Mori, A., Katoh, R., Everett, L. A., Kohn, L. D. & Green, E. D. (2000). Pendrin, the protein encoded by the Pendred syndrome gene (PDS), is an apical porter of iodide in the thyroid and is regulated by thyroglobulin in FRTL-5 cells. *Endocrinology,* Vol. 141, No 2, (February 2000), pp. 839-845, ISSN 0013-7227

Russo, D., Manole, D., Arturi, F., Suarez, H. G., Schlumberger, M., Filetti, S. & Derwahl, M. (2001). Absence of sodium/iodide symporter gene mutations in differentiated human thyroid carcinomas. *Thyroid,* Vol. 11, No 1, (January 2001), pp. 37-39, ISSN 1050-7256

Saito, T., Endo, T., Kawaguchi, A., Ikeda, M., Katoh, R., Kawaoi, A., Muramatsu, A. & Onaya, T. (1998). Increased expression of the sodium/iodide symporter in papillary thyroid carcinomas. *Journal of Clinical Investigation,* Vol. 101, No 7, (July 1998), pp. 1296-1300, ISSN 00219738

Schmutzler, C., Brtko, J., Winzer, R., Jakobs, T. C., Meissner-Weigl, J., Simon, D., Goretzki, P. E. & Kohrle, J. (1998). Functional retinoid and thyroid hormone receptors in human thyroid-carcinoma cell lines and tissues. *International Journal of Cancer,* Vol. 76, No 3, (May 1998), pp. 368-376, ISSN 0020-7136

Schmutzler, C. & Kohrle, J. (2000). Retinoic acid redifferentiation therapy for thyroid cancer. *Thyroid,* Vol. 10, No 5, (October 2000), pp. 393-406, ISSN 1050-7256

Schmutzler, C., Winzer, R., Meissner-Weigl, J. & Kohrle, J. (1997). Retinoic acid increases sodium/iodide symporter mRNA levels in human thyroid cancer cell lines and suppresses expression of functional symporter in nontransformed FRTL-5 rat thyroid cells. *Biochemical and Biophysical Research Communications,* Vol. 240, No 3, (November 1997), pp. 832-838, ISSN 0006-291X

Schreck, R., Schnieders, F., Schmutzler, C. & Köhrle, J. (1994). Retinoids stimulate type I 5'-deiodinase activity in human follicular thyroid carcinoma cell lines. *Journal of Clinical Endocrinology and Metabolism,* Vol. 79, No 3, (September 1994), pp. 791-798, ISSN 0021-972X

Shen, W. T. & Chung, W. Y. (2005). Treatment of thyroid cancer with histone deacetylase inhibitors and peroxisome proliferator-activated receptor-gamma agonists. *Thyroid,* Vol. 15, No 6, (June 2005), pp. 594-599, ISSN 1050-7256

Shen, Z. X., Chen, G. Q., Ni, J. H., Li, X. S., Xiong, S. M., Qiu, Q. Y., Zhu, J., Tang, W., Sun, G. L., Yang, K. Q., Chen, Y., Zhou, L., Fang, Z. W., Wang, Y. T., Ma, J., Zhang, P., Zhang, T. D., Chen, S. J., Chen, Z. & Wang, Z. Y. (1997). Use of arsenic trioxide (As2O3) in the treatment of acute promyelocytic leukemia (APL): II. Clinical efficacy and pharmacokinetics in relapsed patients. *Blood,* Vol. 89, No 9, (May 1997), pp. 3354-3360., ISSN 0006-4971

Sherman, E., Fury, M., Tuttle, R., Ghossein, R., Stambuk, H., Baum, M., Lisa, D., Su, Y., Shaha, A. & Pfister, D. (2009). Phase II study of depsipeptide (DEP) in radioiodine (RAI)-refractory metastatic nonmedullary thyroid carcinoma. . *Proceedings - American Society of Clinical Oncology,* Vol. 27, No 15s, 2009), pp. 6059, ISSN 1081-0641

Short, S., Suovuori, A., Cook, G., Vivian, G. & Harmer, C. (2004). A phase II study using retinoids as redifferentiation agents to increase iodine uptake in metastatic thyroid cancer. *Clin Oncol (R Coll Radiol)*, Vol. 16, No 8, (December 2004), pp. 569-574, ISSN 0084-5353

Simon, D., Koehrle, J., Reiners, C., Boerner, A. R., Schmutzler, C., Mainz, K., Goretzki, P. E. & Roeher, H. D. (1998). Redifferentiation therapy with retinoids: therapeutic option for advanced follicular and papillary thyroid carcinoma. *World Journal of Surgery*, Vol. 22, No 6, (June 1998), pp. 569-574, ISSN 0364-2313

Simon, D., Köhrle, J., Schmutzler, C., Mainz, K., Reiners, C. & Roher, H. (1996). Redifferentiation therapy of differentiated thyroid carcinoma with retinoic acid: basics and first clinical results. *Experimental and Clinical Endocrinology & Diabetes*, Vol. 104 Suppl 4, No, 1996), pp. 13-15, ISSN 0947-7349

Simon, D., Korber, C., Krausch, M., Segering, J., Groth, P., Gorges, R., Grunwald, F., Muller-Gartner, H. W., Schmutzler, C., Kohrle, J., Roher, H. & Reiners, C. (2002). Clinical impact of retinoids in redifferentiation therapy of advanced thyroid cancer: final results of a pilot study. *European Journal of Nuclear Medicine and Molecular Imaging*, Vol. 29, No 6, (June 2002), pp. 775-782, ISSN 1619-7070

Smith, V. E., Read, M. L., Turnell, A. S., Watkins, R. J., Watkinson, J. C., Lewy, G. D., Fong, J. C., James, S. R., Eggo, M. C., Boelaert, K., Franklyn, J. A. & McCabe, C. J. (2009). A novel mechanism of sodium iodide symporter repression in differentiated thyroid cancer. *Journal of Cell Science*, Vol. 122, No Pt 18, (September 2009), pp. 3393-3402, ISSN 1477-9137

Sodre, A. K., Rubio, I. G., Galrao, A. L., Knobel, M., Tomimori, E. K., Alves, V. A., Kanamura, C. T., Buchpiguel, C. A., Watanabe, T., Friguglietti, C. U., Kulcsar, M. A., Medeiros-Neto, G. & Camargo, R. Y. (2008). Association of low sodium-iodide symporter messenger ribonucleic acid expression in malignant thyroid nodules with increased intracellular protein staining. *Journal of Clinical Endocrinology and Metabolism*, Vol. 93, No 10, (October 2008), pp. 4141-4145, ISSN 0021-972X

Soh, E. Y., Duh, Q. Y., Sobhi, S. A., Young, D. M., Epstein, H. D., Wong, M. G., Garcia, Y. K., Min, Y. D., Grossman, R. F., Siperstein, A. E. & Clark, O. H. (1997). Vascular endothelial growth factor expression is higher in differentiated thyroid cancer than in normal or benign thyroid. *Journal of Clinical Endocrinology and Metabolism*, Vol. 82, No 11, (November 1997), pp. 3741-3747, ISSN 0021-972X

Srinivas, S. & Feldman, D. (2009). A phase II trial of calcitriol and naproxen in recurrent prostate cancer. *Anticancer Research*, Vol. 29, No 9, (September 2009), pp. 3605-3610, ISSN 1791-7530

Stepien, T., Krupinski, R., Sopinski, J., Kuzdak, K., Komorowski, J., Lawnicka, H. & Stepien, H. (2010). Decreased 1-25 dihydroxyvitamin D3 concentration in peripheral blood serum of patients with thyroid cancer. *Archives of Medical Research*, Vol. 41, No 3, (April 2010), pp. 190-194, ISSN 1873-5487

Tanaka, K., Inoue, H., Miki, H., Masuda, E., Kitaichi, M., Komaki, K., Uyama, T. & Monden, Y. (1997). Relationship between prognostic score and thyrotropin receptor (TSH-R) in papillary thyroid carcinoma: immunohistochemical detection of TSH-R. *British Journal of Cancer*, Vol. 76, No 5, (May 1997), pp. 594-599, ISSN 0007-0920

Tanaka, T., Umeki, K., Yamamoto, I., Sugiyama, S., Noguchi, S. & Ohtaki, S. (1996). Immunohistochemical loss of thyroid peroxidase in papillary thyroid carcinoma:

strong suppression of peroxidase gene expression. *Journal of Pathology*, Vol. 179, No 1, (May 1996), pp. 89-94, ISsN 0022-3417

Temple, R., Berman, M., Robbins, J. & Wolff, J. (1972). The use of lithium in the treatment of thyrotoxicosis. *Journal of Clinical Investigation*, Vol. 51, No 10, (October 1972), pp. 2746-2756, ISSN 0021-9738

Tepmongkol, S., Keelawat, S., Honsawek, S. & Ruangvejvorachai, P. (2008). Rosiglitazone effect on radioiodine uptake in thyroid carcinoma patients with high thyroglobulin but negative total body scan: a correlation with the expression of peroxisome proliferator-activated receptor-gamma. *Thyroid*, Vol. 18, No 7, (July 2008), pp. 697-704, ISSN 1050-7256

Tuncel, M., Aydin, D., Yaman, E., Tazebay, U. H., Guc, D., Dogan, A. L., Tasbasan, B. & Ugur, O. (2007). The comparative effects of gene modulators on thyroid-specific genes and radioiodine uptake. *Cancer Biotherapy & Radiopharmaceuticals*, Vol. 22, No 3, (June 2007), pp. 443-449, ISSN 1084-9785

Vadysirisack, D. D., Venkateswaran, A., Zhang, Z. & Jhiang, S. M. (2007). MEK signaling modulates sodium iodide symporter at multiple levels and in a paradoxical manner. *Endocrine-related Cancer*, Vol. 14, No 2, (June 2007), pp. 421-432, ISSN 1351-0088

van Herle, A. J., Agatep, M. L., Padua III, D. N., Totanes, T. L., Canlapan, D. V., van Herle, H. M. L. & Juillard, G. J. F. (1990). Effects of 13 cis-retinoic acid on growth and differentiation of human follicular carcinoma cells (UCLA RO 82 W-1) in vitro. *Journal of Clinical Endocrinology and Metabolism*, Vol. 71, No, 1990), pp. 755-763, ISSN 0021972X

Venkataraman, G. M., Yatin, M., Marcinek, R. & Ain, K. B. (1999). Restoration of iodide uptake in dedifferentiated thyroid carcinoma: relationship to human Na+/I-symporter gene methylation status. *Journal of Clinical Endocrinology and Metabolism*, Vol. 84, No 7, (July 1999), pp. 2449-2457, ISSN 0021-972X

Vivaldi, A., Miasaki, F. Y., Ciampi, R., Agate, L., Collecchi, P., Capodanno, A., Pinchera, A. & Elisei, R. (2009). Re-differentiation of thyroid carcinoma cell lines treated with 5-Aza-2'-deoxycytidine and retinoic acid. *Molecular and Cellular Endocrinology*, Vol. 307, No 1-2, (August 2009), pp. 142-148, ISSN 1872-8057

Wan, Y. (2010). PPARgamma in bone homeostasis. *Trends in Endocrinology and Metabolism*, Vol. 21, No 12, (December 2010), pp. 722-728, ISSN 1879-3061

Wang, C., Zhong, W., Chang, T., Lai, S. & Tsai, Y. (2003). Lovastatin, a 3-hydroxy-3-methylglutaryl coenzyme A reductase inhibitor, induces apoptosis and differentiation in human anaplastic thyroid carcinoma cells. *Journal of Clinical Endocrinology and Metabolism*, Vol. 88, No 7, (July 2003), pp. 3021-3026, ISSN 0021972X

Wang, C. Y., Shui, H. A. & Chang, T. C. (2010). In vivo evidence of duality effects for lovastatin in a nude mouse cancer model. *International Journal of Cancer*, Vol. 126, No 2, (January 2010), pp. 578-582, ISSN 1097-0215

Wang, Z. F., Liu, Q. J., Liao, S. Q., Yang, R., Ge, T., He, X., Tian, C. P. & Liu, W. (2011). Expression and correlation of sodium/iodide symporter and thyroid stimulating hormone receptor in human thyroid carcinoma. *Tumori*, Vol. 97, No 4, (July-August 2011), pp. 540-546, ISSN 0300-8916

Wangemann, P., Itza, E. M., Albrecht, B., Wu, T., Jabba, S. V., Maganti, R. J., Lee, J. H., Everett, L. A., Wall, S. M., Royaux, I. E., Green, E. D. & Marcus, D. C. (2004). Loss of KCNJ10 protein expression abolishes endocochlear potential and causes deafness in Pendred syndrome mouse model. *BMC Medicine*, Vol. 2, No 20, (August 2004), pp. 30, ISSN 1741-7015

Wapnir, I. L., van de Rijn, M., Nowels, K., Amenta, P. S., Walton, K., Montgomery, K., Greco, R. S., Dohan, O. & Carrasco, N. (2003). Immunohistochemical profile of the sodium/iodide symporter in thyroid, breast, and other carcinomas using high density tissue microarrays and conventional sections. *Journal of Clinical Endocrinology and Metabolism*, Vol. 88, No 4, (April 2003), pp. 1880-1888, ISSN 0021-972X

Wolff, J. (2005). What is the role of pendrin? *Thyroid*, Vol. 15, No 4, (April 2005), pp. 346-348, ISSN 1050-7256

Wolff, J. & Chaikoff, I. L. (1948). The inhibitory action of excessive iodide upon the synthesis of diiodotyrosine and of thyroxine in the thyroid gland of the normal rat. *Endocrinology*, Vol. 43, No 3, (September 1948), pp. 174-179, ISSN 0013-7227

Woyach, J. A., Kloos, R. T., Ringel, M. D., Arbogast, D., Collamore, M., Zwiebel, J. A., Grever, M., Villalona-Calero, M. & Shah, M. H. (2008). Lack of therapeutic effect of the Histone Deacetylase Inhibitor Vorinostat in Patients with Metastatic Radioiodine-Refractory Thyroid Carcinoma. *Journal of Clinical Endocrinology and Metabolism*, Vol. 94, No 1, (January 2008), pp. 164-170, ISSN 0021-972X

Xing, M. (2007). Gene methylation in thyroid tumorigenesis. *Endocrinology*, Vol. 148, No 3, (March 2007), pp. 948-953, ISSN 0013-7227

Zarnegar, R., Brunaud, L., Kanauchi, H., Wong, M., Fung, M., Ginzinger, D., Duh, Q. & Clark, O. (2002). Increasing the effectiveness of radioactive iodine therapy in the treatment of thyroid cancer using Trichostatin A, a histone deacetylase inhibitor. *Surgery*, Vol. 132, No 6, (December 2002), pp. 984-990, ISSN 0039-6060

Zhang, M., Guo, R., Xu, H. & Li, B. (2011). Retinoic acid and tributyrin induce in-vitro radioiodine uptake and inhibition of cell proliferation in a poorly differentiated follicular thyroid carcinoma. *Nuclear Medicine Communications*, Vol. 32, No 7, (April 2011), pp. 605-610, ISSN 1473-5628

Zhang, Y., Jia, S., Liu, Y., Li, B., Wang, Z., Lu, H. & Zhu, C. (2007). A clinical study of all-trans-retinoid-induced differentiation therapy of advanced thyroid cancer. *Nuclear Medicine Communications*, Vol. 28, No 4, (April 2007), pp. 251-255, ISSN 0143-3636

Zhong, W. B., Liang, Y. C., Wang, C. Y., Chang, T. C. & Lee, W. S. (2005). Lovastatin suppresses invasiveness of anaplastic thyroid cancer cells by inhibiting Rho geranylgeranylation and RhoA/ROCK signaling. *Endocrine-related Cancer*, Vol. 12, No 3, (September 2005), pp. 615-629, ISSN 1351-0088

13

Using γ-Camera to Evaluate the *In Vivo* Biodistributions and Internal Medical Dosimetries of Iodine-131 in Thyroidectomy Patients

Sheng-Pin Changlai[1], Tom Changlai[1] and Chien-Yi Chen[2,3]
[1]*Department of Nuclear Medicine, Lin Shin Hospital, Taichung,*
[2]*School of Medical Imaging and Radiological Sciences,*
[3]*Department of Medical Image, Chung Shan Medical University Hospital, Chung Shan Medical University, Taichung, Taiwan, ROC*

1. Introduction

Seidlin, Oshry and Yallow first examined the feasibility of using radioactive iodine, ^{131}I, to treat thyroid carcinoma in 1948. Medical professionals have since adopted ^{131}I extensively to treat both benign and malignant thyroid diseases (Rosario et al., 2004; Chen et al., 2003; Berg et al., 1996). ^{131}I is commonly used in ablative or adjuvant therapy after thyroid carcinoma treatment, which often requires total or near-total thyroidectomy (Chen et al., 2003). Large doses of ^{131}I are routinely administered to patients to treat thyroid remnants at Chung-Shan Medical University Hospital (CSMUH); however, research on the effective half-life (T_{eff}) in the whole-body, thyroid and other organs *in vivo* has been lacking (CSMUH, 2005). Therefore, this study seeks to yield clear scintigraphic images using γ-camera.

1.1 T_{eff} by International Commission on Radiological Protection 30 (ICRP 30)

It is important to evaluate the T_{eff} of the whole-body and each organ in order to calculate the internal medical dosimetries in patients. Many studies have reported and recommended both the short-term 12-day biological half-life (T_{bio}) and the long-term 120-day T_{bio} of ^{131}I (ICRP 30, 1978). Nonetheless, not all of the values necessarily apply directly to patients without normal functioning thyroids or who have partially removed thyroid glands; the T_{eff} of ^{131}I in patients who have undergone total or near-total thyroidectomy differs significantly from that of normal people (ICRP 30, 1978).

Because the body compartments that store iodine in patients who have undergone total or near-total thyroidectomy are smaller, the T_{eff} of ^{131}I is shorter considering both physical decay and biological elimination (North et al., 2001). The T_{eff} of ^{131}I in various organs, including residual normal and neoplastic thyroid tissues, breast, liver, salivary glands and stomach, needs to be evaluated in order to calculate the internal medical doses and graph the time-activity curves (TAC). Prior studies have used NaI(Tl), an ion chamber and calculation models to evaluate the iodine uptake in the neck using whole-body scans (WBSs) (North et al., 2001; Samuel and Rajashekharrao, 1994; Snyder et al., 1983). However, the activities of the whole-body, thyroid remnant and other organs have not been analyzed to re-evaluate the biodistributions, T_{eff} or internal medical doses in Taiwanese patients.

1.2 Nuclear properties of radioiodine ^{131}I

While the knowledge of radiation dosimetry in most organs are not yet thorough, the investigation of the radiation dosimetry in the thyroid using radioiodine, particularly the ^{131}I isotope, has been extensive. North et al. (2001) have derived the age-dependent absorbed doses in the thyroid. ^{131}I is generated by neutron irradiation of tellurium dioxide in a nuclear reactor. ^{131}I then decays to form stable ^{131}Xe with a half-life of 8.04 days, during which it emits 606 keV (maximum) and 191 keV (mean) β-particles as well as 364.5 keV and 637 keV γ-rays of 81.7% abundance (Shieley & Lederer, 1978). The β-particles (β_3) are maximal in abundance at 63.9 keV and 89.9% per transition. The fraction of β-particles absorbed is assumed to be 1, but it varies according to the energy of photon; the actual maximum energy absorbed is 172 keV Bq^{-1} s^{-1}. ^{131}I is administered post-operation: 1) to minimize recurrence because the β-particles may destroy microscopic carcinoma; 2) because the 364.5 keV γ-rays allow post-ablative ^{131}I to detect occult metastases; 3) to ablate residual normal thyroid tissue.

2. Materials and method

Five female patients of 41±4.4 years of age who weighed at 54.6±5.4 kg were diagnosed with papillary thyroid cancer during routine physical examinations from 2002 to 2004 in central Taiwan. All patients had differentiated carcinoma of the thyroid treated by total thyroidectomy followed by 1100 MBq ^{131}I therapy administered by the Department of Nuclear Medicine at Chung-Shan Medical University Hospital (CSMUH). **Table 1** displays the characteristics of the five patients where no evidence of neck lymph node or distant metastases was present. The patients were treated with ^{131}I and WBSs were conducted using a γ-camera at 6 weeks post-operation. Written informed consent for further whole-body studies was obtained from all patients. Medical professionals conducted this study with the approval from CSMUH Institutional Review Board (IRB).

Case no	Gender	age	Weight (kg)	Syndrome	status of remnant
1	Female	37	55	papillary thyroid cancer	Complete ablation
2	Female	37	58	papillary thyroid cancer	minimal residual
3	Female	38	41	papillary thyroid cancer	minimal residual
4	Female	46	57	papillary thyroid cancer	Complete ablation
5	Female	47	62	papillary thyroid cancer	complete ablation

Table 1. The characteristics of the five patients who underwent whole-body scans (WBSs) at Chung-Shan Medical University Hospital (CSMUH).

2.1 ^{131}I capsules

Syncor International Corporation manufactured and delivered carrier-free ^{131}I-NaI capsules in a single batch. Medical professionals administered ^{131}I capsules to the patients. Each dose exceeded 99.9% radionuclide purity and 95% radiochemical purity. Verified by spot checks, the coefficient of variance (%CV) between capsules in a single batch did not exceed 1.0% (CSMUH, 2005). Furthermore, the ^{131}I-NaI capsules were ingested orally at CSMUH to minimize the radioactivity released into the environment during handling, compared to the high specific activity if sodium iodine were administered in liquid solutions.

2.2 Image acquisitions

Nuclear medicine physicians treated patients who had undergone thyroidectomy with 100 MBq (29.5 mCi) ^{131}I six weeks after surgery when thyroid medications were discontinued. The patients then return for *in vivo* WBSs in a week. No drugs containing iodine or radiographic contrast agents were administered to the patients prior to the WBSs. The patients were given a light breakfast and asked to urinate on day 1 before the WBSs. At the end of day 1, the patients were discharged after the health physicist had verified that the patient's whole-body retention of ^{131}I is within the regulatory limit set by the governing body (CSMUH, 2005; Rosario et al., 2004; United States Nuclear Regulatory Commission, 1997), which allows the patients to have an external dose rate of under 50 μSv (5 mrem) per hour at a distance of 1 meter. The number of pixels was maintained constant over all subsequent images and the same regions of interest (ROIs) were captured in all scans.

2.3 *In vivo* WBS via E-CAM γ-camera

Medical Physicists drew ROIs to quantify the ^{131}I radioactivity uptake in various organs. *In vivo* WBSs were performed using a Canberra 7350-PE collimator connected to a 19-inch high × 13-inch wide × 5/8-inch thick NaI(Tl) crystal Siemens E-CAM γ-camera positioned at a fixed distance of 5 centimeters from the patient's body (Siemens, 1998). **Figure 1** displays the scintigraphic images from the 20-minute WBSs of patient case no 4. An experienced nuclear medicine professional analyzed the images and selected the thigh to subtract the background (Chen et al., 2003). Quality assurance, regular quality controls and energy peak calibration of the NaI(Tl) detector were performed and energy resolution test results were calibrated daily by the CSMUH staff (CSMUH, 2005; Siemens, 1998). To ensure the drop in uptake by the lesion following therapeutic dose administration was not related to increased γ-dead-time, the linearity of the E-CAM counting rate was calibrated for the radioactivity range encountered. Medical physicists determined the T_{eff} of each organ by linearly regressing and then dividing the natural logarithm of the dose injected (%ID) into the whole-body at hour 24. **Figure 2** displays the time-activity curves (TACs) of representative ROIs from the bladder, the brain, kidneys, the liver, lower large intestine (LLI), the thigh, the thyroid remnant and the whole-body of a 46 year-old female patient. The area under the corresponding fitted curve is also calculated.

2.4 Effective and biological half-life (T_{eff} and T_{bio})

Medical professionals used γ-camera to collect the activity of each organ *in vivo* and generated the TACs for dosimetric calculations. The sum of the organ counts was subtracted from the whole-body counts. Both biological elimination and physical decay account for the ^{131}I activity decay in thyroidectomy patients. T_{eff} is evaluated using the formula,

$$\frac{1}{T_{eff}} = \frac{1}{T_{bio}} + \frac{1}{T_{phy}} \quad (1)$$

where T_{phy} is the physical half-life (T_{phy}) of ^{131}I which is 8.04 days (Pacilio et al., 2005; Shieley and Lederer, 1978).

The activity (A_i) is measured at different times (T_i) to re-estimate the T_{eff},

$$A_i = A_0 e^{-\frac{\ln 2}{T_{eff}} Ti} \quad (2)$$

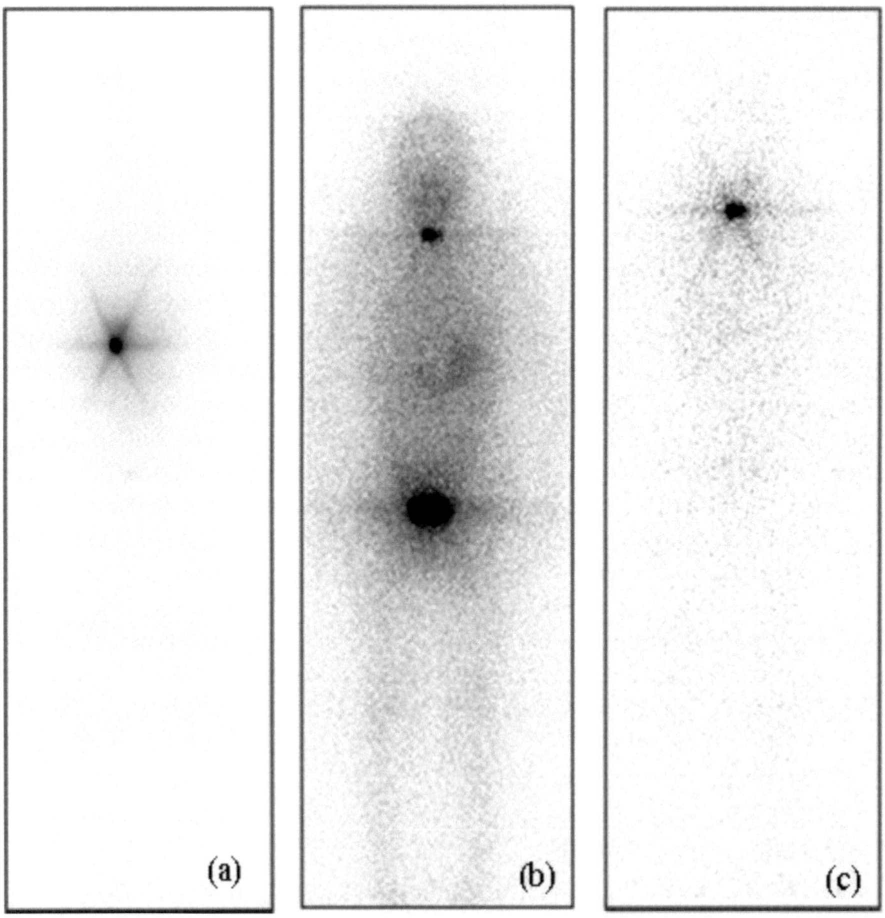

Fig. 1. The anterior whole-body scans of a 46-year-old female patient (case no 4) in (a) 3 hours (b) 46 hours and (c) 142 hours after ^{131}I administration.

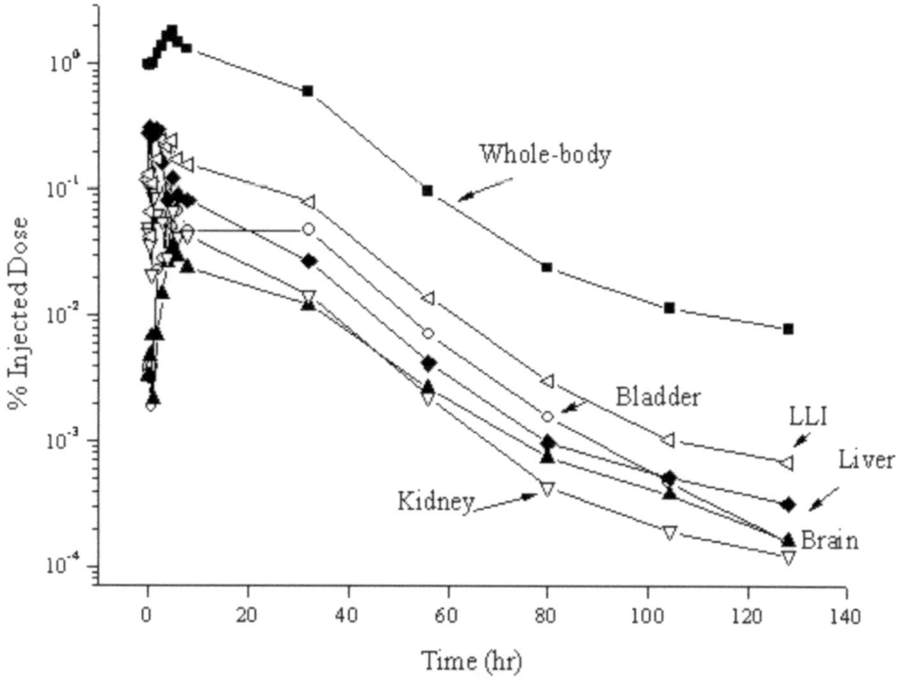

Fig. 2. The time-activity curves (TACs) for the whole-body and each organ calculated from direct measurements of the 46-year-old female patient in organ-specific ROIs without decay correction. ■ represents the whole-body; △, LLI; ○, the bladder; ◆, the liver; ▲, the brain; ▽, the kidneys. The area under the curve is obtained using the trapezoidal rule from the origin to the last activity measured and the T_{eff} is used to evaluate the remaining area under the TAC to infinity for dosimetric calculations.

2.5 Data analysis

The radioiodine ingested by the patients is completely absorbed by the stomach into blood and does not pass through other compartments of the gastrointestinal tract (ICRP 26, 1990). The first scan was performed 2 hours after treatment, and therefore the regressed data were normalized to 100% on day 2. A_0 is the activity of each organ on day 2. A_i is the cumulative activity (sum of all nuclear transitions) in source organ letter i (μCi h or MBq s), and it can be determined by various *in vivo* scanned pixels under the assumed conditions. Computer counts for each ROI were converted into activity. The weighted mean (A_w) of A_i is (Pan and Chen, 2001; Stabin et al., 1999; Saha, 1997),

$$A_w = \frac{\sum W_i A_i}{\sum W_i} \tag{3}$$

where the weighting factor (W_i) is obtained from the percentage standard deviation ($\%\sigma_i$) and the standard error (σ_i):

$$\sigma_i = \sqrt{A_i} \tag{4}$$

$$\sigma_i \% = (100\sqrt{A_i})\% \quad (5)$$

$$W_i = \sigma_i^{-2} \quad (6)$$

The weighted standard error ($\sigma(A_w)$) is

$$\sigma(A_w) = (\sum W_i)^{-1/2} \quad (7)$$

Table 2 displays the re-estimated T_{eff} for the whole-body and each organ from the five Taiwanese female patients using the gradient of the linear regression of normalized residual activity.

2.6 Internal dosimetric calculations

While internal dosimetric calculations as a result of radioiodine therapy depend on the biodistribution of ^{131}I in the whole-body, thyroid remnant and each organ, biodistribution is characterized by the rate of uptake and clearance. TACs were generated in the anterior positions of the brain, kidneys, liver, LLI, thigh, thyroid remnant, the whole-body and in the posterior position of the kidney (Chen et al., 2003). The Medical Internal Radiation Dose (MIRD) committee of the Society of Nuclear Medicine used the MIRDOSE 3 software to determine the radiation dose of each target organ (Sajjad et al., 2002; Stabin et al., 1999; Stabin, 1996; Loevinger et al., 1988; Cristy and Eckerman, 1987). The reference phantom selected from MIRDOSE 3 was a 57 kg adult female phantom. The residence time (τ_h) of the whole-body and source organs were fitted by mono-exponential curves based on the pixels of an image captured by Simens E-CAM γ-camera at CSMUH (Stabin, 1996).

The area under the curve of each TAC was measured in two ways.

1. Trapezoidal rule (Parsey et al., 2005):

$$\tau_h = \frac{1}{2}\int_i^n f(t_i)dt + \int_n^\infty f(t_i)e^{-\lambda_{eff} t_i}dt \quad (8)$$

where $f(t_i)$ = ID/100 and is the cumulative activity (A_i) for any source organ divided by the total activity A_0 administered to the patient at time t (Stabin et al., 1999).

2. The remaining area under the TAC to infinity was determined by the exponential drop in the remaining activity.

The effective dose equivalent (EDE), measured in mGy, in any target organ is,

$$EDE = \frac{kA_i \sum_i n_i E_i f_i}{m} \quad (9)$$

where n_i is the number of decays with energy E_i emitted per nuclear transition of ^{131}I; E_i, the energy per disintegration (MeV); f_i, the fraction of the radiation energy absorbed by the target; m, the mass of the target organ (kg); k, the constant of proportionality (Gy kg/MBq s MeV).

Source organ	Residence Times (h)[a]			
	minimum	Maximum	AVG	SD
Bladder	0.26	2.30	1.02	0.54
Brain	0.43	4.29	1.34	1.18
Kidneys	0.92	4.43	1.70	1.09
Liver	1.53	4.11	2.16	1.14
LLI	2.83	5.74	3.88	1.15
Remainder	8.70	361	87.6	109
Thy(net)	0.16	24.7	6.58	7.30
WB	5.67	44.6	28.8	16.0

[a]AVG stands for average; [b]SD, standard deviation.

Table 2. The average half-life (h) of ^{131}I in each source organ.

3. Results and discussion

Figure 1 displays radioactivity distribution in the ROIs of a 46-year-old female patient (case no 4) in (a) 3 hours (b) 46 hours and (c) 142 hours after ^{131}I administration. That most of the activity was distributed to the LLI and the thyroid on day 1 indicates the typical distribution of ^{131}I. The blood activity outside by ROIs was not measured. Instead, the activity was determined by subtracting the activity sum of all organs from the whole-body activity. Medical professionals entered the activity into MIRDOSE 3 as the "remainder of the body" and learned that the brain takes up the least. Furthermore, **Table 2** displays the maximum, minimum and the T_{eff} of all five Taiwanese patients. Moreover, **Table 3** and **Figure 2** display the *in vivo* mean τ_h of the thyroidectomy patients obtained by the γ-camera in various intervals after the ^{131}I administration.

Source organ	Residence Times (h)[a]			
	minimum	Maximum	AVG	SD
Bladder	0.26	2.30	1.02	0.54
Brain	0.43	4.29	1.34	1.18
Kidneys	0.92	4.43	1.70	1.09
Liver	1.53	4.11	2.16	1.14
LLI	2.83	5.74	3.88	1.15
Remainder	8.70	361	87.6	109
Thy(net)	0.16	24.7	6.58	7.30
WB	5.67	44.6	28.8	16.0

[a]Uptake values are not corrected for physical decay. The results are from a fitted line of five female patients.

Table 3. The calculated ^{131}I residence times (h) using whole-body planar images.

3.1 Biodistributions and dosimetry

Because the information on the T_{eff} of ^{131}I in the thyroid, as well as other organs, of total or near-total thyroidectomy patients is limited, this study estimates the radiation dose absorbed as a result of ^{131}I administration. The biodistribution pattern of ^{131}I was computed from 14 sequential WBSs of the five female patients. Having fitted the ratio of the activities in individual organs (A_i) after the exponential decay to the first whole-body (A_0) decay in **Equation 2**, medical professionals determined the T_{eff} values of these organs. The regional concentrations of ^{131}I changed significantly from hour 1 to hour 4. **Figure 1** shows that a moderate level of background activity remained evident for 32 hours of observation. Furthermore, **Figure 2** shows that the areas known to contain high concentrations of ^{131}I, such as LLI and the liver, exhibited increasing activity. The amount of diagnostic ^{131}I retained by patient no 4 dropped to 1.54% of the initial administered dose after 7 hours, and it did not rise after this initial decline. Whole-body images in **Figure 2** demonstrate persistently high LLI and liver uptake as well as lower brain, kidney and bladder uptake. **Figure 2** also displays the TACs for the whole-body, the bladder, the brain, LLI, the liver and the kidney; it shows that the rate of LLI activity appears to be particularly clean and slow. The biodistribution in the gallbladder, the colon and the esophagus could not be analyzed primarily because the number of pixels and counting statistics were too small. The thyroid remnant uptake in Patient No. 4 declined from 3.69% to 1.54% on day 1, whereas the uptake in the other organs began to fall rapidly at day 2. **Table 4** displays the internal

Source organ	Internal dosimetry (mGy/MBq)			
	Minimum	Maximum	AVG	S D
Adrenal	0 .040	1 .34	0 .35	0 .40
Brain	0 .039	0 .71	0 .21	0 .20
Breasts	0 .027	1 .09	0 .27	0 .33
Gallbladder Wall	0 .040	1 .32	0 .34	0 .39
LLI Wall[a]	0 .96	2 .94	2 .00	0 .67
Small Intestine	0 .051	1 .35	0 .36	0 .40
Stomach	0 .038	1 .34	0 .34	0 .40
ULI Wall[b]	0 .042	1 .40	0 .36	0 .40
Heart Wall	0 .034	1 .34	0 .33	0 .40
Kidneys	0 .22	2 .04	0 .89	0 .46
Liver	0 .064	0 .79	0 .32	0 .20
Lungs	0 .032	1 .25	0 .31	0 .38
Muscle	0 .033	1 .21	0 .29	0 .36
Ovaries	0 .07	1 .46	0 .41	0 .42
Pancreas	0 .04	1 .39	0 .35	0 .41
Red Marrow	0 .038	1 .29	0 .32	0 .38
Bone Surfaces	0 .037	1 .38	0 .34	0 .41
Skin	0 .026	1 .03	0 .25	0 .31
Spleen	0 .037	1 .32	0 .34	0 .39
Thymus	0 .032	1 .28	0 .31	0 .39
Thyroid	0 .029	1 .19	0 .29	0 .38
Urine Bladder Wall	0 .042	1 .29	0 .31	0 .42
Uterus	0 .048	1 .42	0 .36	0 .42
Total body	0 .038	1 .20	0 .31	0 .36
Eff Dose Equiv.[c]	0 .11	1 .42	0 .49	0 .37
Eff Dose[c]	0 .16	1 .49	0 .55	0 .38

[a]LLI stands for lower large intestine; [b]ULI, upper large intestine.
[c]The units for effective dose and effective dose equivalent are mGy/MBq.

Table 4. The estimated amount of radiation dose absorbed (mGy/MBq) as a result of ^{131}I administration.

dosimetric evaluations (mGy/MBq) evaluated from each patient's TACs using MIRDOSE 3 and states the radiation dose absorbed by each organ. The three organs with the highest exposures were the LLI wall, the kidneys and the ovaries.

3.2 T_{eff} of whole-body and other organs

According to **Equation 1**, T_{eff} was determined by the biological elimination and physical decay of ^{131}I activity (Chen et al., 2003; Stabin et al., 1999; Berg et al., 1996; Stabin 1996; Synder et al., 1983). An important step in generating the TACs and determining the dose required for thyroidectomy patients is to calculate the exact T_{eff} of each organ of interest. Dunning and Schwarz (1981) determined that large uncertainties might be primarily associated with the patient's age, and the physiological and metabolic characteristics of each organ.

Using planar images to analyze data yields conservative estimates of activities because the large ROIs include overlying tissues, as displayed in **Figure 1**. The T_{eff} of ^{131}I for Graves' disease is 5.0±0.16 days (s.d. = 1.3); toxic nodular goiter, 6.0±0.12 days (s.d = 1.2) as reported by Berg et al. (1996). **Figure 2** shows that ^{131}I-NaI was clearing from the whole-body at an T_{eff} of 22.7±16.3 hour, which is consistent with that obtained by Pacilio et al. (2005), who also found that the median and mean (±1 standard deviation) T_{bio} distribution of 225 ablation treatments were 0.63 days and 0.70±2.25 days, respectively. In this study, the whole-body T_{eff} values of five female patients who have undergone a total or near-total thyroidectomy ranged from 15.4 to 175.4 hours and T_{bio} was 31.9±4.8 hours. These data correlated well with 2.18±1.45 days of complete ablation patients, reported by Samuel and Rajashekharrao (1994) as displayed in **Table 5**. Samuel and Rajashekharrao (1994) also reported ranges of 0.83 to 3.7 day for complete ablation patients and 1.6 to 5.0 days for partial ablation patients; these numbers are also displayed in **Table 5**. Furthermore, Samuel and Rajashekharrao (1994) employed a portable β-γ exposure rate meter to measure the ^{131}I activity in residual thyroid tissue in the neck region directly in order to evaluate the T_{eff} of ^{131}I. Using γ-camera *in vivo* at CSMUH may yield more precise results than using a portable β-γ exposure rate meter. North et al. (2001) obtained an T_{eff} of 0.71 days in complete ablation patients who received 1.7-13 GBq of ^{131}I, which is greater than the 1100 MBq dose in this study. Furthermore, this study included only five patients, and therefore the results should be considered as preliminary estimates only. Although the patients were all female, the biodistribution is not expected to differ significantly due to gender.

3.3 Internal medical dosimetry

The MIRDOSE 3 software can be used to determine the effective dose as defined by ICRP 23. Internal medical dosimetry was conducted for each subject independently, and the results were averaged. **Table 4** displays the average dose amount absorbed by the six principal target organs in the five female patients. LLI absorbed the most radiation (2.00±0.67 mGy/MBq), ranging from 0.96 to 2.94 mGy/MBq; the kidney (0.89±0.46 mGy/MBq), second; the ovaries (0.41±0.42 mGy/MBq), third. The species as well as physiological and metabolic characteristics may account for the differences. These τ_h obtained from the fitted lines of individual organs were highest in the LLI wall (3.88±1.15 hours) and then in the liver (2.16±1.14 hours), as displayed in **Table 3**. Self-dose, according to MIRDOSE 3, was the main contributor to the dose absorbed by all of the organs listed in Table 4. The effective dose was 0.55±0.38 mGy/MBq and effective dose equivalent was 0.49±0.37 mGy/MBq, which did not include the effective dose of the thyroid remnant, and was lower the 16.00 mSv/MBq reported by Weng et al. (1989), who determined the values by either EDE per radiopharmaceutical drug or an published procedure of data in Kaohsiung from 1977 to 1988.

Pathology	Therapeutic dose (^{131}I)	Effective Half-Life (day)	Method	Reference
Thyroidectomy	1.1 GBq	22.7±16.3 (hr)	E-CAM γ-camera	This work
Extrathyroidal	1.22 GBq	0.32	Model	USNRC, 1997
Complete ablation	3.4 ± 2.4 GBq	2.18 ± 1.45	Exposure rate meter	Samuel, and Rajashekharrao, 1994
Thyroid cancer	3.7-7.4 GBq	2.2± 0.8	γ-camera	Mathieu, 1996
Total lobectomy	1.1 GBq	5	Rectilinear scanner	Synde, 1983
Grave's disease	0.5 MBq	5.0± 1.56	2-inch NaI neck uptake	Berg, 1996
Toxic nodular goiter	0.5 MBq	6.0± 1.2	2-inch NaI neck uptake	Berg, 1996
Normal, Adults	Trace amount	T_{bio} =120 T_{bio} =12	Model	ICRP 30

Table 5. The effective half-life of ^{131}I for whole-body therapy.

Beekhuis et al. (1988) found large variations among medical internal doses across hospitals that apply various radioactivity dose levels in similar investigations (Beekhuis et al., 1988). Furthermore, Beekhuis et al. (1988) established that EDEs were rough estimates of real radiation burdens. The dose required for ablation is directly related to the mass of the remnant, thus using US, CT or MRI to evaluate organ and tumor mass yields more accurate and reproducible results (Rosario et al., 2004). Published reports by Comtois et al. (1993) also strongly asserted that 1100 MBq of ^{131}I, the dose applied in this study, can ablate residual thyroid tissues completely. Moreover, the 1100 MBq dose reduces the financial burden on the patients who no longer require hospitalization (CSMUH, 2005).

4. Conclusion

To our knowledge, this study is the first attempt to re-calculate biodistributions, T_{eff} and the internal medical dosimetric data for Taiwanese female ^{131}I patients. The T_{eff} for the thyroid was 22.7±16.3 hours and for the whole-body was 69.5±70.9 hours. **Table 5** shows that the results differ significantly from those reported by ICRP 30, but are consistent with Samuel and Rajashekharrao's (1994) 2.18±1.45 days for patients who exhibited complete ablation. Despite the consideration of thyroid remnant, the medical internal doses in this study were highest in LLI, 2.00±0.67 mGY/MBq, and second highest in the kidney, 0.89±0.46 mGy/MBq as determined by using the trapezoidal rule to evaluate the area under the TACs. Based on an effective dose of 0.55±0.38 mGy/MBq for the five thyroidectomy patients at CSMUH, the biodistributions and T_{eff} can be easily estimated from medical images obtained using Siemens E-CAM coincidence γ-camera. 1100 MBq of ^{131}I could be safe and sufficient to administer to total thyroidectomy patients.

5. Acknowledgements

Lin Shin Hospital and its staff provided financial support under Contract Number: LSRP099007.

6. References

Beekhuis, H. (1988). Population radiation absorbed dose from nuclear medicine procedures in the Netherlands. *Health Phys.* Vol. 54, pp287-291, ISSN 0017-9078

Berg, G. E. B. et. al. (1996). Iodine-131 Treatment of Hyperthyroidism: Significance of Effective Half-life Measurements. *J. Nucl. Med.* Vol. 37(2), pp228-232, ISSN 0161-5505

Chen, C.Y. et al., (2003). Effective half-life of ^{131}I of whole-body and individual organs for thyroidectomy patient using scintigraphic images of camera. *Chung Shan Med. J.* Vol. 14(2), pp557-565, ISSN 1680-3108

Chen, C. Y. & Pan, L. K. (2001). Trace elements of race elements of Taiwanese Dioscorea Spp. Using neutron activation analysis. *Food Chem.* Vol. 72, pp255-260, ISSN 0278-6915

Comtois, R.; Theriault, C. & Vecchio, P. D. (1993). Assessment of the efficacy of iodine-131 for thyroid ablation. *J. Nucl. Med.* Vol. 34, pp1927-1930, ISSN 0161-5505.

Cristy, M. & Eckerman, K., (1987). Specific absorbed fractions of energy at various ages from internal photon sources. *ORNL/TM-8381/VII.* P.7-29. Oak Ridge National Laboratory, Oak Ridge, Tenn. USA

Department of Nuclear Medicine, Chung Shan Medical University Hospital, (2005). Introduction to Radiation Safety in Nuclear Medicine. Chung Shan Medical University Guide. *Chung Shan Medical University Hospital* Taiwan, ROC.

Dunning, Jr. D. E. & Schwarz, G. (1981). Variability of Human Thyroid Characteristics and Estimates of Dose from Ingested ^{131}I. *Health Phys.* Vol. 40(1), pp. 661-675, ISSN 0017-9078

International Commission on Radiological Protection, (1990). Report of the task group on reference man. *ICRP Publication 26.* Pergamon Press, Oxford. USA

International Commission on Radiological Protection, (1978). Limits for intakes of radionuclides by workers. ICRP Publication 30 (Part 1). Pergamon Press, Oxford. USA

Loevinger, R.; Budinger, T. & Watson E., (1988). *MIRD primer for absorbed dose calculations.* Society of Nucl Med, New York, USA.

North, D.L. et al, (2001). Effective Half-Life of ^{131}I in Thyroid Cancer Patients. *Health Phys.* Vol. 81(3), pp.325-329, ISSN 0017-9078.

Rosario, P. W. S. et al., (2004). Efficacy of low and high ^{131}I doses for thyroid remnant ablation in patients with differentiated thyroid carcinoma based on post-operative cervical uptake. *Nucl. Med. Commun.* Vol. 25, pp.1077-1081, ISSN 0143-3636.

Saha G.B., (1997). *Fundamentals of Nuclear Pharmacy.* 4th ed. P27. ISBN 0-387-98341-4 Springer USA.

Samuel, A. M. & Rajashekharrao, B. (1994). Radioiodine Therapy for Well-Differentiated Thyroid Cancer: A Quantitative Dosimetric Evaluation for Remnant Thyroid Ablation After Surgery. J. *Nucl. Med.* Vol. 35(12), pp,1944-1950, ISSN 0161-5505.

Seidlin, S.; Oshry, E. & Yallow, A. A. (1948). Spontaneous and experimentally induced uptake of radioactive iodine in metastases from thyroid carcinoma. *J. Clin. Endocrinol. Metab.* Vol 8, pp. 423- 425, ISSN 0021-972X.

Shieley, V. S. & Lederer. C. M. (1978) *Table of isotopes*, Wiley-interscience Publishing Co., ISBN New York, USA

Siemens Medical Systems Inc, (1998). E. *CAM Dual-Detector System, Addendum #52 54 417 Rev. 01.* Hoffman Estates IL USA.

Snyder, J. et al. (1983). Thyroid Remnants Ablation: Questionable Pursuit of all ill-defined Goals. *J. Nucl. Med.* Vol.24(8), pp. 659-665, ISSN 0161-5505

Stabin, M. G. et al., (1999). Radiation dosimetry in nuclear medicine. *Appl. Radiat. Isot.* Vol.50, pp. 73-87, ISSN 0969-8043

Stabin, M. G., (1996). MIRDOSE: Personal computer software for internal dose assessment in nuclear medicine. *J. Nucl. Med.* Vol.37, pp. 538-546, ISSN 0161-5505

Taylor, D. M., (2000). Generic models for radionuclide dosimetry: ^{11}C-, ^{18}F- or ^{75}Se-labelled amino acids. *Appl. Radiat. Isot.* Vol.52, pp. 911-922, ISSN 0969-8043

U.S. Nuclear Regulatory Commission, (1997). Code of federal regulations: Release of patients administered radioactive material. *U.S. Government Printing Office*; Regulatory guide 8.39. Washington, DC. USA

Weng, P. S. et al., (1989). Effective dose equivalent from nuclear medicine procedures in South Taiwan. *Nucl. Sci. J.* Vol.26(4), pp. 318-324, ISSN 0029-5647

14

Thyroid Cancer: The Evolution of Treatment Options

Hitoshi Noguchi
Noguchi Thyroid Clinic and Hospital Foundation
Japan

1. Introduction

Joseph Stalin once said that one death is a tragedy but a million deaths is a statistic. Medical textbooks present percentages and p values, but medical professionals must deal with one death at a time. Textbooks are read in preparation for the profession. The purpose of this chapter is to bridge the gap by presenting an historical overview of the various controversies in the field of thyroid cancer that shaped our current knowledge and thereby assist the student in grasping the underlying structure beneath the vast amount of sometimes conflicting data.

A student new to the arena may be surprised at finding the candy box assortment of colorful characters engaged in lively debate within the outwardly staid community. These people are passionate about the arcane details of thyroid carcinoma, a narrow specialty about which most students of medicine are indifferent. But the history of this field is fraught with debate, controversy, confrontations and a legacy of brave souls who dared to fight against the tide.

The current opinions, as of 2011, regarding the treatment of differentiated thyroid cancer can roughly be divided into two groups, those that aggressively promote the adoption of total thyroidectomy with radioiodine ablation followed by periodic screening for biochemical recurrence and those that do not. The latter group usually prefers to perform thyroid lobectomy when the gross tumor is small and limited to one lobe of the thyroid, which would automatically rule out post-surgical ablation and the use of recombinant-TSH to screen for thyroglobulin. The option of lobectomy, although still resisted by many in the field, was finally adopted in the 2009 version of the guideline for the treatment of differentiated thyroid carcinoma by the American Thyroid Association[1)], but only for tumors measuring 10 millimeters or less. The following year, Sonkar et al[2)] wrote an article titled "Papillary Thyroid Carcinoma: Debate at Rest" writing that "the controversy regarding the extent of thyroidectomy in papillary thyroid carcinoma is relatively settled" with total thyroidectomy and radioiodine ablation being the preferred option for all but the smallest tumors. This announcement, however, proved premature. The 2010 version of the Japanese guideline for the treatment of thyroid tumors declared that papillary carcinomas as large as 30 millimeters were candidates for lobectomy when they were limited to one lobe of the thyroid with little or no extra-capsular invasion and gross lymph node involvement[3)]. As for papillary carcinoma less than 10 millimeters, some Japanese surgeons are proposing that observation without surgery may be sufficient[4]. The journey that lead to this schism and how it relates to the current therapeutic options is explained in this chapter as well as the most likely course that future therapy may take.

2. The maverick

Thyroid surgery was a dangerous endeavor in the 19th century and the French Academy of Medicine officially condemned the practice, but with the introduction of anesthesia, antisepsis techniques and hemostatic forceps, the prognosis improved dramatically. Billroth reported a mortality rate of 40% early in his career which fell to 8% in the 1870s[5]. Kocher reported a reduction in mortality from 12.6% to 0.2% from the 1870s to the end of the 19th century[6]. Successful thyroidectomy lead to the discovery of postoperative hypothyroidism which in turn elucidated the true function of the normal thyroid gland[7]. Klein reported on loss of voice due to injury to the recurrent laryngeal nerves during the removal of goiter[8]. Tetany was observed in patients who underwent total thyroidectomy, but it was only with the concerted efforts of multiple investigators around the turn of the century that damage to the parathyroid glands was found to be responsible for this condition[9]. Eventually, these discoveries lead to the reduction of surgical complications in thyroid surgery.

Medical progress has advanced on a precarious balance between the pressing need for immediate solutions and the effort to keep harmful options out of the field. Pioneers of medicine made courageous, sometimes reckless, forays into uncharted territory to which we owe our current technology. But once the frontier was conquered and patient survival improved, more attention was paid to the tradeoffs of treatment, such as compromised quality of life, and efforts were made to diminish them. Surgery in particular has progressed, over the past half century, in the direction of reducing the extent of dissection and thereby lowering the risk of complications.

George "Barney" Crile Jr. stands out as the man who set the field of surgery onto this course. Father of the celebrated journalist George Crile III and son of the venerated founding member of the Cleveland Clinic, George Crile Sr., he is something of an unsung hero of modern surgery. Surgery for thyroid carcinoma of his time, called the "block dissection" or "conventional radical neck dissection", usually sacrificed the sternocleidomastoid muscle, often the accessory nerve and sometimes the inframandibular branch of the facial nerve. He wrote in 1957 "The deformities and dysfunctions which ensue are tragic consequences to teen-age girls and young women who are most commonly affected by papillary cancers of the thyroid. Loss of contour of the neck, paralysis of the muscles of the lower face, shoulder drop, later arthritic changes in the shoulder girdle, hoarseness from unilateral laryngeal nerve injuries, stridor from bilateral injuries, and tetany are serious and often permanent complications. The surgeon who inflicts them must be prepared to defend his position by incontrovertible proof of a higher rate of cure."[10] He argued that there was none. He was one of the first surgeons ever to promote the idea that "the less surgery the better", and he campaigned vigorously for the abandonment of the classic block dissection. His ideas on thyroid cancer surgery, and later breast cancer surgery, were reluctantly but steadily adopted by the surgical community and have since shaped the evolution of surgical treatment.

It would be easier to compose a narrative if the history of thyroid surgery were a linear progression from "conventional radical neck dissection" to less and less invasive procedures. But the story is more muddled, partly due to the particular characteristics of the organ and also due to entrenched positions of opinionated surgeons and oncologists. The trajectory was also confounded by the periodic infusion of breathtaking new technology for which there was widespread but misguided enthusiasm. There was no consensus for the optimum surgical procedure for thyroid cancer surgery in the early to mid-twentieth century. If the gross tumor was limited to one lobe, some surgeons performed lobectomy, some lobectomy with isthmus, some lobectomy with isthmus and a part of the opposing lobe and some insisted on total thyroidectomy. A few even dared to perform partial lobectomy and preserved most of the thyroid. The extent of lymph node dissection also varied greatly[11)]. Early on, metastasis to the lymph nodes in the neck were mistaken for embryological migration error termed "lateral aberrant thyroid" and believed not to require surgery. Conventional radical dissection may have been a backlash against this initial complacency[12)].

During the time Crile was battling conventional radical dissection, others were arguing for more radical surgery. Clark et al performed serial sections of the whole thyroid. He found intraglandular dissemination in 58% of the 79 cases he studied[13)]. Similar studies by Black et al found multicentricity in 20%[14)], and Underwood et al found contralateral lobe involvement in 32% of cases studied[15)]. Each of these authors advocated total thyroidectomy or more based on their findings. However, Tollefsen, citing these works and others, compared them to the actual clinical recurrence rate in the opposite lobe. He pointed out that his recurrence rate was 3.7% and even Black, a proponent of radical surgery, had reported a recurrence in the opposite lobe in only 7%. In his 1963 report, Tollefsen wrote "The final importance of these histologic observations must rest in the clinical results. All but a small percentage of our patients have remained well for periods up to twenty-five years without clinical recurrence in the remaining lobe. We must, therefore, interpret these histologic cancers in the other lobe as being of slight importance and somewhat analogous to the autopsy incidence of microscopic cancer in the prostate."[16)] It is surprising today to find that a surgeon in New York had already outlined the position taken by Japanese specialists of the twenty-first century half a century previously. Nobody today questions that papillary thyroid carcinoma is very often multi-focal, although some authors argue that microscopic multifocal disease is clinically irrelevant.

3. Stratifications

Care should be taken in reading, and especially in citing, medical reports of this era. Histologic classification and diagnosis did not follow the same criteria as we use today. Statistics were rudimentary and rarely employed anything more sophisticated than simple percentages. Most troublesome of all, such variables as the initial size of the pre-operative tumor or the age of the patient were not taken into account when discussing the merits of one surgical procedure over another. In 1953, Crile reported that patients aged over 40 at initial diagnosis had a poorer prognosis compared to patients aged under 40. He concluded "Since almost all cancers of the thyroid that occur in patients under 40 years of age are of the lowest grade malignancy, the prognosis in this age group is almost universally good if an adequate operation is performed"[17)]. In his 1964 report Tollefsen analyzed 70 fatal cases of papillary thyroid carcinoma and isolated age, initial size of tumor over 5 centimeters, recurrent laryngeal nerve palsy and distant metastasis as indicators of poor prognosis[18]. This was the beginning of the study of risk profiles in thyroid cancer. It was only after the prognostic indicators were clearly identified, and the outcome of treatment was compared among groups with equivalent risk profiles that the debate on surgical procedures rested on firm footing. Statistical techniques such as multivariate analysis were not employed in the study of thyroid cancer until the introduction of practical personal computers in the mid 1980s. Nonetheless, "conventional radical neck dissection" fell out of favor by the early 1970s.

Meanwhile, a remarkable paradigm shift was surrounding the realm of thyroid surgery. The increasing acceptance of iodine prophylaxis markedly decreased the incidence of endemic goiter. Radioiodine and anti-thyroid drugs reduced the number of surgically treated Graves disease. Prior to the development of oral steroid medications, even subacute thyroiditis was often treated by surgery, but this method was completely abandoned. The practice of irradiating children for benign diseases, which apparently increased the incidence of radiation induced thyroid cancer, was no longer performed[19]. Core needle and fine needle biopsies made preoperative differentiation of benign and malignant tumors possible. Due to these developments and others, the number of thyroid operations performed in the Cleveland Clinic fell from 2,700 in the year 1927 to less than 50 in the late 1960s[20]. Thyroid cancer effectively became the last bastion of thyroid surgery.

Imaging modalities also influenced surgery. In the late 1940s, ultrasonography was developed simultaneously in the United States, United Kingdom, Sweden and Japan. Although the earliest machines were cumbersome and impractical, the technology eventually improved to incorporate hand held probes which produced acceptably clear images. Fine needle aspiration biopsy was developed in the 1950s and eventually came into wide acceptance. But the combination of the two did not appear until the 1970s and was not widely used in the diagnosis of thyroid diseases until the 1980s. Computerized axial tomography was commercialized in the mid 1970s and magnetic resonance imaging in the early 80s, but neither machines were initially suitable for the examination of the neck area , CAT scan because of image artifacts from the bones and MRI (then called NMR-CT) because of low resolution. Both imaging technologies developed rapidly and became indispensable tools in the examination of the thyroid by the 1990s. The introduction of these diagnostic tools contributed greatly in the early detection of thyroid cancer and the incidence of thyroid cancer steadily increased[21] while the size of tumor upon discovery steadily decreased after the mid 1980s[3].

Over the years, improvements in anesthesia made it safer for surgeons to take the time to carefully visualize the recurrent laryngeal nerve which was eventually proven to diminish the incidence of paralysis[22]. The same was true for the parathyroid, which when better preserved caused fewer cases of tetany. This meant that total thyroidectomy could be performed with smaller risk of surgical complications.

So if the tumors were smaller but the complications were fewer, was it more logical to perform more conservative surgery or more radical surgery? Although this was not the question that was openly verbalized, this was the general area where the battle lines were drawn. And the debate was closely linked to the question of radioiodine therapy.

The use of radioactive isotope of iodine as a tracer for the thyroid was developed during the 1930s and 40s. Eventually, this lead to the treatment of hyperthyroidism using 131-I[23]. The experimental application of radioiodine on thyroid cancer began almost simultaneously[24]. It was soon established that replacement thyroid hormones should be withdrawn for the duration of this therapy and that healthy thyroid tissues need to be removed for this method to be effective. The use of thyroglobulin to screen for cancer recurrence was developed later[25]. It was then established that thyroglobulin measurements yield no useful information in the follow up of thyroid cancer patients in the presence of residual thyroid tissue[26]. Thus a new rationale for total thyroidectomy was introduced. Thyroid cancer patients would hence forth be given total thyroidectomy not because tumors were found in both lobes, but because it facilitated post-operative screening for recurrence and the treatment of recurrence should any be found. And not only were the thyroid removed surgically, but they were completely eradicated by means of "remnant ablation" using 131-I.

Although some surgeons were initially skeptical about the utility of radioiodine therapy in the treatment of metastatic thyroid carcinoma, the contrarians were eventually silenced as data mounted supporting its efficacy. By the 1970s few argued against the adoption of radioiodine therapy, and consequently total thyroidectomy, on patients with proven distant metastasis. Routine remnant ablation and thyroglobulin screening, however, was a different matter. Once again, superiority of one regimen over the other was frequently argued without stratifying the cases according to various risk factors. In one example, Snyder pointed out in 1983 that the actual effectiveness of routine remnant ablation in reducing morbidity and mortality was not objectively proven due to this reason[27]. In a subsequent issue of the same journal, Riccabona published a letter to the editor which included a survival curve comparing the survival of patients who had undergone radioiodine ablation and patients who had not to show that radioiodine ablation indeed had a positive effect[28]. To this, Snyder replied that this was "yet another testimonial to what has plagued the evaluation of different approaches to the treatment of thyroid cancer patients" and asked "Were Dr. Riccabona's patients randomized as to treatment? Were variables such as age, sex, histological type, histological grade, extent of disease, extent of surgery, and use of thyroid suppression therapy taken into account? What method was used in the detection of postoperative functioning tissue? Was ablation aimed at presumably normal thyroid tissue, or known residual thyroid cancer in the thyroid bed, or extrathyroidal functioning metastasis? Were these variables considered in the survival curve presented?" Few such dialogues were preserved in print, but similar debates occurred frequently in conferences around the world, occasionally accompanied by thunderous arguments and animated gesticulations, throughout the 1980s. Although not entirely as a consequence of such confrontations, the TNM staging system was introduced in 1987, AMES system in 1988, AGES system in 1987 and MACIS system in 1993.

4. Debates

Randomized prospective trials, had they been performed, may have helped settle many of the disputes. But differentiated thyroid carcinoma is an indolent cancer with a low rate of recurrence regardless of the treatment modality and often remains dormant for many years before tangible physical recurrence can be observed. This means that large numbers of patients would have to be followed for a very long time before a definite conclusion could be reached. Thus, the studies on the optimum treatment for thyroid cancer would be left in the hands of prolific surgeons who would showcase their vast surgical experience in retrospective studies involving large numbers of patients. The field of thyroid cancer is littered with retrospective studies of hundreds, sometimes thousands of cases aimed at demonstrating the validity or otherwise of a given procedure. The extent of surgery is one of many controversial subjects that are so studied and there is a number of retrospective studies, properly stratified with AGES, AMES and pTNM, which demonstrate that total or near-total thyroidectomy reduces recurrence rates compared to lobectomy and similar unilateral resections[29)30)31)]. What is often left unsaid is that patients who undergo near-total or total thyroidectomy must receive oral hormone replacement for a lifetime, while the majority of patients who undergo unilateral lobectomy remain euthyroid without medication. As a consequence, the patients who undergo lobectomy tend to have poor retention in retrospective studies because patients tend to stop visiting their doctors when they are feeling well. The difference in retention between patients of near-total or total thyroidectomy and patients of lobectomy is rarely ever mentioned in retrospective studies. But this helps explain why some investigators found no significant difference in recurrence between the two procedures[32)33)].

And on top of all this was the professional bias of individual investigators. In the absence of a randomized trial, doctors generally do not perform treatments they do not believe in, due to which single-institution retrospective studies tend to have poorly structured control groups. Shiro Noguchi performed over ten thousand thyroid surgeries during his career by official record, not counting the thousands he hijacked while nominally assisting or overseeing them. He employed clerks whose sole mission was to stay in contact with his postoperative patients by telephone and mail, and to do detective work to track down their ever changing addresses. As a result, he published a number of long-term retrospective studies with large populations and excellent patient retention. His focus, however, was to prove the validity of prophylactic lymph node dissection. He called his procedure "modified radical neck dissection" even though nearly half of his cases involved only lobectomy. His belief was, if the lymph nodes of the neck were properly excised, neither total thyroidectomy nor remnant ablation were necessary in most low-to-moderate risk cases. His support of lobectomy was only secondary to his belief in prophylactic node dissection. Another prolific surgeon Orlo H. Clark, on the other hand, was a proponent of total thyroidectomy and remnant ablation who also happened to be skeptical about the value of prophylactic lymph node dissection. Naturally, Noguchi's reports expounded on the merits of prophylactic node dissection, but compared results in the absence of remnant ablation. Clark's reports stressed the merits of total thyroidectomy with remnant ablation in the absence of prophylactic node dissection. Clark's arguments against prophylactic lymph node dissection rested on the assumption that the patient would receive remnant ablation. Noguchi did not employ radioiodine therapy in any of his cases with rare exceptions, low risk or otherwise, unless there was proven metastasis on image scans such as sonography, CAT, MRI or scintigraphy because he believed ablation was unnecessary and harmed the quality of life of his patients. Clark did not perform neck dissection unless there was proven metastasis on image scans for the same reason. Both surgeons reported excellent prognosis and low incidence of complications. (The two experts once joined hands to create a "definitive text" on thyroid cancer but the book, not surprisingly, was not a commercial success[34)].) As this example illustrates, each investigator had priorities among different points of controversy that made it difficult to compare the results of one report with another.

Other than the lack of prospective trials, varied patient retention, insufficient risk stratification and professional bias, there was also a linguistic problem. The idea that there is always some dissociation between the "signifier" and the "signified" is a relatively new concept that was not widely accepted among medical professionals of the previous generation. Authors almost never gave any thought to it. Noguchi's use of the term "modified radical neck dissection" was just one example of many idiosyncrasies in the use of terminology that hampered understanding and obstructed progress. One of the more glaring examples was Mazzaferri's use of the word "recurrence". He frequently neglected to make the distinction between "recurrence" and "biochemical recurrence"[35]. In some cases, TSH stimulation produced positive thyroglobulin serum tests in the absence of tangible metastasis on image scans. Recurrence of thyroid cancer was only implied by serum data. Such cases were termed "biochemical recurrence". The assumption was that these test results represented malignant recurrences too small to be visualized. When some doctors heard or read "recurrence" they automatically assumed that there was a detectable physical mass, but Mazzaferri was such an influential and widely cited authority that there would eventually be a school of specialists who used the term "recurrence" interchangeably with "biochemical recurrence". It takes an astute reader to realize that the "recurrence rate" in one citation is not always the same thing as a "recurrence rate" in another.

And then, in 1998, human recombinant TSH was approved for thyroglobulin testing. This was truly a product of advanced molecular biology and a cutting edge drug of a new era. It allowed testing for thyroglobulin without withdrawing replacement thyroid hormones. It would eventually be approved for use in radioiodine therapy, for which it had the same advantage. Unfortunately, the enthusiasm that this drug generated also provided incentive to perform total thyroidectomy where its necessity was still in question.

Under the influence of these persistent obstacles, some researchers continued to hone their investigative strategies with ever more refined study designs. Others seemingly decided to take the kick-in-the-teeth approach. Ito et al performed an observational study of papillary microcarcinoma and found that only 15.9% increased in size beyond the margin of error (3mm or more) and only 3.4% presented novel nodal metastasis after 10 years of observation without treatment[4]. This finding was in line with the data from unsuspected microcarcinomas found in thyroids resected for other reasons[36]. If this is the malignant potential of clinically tangible tumors, the reasoning implied, what is the clinical significance of microscopic intragrandular focci or invisible biochemical recurrence? Granted that there is evidence that post-ablative serum thyroglobulin is a predictor of recurrence in low risk thyroid carcinoma[37], an increasing number of studies suggest that routine ablation does not significantly suppress recurrence in low risk cases[38][39]. Some experts argue that remnant ablation should be performed anyway in order to prevent what little differentiated cancer that may remain from turning into anaplastic carcinoma, which is universally fatal. But the incidence of anaplastic carcinoma in North America where post-surgical ablation is performed routinely is substantially higher than the incidence in Japan where post-surgical ablation is still uncommon, although this difference has been attributed to the higher iodine content of the Japanese diet[40].

Authors on both sides of the debate have pointed out that not all papillary carcinomas are equally indolent. Some grow rapidly and progress more aggressively than others without obvious histological differences. Histological variations such as tall cell variants and columnar cell variants have been identified[41)42)], but many unusually malignant strains cannot be morphologically identified as any different from other examples of papillary carcinoma. How to identify the rare differentiated cancers that are most likely to take a more malignant course is an important and unanswered question. Clinical risk factors are currently the only guide, although some studies on molecular prognostic markers are being performed[43)44)].

Proponents of lobectomy point out that only one recurrent laryngeal nerve is at risk when only one lobe of the thyroid is being resected thus the theoretical risk of nerve palsy is halved[45)]. Proponents of total thyroidectomy insist that the increase in complications is minimal at the hands of an experienced surgeon[46)]. Disagreement over the merits of prophylactic central node dissection is argued along similar lines[47)48)49)]. Experience suggests that the incidence of surgical complications is much more dependent on the proficiency of the surgeon than the type of surgery performed. Experts who are experienced enough to publish large retrospective studies invariably report excellent results regardless of the type of surgery they promote.

5. Where we are

So which is the better option? Is it more practical to allow a small number of recurrences and re-operate on those that recur, or ablate at the first sign of a biochemical recurrence and risk salivary gland damage to prevent re-operation? Is it more economical to periodically check for thyroglobulin with recombinant TSH, or just follow with sonogram and surgically remove the metastasis when they appear? The cost of surgery, radioiodine therapy, image scans and cytology tests vary tremendously in the US, Europe and Japan, to say nothing of the availability of high end care, the social costs of hospitalization, the geographic distance to specialized institutions and the medical legal demands on the doctor. Depending on the location of the patient and the local cost structure of medical care, one option may be more advantageous than another. At the bottom line, the current argument on low risk thyroid cancer is whether or not it is an acceptable tradeoff to allow a minimally increased risk of surgical complications to guard against a minimally increased risk of cancer recurrence when there is no proven difference in prognosis. It is difficult to reach a conclusion because the difference in benefits and demerits are so small, the choice is largely dependent on the preference and socio-economic situation of the patient. Perhaps it is time for this debate to leave the ivory tower and be presented to the patients who are directly affected.

The experts now nearing retirement or who have retired in the past few decades have lived through a vibrant age. Long ago, in an American hospital, two reputable surgeons with conflicting surgical philosophy had an argument in the operating room when, after the initial incision, they found the extent of disease to be not what they expected. Anesthesia was not as stable then as it is today and time was precious. In exasperation, one surgeon punched the other in the face, calmly changed his gloves, and completed the surgery alone while the other lay unconscious on the operating room floor. Such buccaneering days have long since ended. The controversies surrounding thyroid cancer today do not have the consequences of Crile's time when he started his crusade against radical thyroidectomy and radical mastectomy. This is an inevitable result of medical progress. As the prognosis improves and complications diminish, the persisting debates become increasingly pedantic.

Today there are surgical conferences around the world that no longer hold independent sessions for the discussion of thyroid cancer surgery. As sobering as it may sound, fading from attention is the final reward of great medical progress. We cannot be disappointed that the scope of our arguments has become smaller. Our patients are better for it.

If the past is any guide, the future of thyroid cancer treatment will most likely evolve in two major directions. One is the treatment of poorly differentiated and unresponsive cancers. The other is the ever earlier diagnosis and increasingly conservative treatment of low malignancy cancers. Endoscopic and robotic surgery that are seeing wider application in the gastroenterological field are being tested in thyroid surgery. Laser ablation and radio frequency ablation, both of which use specialized needles inserted percutaneously to ablate benign thyroid nodules, are also being tested on a limited sub-group of malignant tumors[50)51)]. If more evidence is accumulated that low-risk papillary cancers are as indolent as some researchers claim, such low invasion techniques may see wider application. The current debate on the choice between total thyroidectomy and lobectomy may seem quaint when, in the future, microcarcinomas are treated with needles tipped with thermal coagulation devises.

Conservative surgery became possible in other fields of oncology partly due to the development of adjuvant chemotherapy. Though conventional chemotherapy is not effective for differentiated thyroid cancer, tyrosine kinase inhibitors hold some promise. This new class of drugs is being tested, with encouraging results, on radioiodine refractory cases[52)], medullary carcinoma[53)] and anaplastic carcinoma[54)]. Combination therapy in the future may produce even better results.

Molecular biology has enhanced our understanding of thyroid cancer greatly. Genetic testing has allowed for early detection of MEN type 2 and prophylactic thyroidectomy[55)]. Tyrosine kinase inhibitors, histone deacetylase inhibitors[56)] and nijmegen breakage syndromes[57)] are being studied as potential new therapies for anaplastic carcinoma. Studies of micro-RNAs have provided some interesting hints in their potential for diagnosis and treatment of cancer[58)]. Further studies may present more focused differentiation of low-risk and high-risk cancers on the molecular level.

6. Summary

In summary, much has been elucidated about thyroid cancer in the past century and a half. We owe our current expertise to those who dared to challenge the status quo. The general direction of the evolution of thyroid cancer treatment has been toward lesser invasion and increasingly tailored therapy as we learned to more correctly differentiate low-risk from high-risk and acquired knowledge and confidence to leave well enough alone. The future will most likely follow this trend, differentiating the risk categories with ever greater accuracy and treating them with increasingly focused therapy. Trends to the contrary are likely to be momentary aberrations or corrections to the course. As prognosis improves and complications diminish, points of controversy in treatment options will be of increasingly smaller universal significance and will inevitably invite greater patient involvement in clinical decision making. There are still frontiers to be conquered in the field of thyroid cancer, though not as wild or lawless as in the past. There will always be room for innovators in the future. One only needs to proceed in the right direction.

(The author is a fourth generation thyroidologist. The Noguchi Thyroid Clinic and Hospital Foundation celebrates its 90th anniversary in 2012.)

7. References

[1] Revised American Thyroid Association Management Guidelines for Patients with Thyroid Nodules and Differentiated Thyroid Cancer, November 2009
[2] Sonkar AA, Rajamanickam S, Singh D. Papillary thyroid carcinoma: debate at rest. Indian J Cancer. 2010 Apr-Jun;47(2):206-16.
[3] Takami H, Ito Y, Okamoto T, Yoshida A. Therapeutic strategy for differentiated thyroid carcinoma in Japan based on a newly established guideline managed by Japanese Society of Thyroid Surgeons and Japanese Association of Endocrine Surgeons. World J Surg. 2011 Jan;35(1):111-21.
[4] Ito Y, Miyauchi A, Inoue H, Fukushima M, Kihara M, Higashiyama T, Tomoda C, Takamura Y, Kobayashi K, Miya A. An observational trial for papillary thyroid microcarcinoma in Japanese patients. World J Surg. 2010 Jan;34(1):28-35.
[5] Shedd DP. Historical landmarks in head and neck cancer surgery, Pittsburg, 1999, American Head and Neck Society
[6] McGreevy PS, Miller FA. Biography of Theodore Kocher, Surgery 65;990, 1969
[7] Ord WM. Report of a committee of the Clinical Society of London nominated December 14, 1883, to investigate the subject of myxoedema. Trans Clin Soc Lond 1888;21 [suppl]
[8] Halsted WS. The operative story of goiter. Johns Hopkins Hosp Rep 19;71, 1920.
[9] Welbourn RB. The history of endocrine surgery. New York, 1990, Praeger Publishers.
[10] Crile G Jr. The Fallacy of the Conventional Radical Neck Dissection for Papillary Carcinoma of the Thyroid. Annals of Surgery. 1957, 145(3) 317-20
[11] Rose RG, Kelsey MP, Russell WO, Ibanez ML, White EC, Clark RL. Follow-Up Study of Thyroid Cancer Treated by Unilateral Lobectomy. Am J Surg 106:494-5001, 1963
[12] Crile G Jr. Adenoma and carcinoma of the thyroid gland, N Eng J Med 249; 585, 1953
[13] Clark RL, White EC, Russell WO. Total Thyroidectomy for Cancer of the Thyroid: Significance of Intraglandular Dissemination. Annals of Surgery. June 1959 149(6):858-866
[14] Black BM, Kirk TA, Woolner LB. Multicentricity of the Papillary Adenocarcinoma of the Thyroid: Influence on Treatment. Jan. 1960. JCEM, vol.20, 130-35
[15] Underwood CR, Ackerman LV, Eckert C. Papillary Carcinoma of the Thyroid: An Evaluation of Surgical Therapy. Surgery April 1958 43(4) 610-21
[16] Tollefsen HR, DeCosse JJ. Papillary carcinoma of the thyroid. Recurrence in the thyroid gland after initial surgical treatment. Am J Surg. 1963 Nov;106:728-34.
[17] Crile G Jr, Hazard JB. Relationship of the age of the patient to the natural history and prognosis of carcinoma of the thyroid. Ann Surg. 1953 Jul;138(1):33-8.
[18] Tollefsen HR, DeCosse JJ, Hutter RV. Papillary Carcinoma of the Thyroid. A clinical and pathological study of 70 fatal cases. Cancer. 1964 Aug;17:1035-44.
[19] Mehta MP, Goetowski PG, Kinsella TJ. Radiation induced thyroid neoplasms 1920 to 1987: a vanishing problem? Int J Radiat Oncol Biol Phys. 1989 Jun;16(6):1471-5.
[20] Crile G Jr. The Way it Was: Sex, Surgery, Treasure, & Travel 1907-1987. Kent State University Press. 1992

[21] Ries LAG, Eisner MP, Kosary CL, et al. SEER Cancer Statistics Review, 1973-1997. Bethesda, MD. National Cancer Institute, 2000.
[22] Kurihara H, Takashi M. Safety of operation and indications for total thyroidectomy. Operation 1981; 35:1077-1086
[23] Sawin CT, Becker DV. Radioiodine and the treatment of hyperthyroidism: the early history. Thyroid. 1997 Apr;7(2):163-76.
[24] Seidlin SM, Rossman I, et al. Radioiodine therapy of metastases from carcinoma of the thyroid; a 6-year progress report. J Clin Endocrinol Metab. 1949 Nov;9(11):1122-37
[25] Herle AJ, Uller RP. Elevated serum thyroglobulin. A marker of metastases in differentiated thyroid carcinomas. J Clin Invest. 1975 Aug;56(2):272-7.
[26] Schlumberger M, Fragu P, Parmentier C, Tubiana M. Thyroglobulin assay in the follow-up of patients with differentiated thyroid carcinomas: comparison of its value in patients with or without normal residual tissue. Acta Endocrinol (Copenh). 1981 Oct;98(2):215-21.
[27] Snyder J, Gorman C, Scanlon P. Thyroid remnant ablation: questionable pursuit of an ill-defined goal. J Nucl Med. 1983 Aug;24(8):659-65.
[28] Riccabona G. Thyroid remnant ablation: questionable pursuit of an ill-defined goal. J Nucl Med. 1984 Jun;25(6):727-8.
[29] Grant CS et al: Local recurrence in papillary thyroid carcinoma: Is extent of surgical resection important? Surgery 104:954, 1988
[30] Hay ID et al: Unilateral total lobectomy: Is it sufficient surgical treatment for patients with AMES low risk papillary thyroid carcinoma? Surgery 124:958, 1998.
[31] Tsang RW et al: The effects of surgery, radioiodine, and external radiation therapy on the clinical outcome of patients with differentiated thyroid carcinoma, Cancer 82:375, 1998.
[32] Shaha AR, Shah JP, Loree TR: Low-risk differentiated thyroid cancer: the need for selective treatment, Ann Surg Oncol 4:328, 1997
[33] Sanders LE, Cady B: Differentiated thyroid cancer: reexamination of risk groups and outcome of treatment, Arch Surg 133:419, 1998
[34] Clark OH, Noguchi S. Thyroid cancer: diagnosis and treatment, Quality Medical Publishing, 2000
[35] Werner & Ingbar's The Thyroid: a fundamental and clinical text, ninth edition. Lippincott, Williams & Wilkins, 2005. pp934-966
[36] Dunki-Jacobs E, Grannan K, McDonough S, Engel AM. Clinically unsuspected papillary microcarcinomas of the thyroid: a common finding with favorable biology? Am J Surg. 2011 May 18.
[37] Pelttari H, Välimäki MJ, Löyttyniemi E, Schalin-Jäntti C. Post-ablative serum thyroglobulin is an independent predictor of recurrence in low-risk differentiated thyroid carcinoma: a 16-year follow-up study. Eur J Endocrinol. 2010 Nov;163(5):757-63. Epub 2010 Sep 2.
[38] Sacks W, Fung CH, Chang JT, Waxman A, Braunstein GD. The effectiveness of radioactive iodine for treatment of low-risk thyroid cancer: a systematic analysis of the peer-reviewed literature from 1966 to April 2008. Thyroid. 2010 Nov;20(11):1235-45.
[39] Vaisman F, Shaha A, Fish S, Tuttle R. Initial therapy with either thyroid lobectomy or total thyroidectomy without radioactive iodine remnant ablation is associated with very low rates of structural disease recurrence in properly selected patients with

differentiated thyroid cancer. Clin Endocrinol (Oxf). 2011 Feb 8. doi: 10.1111/j.1365-2265.2011.04002.x.
[40] Ain KB. Anaplastic thyroid carcinoma: behavior, biology, and therapeutic approaches. Thyroid. 1998 Aug;8(8):715-26.
[41] Rosai J: Papillary carcinoma, Monogr Pathol 35:138, 1993
[42] Hamzany Y, Soudry E, Strenov Y et al. Early death from papillary thyroid carcinoma. Am J Otolaryngol. 2011 Jun 7.
[43] Balta AZ, Filiz AI, Kurt Y et al. Prognostic value of oncoprotein expressions in thyroid papillary carcinoma. Med Oncol. 2011 May 6.
[44] Yip L, Kelly L, Shuai Y et al. MicroRNA Signature Distinguishes the Degree of Aggressiveness of Papillary Thyroid Carcinoma. Ann Surg Oncol. 2011 Jul;18(7):2035-41. Epub 2011 May 3.
[45] Hassanain M, Wexler M. Conservative management of well-differentiated thyroid cancer. Can J Surg. 2010 Apr;53(2):109-18.
[46] Ruan DT, Clark OH. Is total thyroidectomy the procedure of choice for low-risk papillary thyroid cancer? Nat Clin Pract Endocrinol Metab. 2008 Mar;4(3):128-9. Epub 2007 Dec 4.
[47] Kutler DI, Crummey AD, Kuhel WI. Routine central compartment lymph node dissection for patients with papillary thyroid carcinoma. Head Neck. 2011 Mar 17. doi: 10.1002/hed.21728.
[48] Shaha AR. Prophylactic central compartment dissection in thyroid cancer: a new avenue of debate. Surgery. 2009 Dec;146(6):1224-7.
[49] Shindo M, Stern A. Total thyroidectomy with and without selective central compartment dissection: a comparison of complication rates. Arch Otolaryngol Head Neck Surg. 2010 Jun;136(6):584-7.
[50] Papini E, Guglielmi R, Hosseim G et al. Ultrasound-Guided Laser Ablation of Incidental Papillary Thyroid Microcarcinoma: A Potential Therapeutic Approach in Patients at Surgical Risk. Thyroid. 2011 May 19.
[51] Jung Hwan Baek et al. Locoregional control of metastatic well differentiated thyroid cancer in the neck by ultrasonography-guided radiofrequency ablation. Unpublished manuscript.
[52] Pacini F, Brilli L, Marchisotta S. Targeted therapy in radioiodine refractory thyroid cancer. Q J Nucl Med Mol Imaging. 2009 Oct;53(5):520-5.
[53] Sugawara M, Geffner DL, Martinez D et al. Novel treatment of medullary thyroid cancer. Curr Opin Endocrinol Diabetes Obes. 2009 Oct;16(5):367-72.
[54] Kapiteijn E, Schneider TC, Morreau H et al. New treatment modalities in advanced thyroid cancer. Ann Oncol. 2011 Apr 6.
[55] Wohllk N, Schweizer H, Erlic Z et al. Multiple endocrine neoplasia type 2. Best Pract Res Clin Endocrinol Metab. 2010 Jun;24(3):371-87.
[56] Catalano MG et al. Valproic acid, a histone deacetylase inhibitor, enhances sensitivity to doxorubicin in anaplastic thyroid cancer cells. J Endocrinol. 2006 Nov;191(2):465-72.
[57] Okamoto N, Takahashi A, Ota I et al. siRNA targeted for NBS1 enhances heat sensitivity in human anaplastic thyroid carcinoma cells. Int J Hyperthermia. 2011;27(3):297-304.
[58] Pallante P, Visone R, Croce CM, Fusco A. Deregulation of microRNA expression in follicular-cell-derived human thyroid carcinomas. Endocr Relat Cancer. 2010 Jan 29;17(1):F91-104. Print 2010 Mar.